Hematology Laboratory in the Digital and Automation Age

Editors

OLGA POZDNYAKOVA
CARLO BRUGNARA

CLINICS IN LABORATORY MEDICINE

www.labmed.theclinics.com

Editor-In-Chief
MILENKO TANASIJEVIC

September 2024 • Volume 44 • Number 3

ELSEVIER

1600 John F. Kennedy Boulevard • Suite 1800 • Philadelphia, Pennsylvania, 19103-2899

http://www.theclinics.com

CLINICS IN LABORATORY MEDICINE Volume 44, Number 3
September 2024 ISSN 0272-2712, ISBN-13: 978-0-443-29394-8

Editor: Taylor Hayes
Developmental Editor: Akshay Samson

Reprints. For copies of 100 or more, of articles in this publication, please contact the Commercial Reprints Department, Elsevier Inc., 360 Park Avenue South, New York, New York 10010-1710. Tel. 212-633-3874, Fax: 212-633-3820, E-mail: reprints@elsevier.com.

Clinics in Laboratory Medicine (ISSN 0272-2712) is published quarterly by Elsevier Inc., 360 Park Avenue South, New York, NY 10010-1710. Months of issue are March, June, September, and December. Business and Editorial offices: 1600 John F. Kennedy Blvd., Suite 1800, Philadelphia, PA 19103-2899. Periodicals postage paid at NewYork, NY and additional mailing offices. Subscription prices are $300.00 per year (US individuals), $100.00 per year (US students), $374.00 per year (Canadian individuals), $100.00 per year (Canadian students), $416.00 per year (international individuals), $185.00 (international students). For institutional access pricing please contact Customer Service via the contact information below. Foreign air speed delivery is included in all Clinics subscription prices. All prices are subject to change without notice. Orders, claims, and journal inquiries: Please visit our Support Hub page https://service.elsevier.com for assistance.

Clinics in Laboratory Medicine is covered in *EMBASE/Exerpta Medica, MEDLINE/PubMed (Index Medicus), Cinahl, Current Contents/Clinical Medicine, BIOSIS and ISI/BIOMED.*

Contributors

EDITOR-IN-CHIEF

MILENKO TANASIJEVIC, MD, MBA
Visiting Scholar and Mentor, The Wyss Institute at Harvard University, Vice Chair of Clinical Pathology and Associate Professor, Brigham and Women's Hospital, Founder, LabDx Advising, LLC, Boston, Massachusetts, USA

EDITORS

OLGA POZDNYAKOVA, MD, PhD
Director, Division of Hematopathology, Professor, Department of Pathology and Laboratory Medicine, The Hospital of the University of Pennsylvania, University of Pennsylvania, Philadelphia, Pennsylvania, USA

CARLO BRUGNARA, MD
Director, Hematology and Coagulation Laboratories, Department of Laboratory Medicine, Boston Children's Hospital, Professor of Pathology, Harvard Medical School, Boston, Massachusetts, USA

AUTHORS

ARCHANA M. AGARWAL, MD
Professor, Department of Pathology, University of Utah, Medical Director, Special Hematology, and Hematopathology, ARUP Laboratories, University of Utah Health, Salt Lake City, Utah, USA

AHMAD AL-ATTAR, PhD, ASCP(SCYM)
Director, Flow Cytometry Laboratory, University of Louisville Health, Louisville, Kentucky, USA

KELLY A. BOWERS, DO, MPH
Associate Staff, Department of Pathology and Laboratory Medicine, Cleveland Clinic, Cleveland, Ohio, USA

SABRINA BUORO, PhD
Director, Centro Regionale di Coordinamento della Medicina di Laboratorio, Milan, Italy

ADAM CUKER, MD, MS
Chief, Section of Hematology, Director, Associate Professor, Departments of Medicine and Pathology and Laboratory Medicine, Perelman School of Medicine, University of Pennsylvania Hospital, University of Pennsylvania, Philadelphia, Pennsylvania, USA

ALEXIS DADELAHI, PhD
Fellow, Immunology, Department of Pathology, University of Utah, ARUP Laboratories, Salt Lake City, Utah, USA

DANIEL C. DEES, DCLS, MLS(ASCP)
Medical Director, Clinical Hematology, Brigham and Women's Hospital, Lecturer, Harvard Medical School, Boston, Massachusetts, USA

EMMANUEL J. FAVALORO, PhD, FFSC (RCPA)
Principle Medical Scientist and Scientific Lead for Research, Haematology, Sydney Centres for Thrombosis and Haemostasis, Institute of Clinical Pathology and Medical Research (ICPMR), NSW Health Pathology, Westmead Hospital, Adjunct Professor, School of Dentistry and Medical Sciences, Faculty of Science and Health, Charles Sturt University, Wagga Wagga, Adjunct Professor, School of Medical Sciences, Faculty of Medicine and Health, University of Sydney, Westmead Hospital, Westmead, New South Wales, Australia

ANDREW L. FRELINGER III, PhD
Director, Center for Platelet Research Studies, Dana-Farber/Boston Children's Cancer and Blood Disorders Center, Boston Children's Hospital, Boston, Massachusetts, USA

ROBERT C. GOSSELIN, CLS
Volunteer Staff, Thrombosisand Hemostasis Center, University of California, Davis Health System, Sacramento, California, USA

CONNOR M. HARTZELL, MD
Resident Physician, Department of Pathology, Microbiology and Immunology, Vanderbilt University Medical Center, Nashville, Tennessee, USA

BRANDON M. HENRY, MD
Researcher, Clinical Laboratory, Division of Nephrology and Hypertension, Cincinnati Children's Hospital Medical Center, Cincinnati, Ohio, USA

GIOVANNI INSUASTI-BELTRAN, MD
Associate Professor of Pathology, Wake Forest University, Winston-Salem, North Carolina, USA

TAYLOR JACKSON, DO
Resident, Department of Pathology University of Utah, ARUP Laboratories, Salt Lake City, Utah, USA

NICHOLAS E. LARKEY, PhD
Assistant Professor, Department of Pathology, Division of Clinical Chemistry, University of Virginia Health, Charlottesville, Virginia, USA

JOSHUA E. LEWIS, MD, PhD
Fellow, Department of Pathology, Brigham and Women's Hospital, Boston, Massachusetts, USA

LEO LIN, MD, PhD
Assistant Professor, Department of Pathology, University of Utah, Associate Director, Research and Innovation, Medical Director, Immunologic Flow Cytometry, Immunology, ARUP Laboratories, Immunology Medical Director, PharmaDx, Research and Innovation ARUP Laboratories, Salt Lake City, Utah, USA

GIUSEPPE LIPPI, MD
Director, Professor, Section of Clinical Biochemistry, School of Medicine, University of Verona, University Hospital of Verona, Verona, Italy

EMILY F. MASON, MD, PhD
Associate Professor, Department of Pathology, Microbiology and Immunology, Vanderbilt University Medical Center, Nashville, Tennessee, USA

MEGAN O. NAKASHIMA, MD
Staff Hematopathologist and Hematopathology Fellowship Director, Department of Pathology and Laboratory Medicine, Cleveland Clinic, Cleveland, Ohio, USA

DAVID P. NG, MD
Assistant Professor, Department of Pathology, University of Utah, Medical Director, Hematopathology, Director, Applied Artificial Intelligence and Bioinformatics, Medical Director, Hematologic Flow Cytometry, ARUP Laboratories, Salt Lake City, Utah, USA

ALAN A. NGUYEN, MD
Physician, Division of Immunology, Boston Children's Hospital, Harvard Medical School, Boston, Massachusetts, USA

IFEYINWA E. OBIORAH, MD, PhD
Assistant Professor, Department of Pathology, Division of Hematopathology, University of Virginia Health, Charlottesville, Virginia, USA

LEONARDO PASALIC, FRCPA, FRACP, PhD
Staff Specialist, Laboratory Haematologist, Clinical Haematologist, Group Leader Platelet Research Laboratory, Haematology, Sydney Centres for Thrombosis and Haemostasis, Institute of Clinical Pathology and Medical Research (ICPMR), NSW Health Pathology, Westmead Hospital, Clinical Senior Lecturer, Westmead Clinical School, University of Sydney, Westmead, New South Wales, Australia

CRAIG D. PLATT, MD, PhD
Assistant Professor, Division of Immunology, Boston Children's Hospital, Harvard Medical School, Boston, Massachusetts, USA

OLGA POZDNYAKOVA, MD, PhD
Director, Division of Hematopathology, Professor, Department of Pathology and Laboratory Medicine, The Hospital of the University of Pennsylvania, University of Pennsylvania, Philadelphia, Pennsylvania, USA

ANTON V. RETS, MD, PhD
Associate Professor, Department of Pathology, University of Utah, Medical Director, Hematopathology, Medical Director, Immunohistochemistry and Histology, ARUP Laboratories, University of Utah School of Medicine, University of Utah Health, Salt Lake City, Utah, USA

AARON C. SHAVER, MD, PhD
Associate Professor, Director, Vanderbilt Flow Cytometry Laboratory, Department of Pathology, Microbiology and Immunology, Vanderbilt University Medical Center, Nashville, Tennessee, USA

RYAN C. SHEAN, DO
Pathology Resident, Department of Pathology, University of Utah School of Medicine, ARUP Laboratories, Salt Lake City, Utah, USA

ELOÍSA URRECHAGA, PhD
Senior Consultant in Clinical Laboratory, Hematology Laboratory, Galdácano Hospital, Galdakao, Vizcaya, Spain

MARGARET C. WILLIAMS, MD
Assistant Professor, Department of Pathology, University of Utah School of Medicine, ARUP Laboratories, Salt Lake City, Utah, USA

Contents

> The evolution of complete blood count (CBC) methodology from manual calculations to sophisticated high throughput hematology analyzers is the focus of this article. In recent years, hematology testing has greatly benefitted from the combination of various technologies with automated neural networks. In addition to an increasing complexity of the laboratory instrumentation, there is a demand on point of care CBC testing with its benefits and drawbacks. This article highlights exciting advancements of hematology testing from the past to the present and into the future.

> Myelodysplastic syndromes (MDS) present with polymorphic and non-specific diagnostic features Research parametersfrom hematology analyzers may be useful to discriminate MDS-related cytopenia.Parameters such as Neu X (related to the cytoplasmic complexity) and Neu Y (related to nucleic acid content) show promise to detect dysplasia of MDS and aid to recognize MDS from cytopenias of other etiologies.

> A leukocyte differential of peripheral blood can be performed using digital imaging coupled with cellular pre-classification by artificial neural networks. Platelet and erythrocyte morphology can be assessed and counts estimated. Systems from a single vendor have been used in clinical practice for several years, with other vendors' systems, in a development. These systems perform comparably to traditional manual optical microscopy, however, it is important to note that they are designed and intended to be operated by a trained morphologist. These systems have several benefits including increased standardization, efficiency, and remote-review capability.

> The clinical analysis of urine has classically focused on conventional chemical-based urinalysis and urine microscopy. Contemporary advances in both analysis subsets have started to employ new technologies such as automated image analysis, flow cytometry, and mass spectrometry. In addition to new detection technologies, current analyzers have incorporated

more advanced imaging, automated sample handing, and machine learning analyses into their workflow. The most advanced semiautomated analyzers can be interfaced with hospital medical record systems, and in the point-of-care setting, smartphones can be used for image analysis. This review will discuss current technological advancements in the field of urinalysis and urine microscopy.

Body fluid analysis has become a critical component of diagnostic and clinical decision-making for a wide spectrum of human pathologies. An automated microscope, a high-quality digital camera, and a software designed to identify and automatically preclassify cells and other features in stained smears comprise the most recent generation of digital morphologic analyzers. The time necessary for expert operator reclassification is another aspect that must be considered at this stage of development, because identifying and sorting distinct elements in body fluids still necessitates the involvement of an expert morphologist.

Evaluation of bone marrow aspirate smear and trephine biopsy specimens is critical to the diagnosis of benign and malignant hematologic conditions. Digital pathology has the potential to revolutionize bone marrow assessment through implementation of artificial intelligence for assisted and automated evaluation, but there remain many barriers toward this implementation. This article reviews the current state of digital evaluation of bone marrow aspirate smears and trephine biopsies, recent research using machine learning models for automated specimen analysis, an outline of the advantages and barriers facing clinical implementation of artificial intelligence, and a potential vision of artificial intelligence-associated bone marrow evaluation.

Hemoglobin (Hb) disorders are among the most prevalent inherited diseases. Despite a limited number of involved genes, these conditions represent a broad clinical and prognostic spectrum. The menu of laboratory tests is extensive. From widely available modalities, for example, complete blood count to rather sophisticated molecular technologies, the investigation of Hb disorders recapitulates an increasing complexity of laboratory workup in other medical fields. This review highlights a current state of biochemical and molecular investigation of Hb disorders and offers a glimpse on technologies that are yet to be fully embraced in clinical practice.

Automation in clinical flow cytometry has the potential to revolutionize the field by improving processes and enhancing efficiency and accuracy.

Integrating advanced robotics and artificial intelligence, these technologies can streamline sample preparation, data acquisition, and analysis. Automated sample handling reduces human error and increases throughput, allowing laboratories to handle larger volumes with consistent precision. Intelligent algorithms contribute to rapid data interpretation, aiding in the identification of cellular markers for disease diagnosis and monitoring. This automation not only accelerates turnaround times but also ensures reproducibility, making clinical flow cytometry a reliable tool in the realm of personalized medicine and diagnostics.

Andrew L. Frelinger III

Clinical assessment of platelet activation by flow cytometry is useful in the characterization and diagnosis of platelet-specific disorders and as a measure of risk for thrombosis or bleeding. Platelets circulate in a resting, "unactivated" state, but when activated they undergo alterations in surface glycoprotein function and/or expression level, exposure of granule membrane proteins, and exposure of procoagulant phospholipids. Flow cytometry provides the means to detect these changes and, unlike other platelet tests, is appropriate for measuring platelet function in samples from patients with low platelet counts. The present review will focus on flow cytometric tests for platelet activation markers.

Emmanuel J. Favaloro and Leonardo Pasalic

The term 'routine coagulation' typically applies to hemostasis tests routinely performed in hematology laboratories, often available 24/7, and potentially ordered urgently. These tests would comprise of the prothrombin time (PT), the PT converted to an international normalized ratio, the activated partial thromboplastin time (often called partial thromboplastin time in North American laboratories) and potentially the thrombin time, the D-dimer assay, and fibrinogen assays. Although other tests could feasibly be offered (testing feasible), there are good reasons for not including all of these other tests in all routine coagulation laboratories.

Daniel C. Dees

This article provides a comprehensive overview of Heparin-Induced Thrombocytopenia (HIT) with an emphasis on laboratory testing and advantages of automation. HIT is a critical condition arising from heparin exposure, leading to a contradictory combination of thrombocytopenia with an increased thrombosis risk. The article discusses HIT's history, clinical presentation, laboratory diagnosis, and management strategies. It highlights the importance of interdisciplinary collaboration for effective diagnosis and treatment, underscoring advancements in technology and targeted therapies that are shaping future approaches to HIT management.

Robert C. Gosselin and Adam Cuker

Direct oral anticoagulants (DOACs) have significant advantages over vitamin K antagonists including lack of need for routine laboratory monitoring. However, assessment of DOAC effect and concentration may be important to guide clinical management including need for DOAC reversal, particularly in acute or emergent situations. In this manuscript, the authors describe tests to screen for DOAC presence and tests that have demonstrated equivalence to gold standard testing for quantifying DOAC exposure. They also discuss the effect of DOACs on other coagulation assays and strategies for monitoring unfractionated heparin in patients with concomitant DOAC exposure.

CLINICS IN LABORATORY MEDICINE

SERIES OF RELATED INTEREST

Advances in Molecular Pathology
Available at: https://www.journals.elsevier.com/advances-in-molecular-pathology

---

THE CLINICS ARE NOW AVAILABLE ONLINE!
Access your subscription at:
www.theclinics.com

Preface

Hematology Laboratory in the Digital and Automation Age

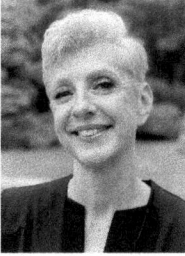

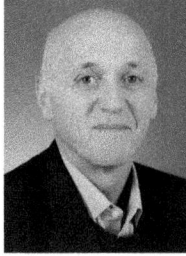

Olga Pozdnyakova, MD, PhD   Carlo Brugnara, MD
Editors

We are delighted to present this issue of *Clinics in Laboratory Medicine* on "Hematology Laboratory in the Digital and Automation Age," a timely and needed update to our previous 2015 contribution (Automated Cell Counters: State of the Art and new directions).

This new issue of *Clinics in Laboratory Medicine* reflects the profound changes that have taken place in Laboratory Medicine in the last decade and highlights the future directions that will soon become mainstream. We discuss recent developments and trends in hematology analyzer, as well as the impact of Artificial Intelligence and digital imaging in classification and identification of cellular blood elements. In coagulation, we examine how routine coagulation has evolved in the new laboratory and discuss testing for heparin-induced thrombocytopenia and novel anticoagulants. This new issue examines the most significant developments in urine and body fluids analyses and in the diagnostics of hemoglobinopathies. A considerable effort has been made in this issue to provide a comprehensive look at the role of flow cytometry in hematology-oncology diagnostics. In dedicated articles, we discuss the implementation of automation in flow cytometry, the diagnostics of malignant hematologic disorders, immunodeficiencies, and red blood cell and platelet disorders.

Clin Lab Med 44 (2024) xiii–xiv
https://doi.org/10.1016/j.cll.2024.06.001
0272-2712/24/© 2024 Published by Elsevier Inc.

labmed.theclinics.com

We would like to thank Elsevier's staff and all our contributors for making this issue possible. We firmly believe that it adds an important goalpost for understanding the evolution and current and future practices of Laboratory Hematology.

Olga Pozdnyakova, MD, PhD
Division of Hematopathology
Department of Pathology and Laboratory Medicine
The Hospital of the University of Pennsylvania
3400 Spruce Street
Office G7.021, Gates Building
Philadelphia, PA 19104, USA

Carlo Brugnara, MD
Hematology and Coagulation Laboratories
Department of Laboratory Medicine
Boston Children's Hospital
Harvard Medical School
300 Longwood Avenue, SK B2-408
Boston, MA 02115, USA

E-mail addresses:
Olga.Pozdnyakova@Pennmedicine.upenn.edu (O. Pozdnyakova)
Carlo.Brugnara@childrens.harvard.edu (C. Brugnara)

Advances in Hematology Analyzers Technology

Ryan C. Shean, DO[a,b,1], Margaret C. Williams, MD[a,b,2],
Anton V. Rets, MD, PhD[a,b,*]

KEYWORDS

- Hematology analyzers • Point of care complete blood count
- Complete blood counttechnology • Complete blood countautomation

KEY POINTS

- Complete blood count (CBC) technology has rapidly progressed from manual counts and calculations to a combination of modern technologies, such as optical, impedance, and flow-based.
- Integration of automated neural networks has significantly improved automated classification of cell populations.
- An increasing demand for point-of-care CBC testing has led to development of more compact instruments with improved characteristics.
- Despite some obstacles, the integration of artificial intelligence in operational workflows is inevitable as it will improve the efficiency of hematology laboratories.

INTRODUCTION

From ancient times, humans have intuitively understood the vital role blood plays in medicine. They observed that the contents change with disease and losing too much is lethal. Despite this, for nearly 5000 years of human history one of the most common procedures surgeons and physicians performed was bloodletting.[1] It was not until 1852 that Karl Vierordt described precise calculation of the concentration of blood cells by spreading a known volume of blood on a microscope slide and manually counting every cell,[2] thus, opening the door for rigorous and systematic analysis of the blood. Although time consuming, clinical utilization soon followed, leading to improved efficiency and the development of the hemocytometer in 1874.[3] Today, the complete blood count (CBC) is the most commonly ordered laboratory test in the world.[4] Manual review of the peripheral blood is useful in the diagnosis of urgently

[a] Department of Pathology, University of Utah School of Medicine, Salt Lake City, UT, USA;
[b] ARUP Laboratories, Salt Lake City, UT, USA
[1] Present address: 15 N Medical Drive E RM 2100, Salt Lake City, UT 84112.
[2] Present address: 500 Chipeta Way, Mail code 115-G04, Salt Lake City, UT 84108-1221.
* Corresponding author. 500 Chipeta Way, Mail code 115-G04, Salt Lake City, UT 84108-1221.
E-mail address: anton.rets@aruplab.com

Clin Lab Med 44 (2024) 377–386
https://doi.org/10.1016/j.cll.2024.04.001
labmed.theclinics.com
0272-2712/24/© 2024 Elsevier Inc. All rights are reserved, including those for text and data mining, AI training, and similar technologies.

actionable and critical conditions, including hemolytic anemia, sickle cell anemia, and leukemia.[5] Hematological analysis is used to guide treatment every day in nearly every practice setting. Ever since manual counts and reviews were first routinely implemented, there has been great interest in automation and improvement as much as safely possible with currently available technologies. In this article, the authors review key historical advancements in hematology analyzers, discuss current state of the art technologies, investigate new point of care (POC) devices, and briefly assess possible future advancements in the hematology laboratory.

HISTORY
Optical Instruments

In 1961 the first attempt to automatically discriminate between blood cell elements was described.[6] The CELLSCAN device was a proof-of-concept instrument designed to identify radiation induced binucleate lymphocytes, which occur at extremely low frequency in the peripheral blood. The instrument used a monochromic photometer to digitize microscope fields of a blood smear into a binary grid of optical densities. "1" represented darker areas, such as nuclei or granules, and "0" indicated lighter areas such as membrane, cytoplasm, or empty space. Solitary 1s were assumed to be noise and converted to 0s, greatly increasing compression efficiency, and allowing a microscope field to be digitized into ~19,000 bits on a rotating loop of magnetic tape. At the computing speed available to the authors processing a single blood smear would require almost a month. While the device was never implemented clinically, it represented foundational work in computerized optical morphologic assessment of hematologic cells. Many of the limitations of this device were because of the technological restrictions of the time. Advancement and development of hematology analyzers continues to be driven by innovations in basic underlying technologies.

Only 5 years later, in 1966, optics, storage, and data processing had advanced enough to make an automatic optical differential of stained hematologic cells a feasible task. The CYDAC cytophotometer used a flying spot microscope and cathode ray tube to digitize a 50x50 micron field into a table of 40,000 8 bit gray scale colorimetric data points.[7] This table was then used to convert a single cell to a vector of manually defined parameter values. Classification vectors of these features were calculated from selected training cells, and closeness of vectors was used to group and differentiate cells in multidimensional parameter space. Discrimination between 4 different types of leukocytes was demonstrated to be possible by computers. The developers presciently noted that automation and refinement of this concept would require capturing more features, as well as more complex processing and decision-making operations.

In 1976, the Hematrack instrument finally automated the time consuming white blood cell (WBC) differential.[8] This device ascribed geometric functions to 3 channel red, green and blue (RGB) color data to produce classification features. Although this significantly increased the amount of data collected, technology again limited discrimination ability. Sacrifices in number of features and therefore discrimination ability were required to characterize cells in a clinically useful timeframe. The final version, working in tandem with a trained technologist to adjudicate unclassifiable cells, was able to do a routine differential count of 100 cells in about 40 seconds. However, reproducibility was poor on automatically classified individual cells: only 55% of cells were placed in the same category on 95% or more occasions, and 20% of repeated cells were placed in the same category less than 70% of the time.[9] The extremely high intra-cell disagreement clearly showed the limitations of feasible data collection and processing algorithms on available hardware. To perform an efficient WBC differential with adequate reproducibility and performance, improvements would be required in scanning, digital signal processing, parameter calculations, and analysis techniques.

Impedance and Optical Flow

As basic optical differentiation techniques developed, advances in flow cytometric technology led to significant and parallel advancements in blood particle counting. In 1953, Crosland-Taylor described a method of counting erythrocytes by examining the optical properties of particles suspended in fluid,[10] while elsewhere the Coulter brothers found that the impedance caused by a cell suspended in fluid passing through an electric current is proportional to size.[11] The development of the first impedance-based cell counters shortly followed, where ideally 1 cell at a time would pass through a current and impedance pulses were used to determine the count and size of cells. From this groundbreaking work, flow-based instruments expanded into clinical and research laboratories.

In 1969, Technicon introduced the SMA-4, which used impedance to measure and report out four parameters (hemoglobin [Hgb], hematocrit, red blood cell [RBC] number, and WBC number). The original version had decent performance but suffered from frequent flow line faults, and required constant assistance from an experienced technician.[12] Additionally, as all original parameters were calculated by impedance, the values were highly sensitive to protein, ethylenediamine tetraacetic acid, and electrolyte concentrations.[13] Despite these limitations, the device was a crucial advancement in mechanization.

The Coulter brothers continuously improved their original counting device, eventually introducing the Coulter Model S.[14] This instrument used impedance in multiple flow channels to count erythrocytes and leukocytes. It also output novel measured and calculated parameters including mean corpuscular volume, mean corpuscular Hgb, and mean corpuscular Hgb concentration (MCHC). These parameters provided a reproducible and precise measure of erythrocyte size and Hgb status, still used widely today in the differential diagnosis of anemia.[15] Overall, it was a cheaper, quicker way of repeatably and reliably quantifying the contents of circulating blood.[16] In 1979, the Coulter brothers debuted the improved Model S+, which reported 12 parameters including red cell distribution width (RDW), introducing a robust and precise method of assessing anisocytosis. The S+ also assessed platelets by counting particles in the 2 to 20 fL volume range. This method was limited by falsely counting RBC fragments as platelets and did not have established linearity below concentrations of 25,000 to 30,000 per μL, which are clinically useful values.[17] However, this was still an accurate and efficient method of calculating platelets in many circumstances. Both devices advanced hematology through formalization of calculated parameters that had previously been manually and subjectively estimated. The utility of these new values for patients and clinicians drove rapid adoption, which spurred further refinement of the techniques used to generate them.

FROM PAST TO PRESENT
ANN-Based Instruments

The very earliest hematology analyzers used optical measurements to detect and classify cells, however, many early papers working on optical discrimination of cells admitted that optics, feature extraction, decision algorithms, and processing power would need to greatly improve before optical classification of leukocytes would be achievable at a clinically useful time scale and cost.[18] Progressive technological improvements, especially in the 80s and 90s, led to the development of automated neural networks (ANNs), for feature extraction and classification, heralding the modern era of automatic hematology analyzers.[19]

In 2001, the first optical ANN based analyzer was developed in Sweden by CellaVision.[20] The first automatic machine vision classifier was the DiffMaster Octavia,[21] but the more automated and precise DM96 saw much wider adoption. The DM96 increased throughput by accepting continuously loaded automatically stained slides.[22] The DM96 scans slides at low power for cells of interest, then acquires high power images of representative fields. The ANN allows the device to quickly and efficiently classify WBCs, although it operates as a decision support system and requires human input for unclassifiable cells.[23] Machine classification followed by digital display has the advantages of reducing technologist eye strain, producing more consistent results, and simplifying training.[24] While manual review of certain slides was still required, the automatic differential decreased turnaround-times (TAT) for simple differentials. Original limitations of this technology included difficulty examining platelets, assessing RBC morphology, and sensitivity to slide preparation techniques.[25] However, new classification models have since been developed and research is ongoing.[26,27]

Another popular ANN based classification instrument manufacturer is Sysmex. This Japanese company has a long history of developing automatic hematology analyzers including an impedance based counter in 1963.[28] In 2013, Sysmex released the DI-60, the first fully integrated digital morphology based hematology analyzer on the market.[29] The device automated sample preparation and analysis with high throughput and excellent performance making Sysmex analyzers highly adopted and well-studied.[30] Successive improvements in gathered features, as well as flags and parameters including blasts[31,32] and RBC abnormalities[33] have made high throughput CBCs with high sensitivity for many critical abnormalities commonplace.

The Mindray MC-100i, a newly developed analyzer, utilizes a deep convolutional network, which leverages modern computational power to allow computers to train and make decisions based off features that cannot be defined by humans. Mindray instruments have good performance compared with other standard hematology analyzers and manual microscopy review.[34] Additionally, other Mindray instruments utilizing deep convolutional networks have shown utility in detecting malaria infected RBCs, even at low levels of parasitemia.[35] This has been a challenging task with previously designed ANN based instruments. Using novel features and decision-making heuristics derived from deep learning techniques has provided a marked improvement for this specific use case. It is likely that deep learning applications for other previously difficult to automate tasks will continue to develop.

Another relatively new analyzer that introduces novel technology is the Scopio Labs X100. A major advance of this instrument is that it captures and analyzes the entire field of a blood smear. Previous analyzers only acquired images of specific cells at the monolayer, which may miss platelet clumps or rare but clinically relevant cells distributed elsewhere on the slide.[30] The X100 utilizes advances in image processing, storage, and deep convolutional learning to classify cells, performing a full smear with differential in around 8 minutes.[36] However, it is still a decision support system where humans are required to help classify the cells. Browser-based operation enables remote review, potentially reducing TAT.[37] The additional power offered by deep convolutional networks allows efficient full field analysis, ameliorating many of the previously described issues with optical peripheral blood smear analysis.

The implementation and use of a variety of digital morphology analyzers from multiple manufacturers, all using proprietary models and techniques has led to international guidelines calling for standardization measures. These platforms show an overall acceptable performance in identification of normal blood cells. However, to assure consistency of validation and clinical implementation of digital morphology analyzers, the International Council for Standardization and Hematology formulated a list of recommendations. These recommendations include implementing public standards for digital image files and guidelines for validation. For example, new flagging parameters or detection models for pathologic cells such as abnormal erythrocytes should be graded in a standardized manner to improve interoperability and allow rigorous comparisons between instruments and techniques.[20]

Point of Care Hematology Analyzers

There is interest from industry and in recent literature regarding POC hematology analyzers. High throughput platforms suffer from several drawbacks that make implementation most efficient at central laboratory facilities including expense, large laboratory footprint, inclusion of complex optics, lasers, and microfluidics that increases maintenance and staff training needs. Also, the hydrodynamic focusing employed by traditional flow cytometry requires a large volume of sheath fluid and reagent handling can become complex and costly. While there are certainly advantages to centralizing instrumentation and expertize, this necessarily increases TATs for external clients and patients. An attractive draw of POC instruments is leveraging the reduction in TAT to make appropriate management decisions based of laboratory results in the clinic during a patient's scheduled appointment.

A novel device that represents advancement in both POC and automated analysis of peripheral blood is the Sight OLO analyzer.[38] This instrument differs from traditional methods by using neither a flow cytometric approach nor a stained slide that can be reviewed by a human technologist. Instead, a very small amount of blood (27uL) is added to a self-sufficient cartridge. In the cartridge, blood cells are diluted onto a suspension matrix where they settle into a monolayer at the focal plane of an optical receiver. Optical data is fed into machine learning classification algorithms to produce a 5-cell differential. The device was shown to be clinically useful for monitoring WBC and absolute neutrophil count (ANC) in both outpatient chemotherapy settings and for routine monitoring of patients on clozapine therapy.[39] When this device was implemented in an outpatient oncology clinic, overall TAT and test utilization, including manual smear reviews, all reduced with no impact on patient safety.[40]

Another new hematology analyzer is the HemoScreen. This device uses a novel viscoelastic focusing technique to create single-file flow of cells using much lower fluid volumes than traditional hydrodynamic focusing. This allows the tabletop device to measure 20 CBC parameters including a 5 part differential and platelet count using artificial intelligence (AI)-assisted machine vision.[41] This analyzer has been directly compared with leading core laboratory analyzers with generally acceptable agreement and reduction in TAT.[42] It can provide rapid evaluation of CBC parameters at lower values making it a suitable alternative to centralized hematology analyzers in a post chemotherapy setting.[43] However, this new technology is not without limitations as in one published report where some abnormal samples were not appropriately identified, including one with 69% blasts.[44] The investigators hypothesized that extreme leukocytosis increased the sample viscosity, which interfered with the novel viscoelastic focusing technology.

Another new POC instrument is the HemoCue WBC DIFF, which performs well at enumerating WBCs and RBCs.[45] The device has a very small platform footprint and can accept as little as 10 μL of blood. The instrument is able to quickly and reliably provide concise and actionable information including total WBC count with lymphocyte and neutrophil differential[46] with good performance on clinically significant samples such as those from severely leukopenic patients.[47] This device is capable of quickly and easily determining if the contents of the blood are grossly abnormal and has a potential use as a screening instrument. However, the device does not count abnormal cells and has a high rate of abnormal cell flagging, which would require a full laboratory analysis.

Another relatively new POC instrument for determining the WBC and ANC is the Athelas One, which accepts ∼3.5 μL of blood and uses a microfluidic test strip that produces a stained monolayer of a known volume and uses computer vision to perform a WBC count and ANC. It shows good correlation with leading core laboratory technology and good linearity even at clinically relevant levels of agranulocytosis.[48] This device is extremely small in size, requires a remarkably low sample volume and is marketed for at home-use.

While there is a clinically driven interest in POC instruments, and they neatly showcase some of the most cutting-edge technologies, there are many factors to be considered before widespread adoption of these devices. A large drawback of POC instruments is up-front and overhead costs. Instead of simply employing a fee for service agreement with a local laboratory, clinics would need to front the purchase price for a new POC instrument. Operational costs would need to be quite low for these instruments to provide economic utility to remote sites. If these devices are not clearly shown to be cost effective, they must demonstrate new clinical benefits that justify the increased cost. Furthermore, POC tests – especially those using capillary sampling with very small volumes of blood are much more susceptible to pre-analytic and analytic errors. An often-remarked benefit of these instruments, which is that they do not need to be operated by trained and regulated laboratorians, further increases the risk of errors. Additionally, none of these machines are capable of multiplexing, meaning tests must be performed serially. In a busy clinic this could prove to be a significant source of delays. When these constraints are combined with the limited test menu of POC platforms it is clear that employment of these devices requires thoughtful consideration and clinical or economic utility must be clearly demonstrated before implementation.[49]

FUTURE DIRECTIONS

Medicine has advanced immensely since the days of leaches and bloodletting. The formalization and automation of manual or subjective parameters led to large gains for patient health and drove widespread adoption of automatic hematology analyzers. Promising new hematology analysis technologies driven by research and industry are on the horizon. Many of the original machine learning instruments used supervised features chosen by humans, such as geometric parameters, to train and classify cells. With further developments in AI and increasingly robust datasets, more complex features, possibly including those humans cannot even detect, may be used to provide better discrimination.[50,51] Many of the recent advancements in non-pathology machine learning technologies, such as ChatGPT, have come from massive and publicly available datasets. However, creating large scale, high quality, and robust hematology training sets is an extremely non-trivial endeavor. The more tasks and differentiation asked of the algorithm, the more data are required indicating a demand for immense training data, especially to leapfrog current technologies. Experienced hematology annotation is time consuming and expensive.[52] The investment required will certainly be spent for proprietary algorithms, but it remains to be seen if there are large high quality publicly available datasets similar to those that drove previous advancements in machine learning.

Robust training data and new input features also have the potential to calculate novel output parameters. Implementation of MCHC and RDW led to improvements in clinical care by replacing previously imprecise and subjective measures with objective measurable values. Machine learning also has the potential to impute clinical utility for any new measures developed. However, despite potential hype and theoretic clinical usefulness, new parameters must be a value-add and have to be bought in from clinical teams. Since many newly designed parameters are proprietary and calculated through different principles and algorithms, they are not easily interchangeable and global application may be difficult. This represents a major challenge for clinical implementation and guideline development.[53] Good quality clinical research to show utility and generalizability will be important.

Overall, ongoing advancements will likely continue to improve the efficiency and utility of the clinical hematology laboratory. The advances in hematology analyzers since the first attempts at rigorous analysis of blood are far too numerous to list, but the course has been dominated by underlying technologies making more robust analysis possible, leading to formalization and standardization of previously subjective, or unknown measures with clinical utility. The greatest next technology to drive future development is machine learning. It is exciting to think about what these new technologies may allow us to do for patients as the field moves forward.

DISCLOSURE

No disclosers from any of the authors to share related to this article.

REFERENCES

1. Parapia LA. History of bloodletting by phlebotomy. Br J Haematol 2008;143(4): 490–5.
2. Green R, Wachsmann-Hogiu S. Development, history, and future of automated cell counters. Clin Lab Med 2015;35(1):1–10.
3. Vembadi A, Menachery A, Qasaimeh MA. Cell cytometry: review and perspective on biotechnological advances. Front Bioeng Biotechnol 2019;7:147.
4. Horton S, Fleming KA, Kuti M, et al. The top 25 laboratory tests by volume and revenue in five different Countries. Am J Clin Pathol 2019;151(5):446–51.
5. Bain BJ. Diagnosis from the blood smear. N Engl J Med 2005;353(5):498–507.
6. Preston K. The CELLSCAN system - T.M. a leucocyte pattern analyzer. In Papers presented at the May 9-11, 1961, western joint IRE-AIEE-ACM computer conference (IRE-AIEE-ACM '61 (Western)). Association for Computing Machinery; New York, NY, 173–183.
7. Prewitt JMS, Mendelsohn ML. The analysis of cell images. Ann N Y Acad Sci 1966;128(3):1035–53.
8. Miller MN. Design and clinical results of hematrak: an automated differential counter. IEEE Trans Biomed Eng 1976;BME-23(5):400–5.
9. Urmston A, Hyde K, Gowenlock Ah, et al. Evaluation of the Hematrak differential leucocyte counter. Clin Lab Haematol 1980;2(3):199–214.
10. Crosland-Taylor PJ. A device for counting small particles suspended in a fluid through a tube. Nature 1953;171(4340):37–8.

11. Coulter WH. Means for counting particles suspended in a fluid. 1953. Available at: https://patents.google.com/patent/US2656508A/en. [Accessed 24 August 2023].

12. Green AE, Middleton VL, Prentis KG, et al. A report on experience with an automatic blood counting machine. J Clin Pathol 1969;22(1):19–27.

13. Lappin TRJ, Lamont A, Nelson MG. An evaluation of the auto analyzer SMA-4. J Clin Pathol 1969;22(1):11–8.

14. Don M. The coulter principle: foundation of an industry. JALA J Assoc Lab Autom 2003;8(6):72–81.

15. Barnard DF, Carter AB, Crosland-Taylor PJ, et al. An evaluation of the Coulter model S. J Clin Pathol Suppl Coll Pathol 1969;3:26–33.

16. Pinkerton PH, Spence I, Ogilvie JC, et al. An assessment of the Coulter counter model S. J Clin Pathol 1970;23(1):68–76.

17. Rowan RM, Fraser C, Gray JH, et al. The coulter counter model S Plus– the shape of things to come. Clin Lab Haematol 1979;1(1):29–40.

18. Harms H, Gunzer U, Aus HM, et al. Computer aided analysis of chromatin network and basophil color for differentiation of mononuclear peripheral blood cells. J Histochem Cytochem Off J Histochem Soc. 1979;27(1):204–9.

19. Lewis JE, Pozdnyakova O. Digital assessment of peripheral blood and bone marrow aspirate smears. Int J Lab Hematol 2023;45(S2):50–8.

20. Kratz A, Lee S hee, Zini G, et al. Digital morphology analyzers in hematology: ICSH review and recommendations. Int J Lab Hematol 2019;41(4):437–47.

21. The history of CellaVision | CellaVision. Available at: https://www.cellavision.com/about/history-cellavision. [Accessed 22 September 2023].

22. Briggs C, Longair I, Slavik M, et al. Can automated blood film analysis replace the manual differential? An evaluation of the CellaVision DM96 automated image analysis system. Int J Lab Hematol 2009;31(1):48–60.

23. Da Costa L. Digital image analysis of blood cells. Clin Lab Med 2015;35(1):105–22.

24. VanVranken SJ, Patterson ES, Rudmann SV, et al. A survey study of benefits and limitations of using CellaVision DM96 for peripheral blood differentials. Clin Lab Sci J Am Soc Med Technol 2014;27(1):32–9.

25. Kratz A, Bengtsson HI, Casey JE, et al. Performance Evaluation of the CellaVision DM96 System: WBC differentials by automated digital image analysis supported by an artificial neural network. Am J Clin Pathol 2005;124(5):770–81.

26. Nakashima MO, Doyle TJ, Phelan-Lewin K, et al. Assessment of semi-quantitative grading of red blood cell abnormalities utilizing images from the CellaVision DM96 compared to manual light microscopy. Int J Lab Hematol 2017;39(5):e110–2.

27. Criel M, Godefroid M, Deckers B, et al. Evaluation of the red blood cell advanced software application on the cellaVision DM96. Int J Lab Hematol 2016;38(4):366–74.

28. Sysmex's history. Available at: https://www.sysmex.co.jp/en/corporate/info/history/index.html. [Accessed 22 September 2023].

29. Kim HN, Hur M, Kim H, et al. Performance of automated digital cell imaging analyzer Sysmex DI-60. Clin Chem Lab Med 2017;56(1):94–102.

30. Lapić I, Miloš M, Dorotić M, et al. Analytical validation of white blood cell differential and platelet assessment on the Sysmex DI-60 digital morphology analyzer. Int J Lab Hematol 2023. https://doi.org/10.1111/ijlh.14101.

31. Petrone J, Jackups R, Eby CS, et al. Blast flagging of the Sysmex XN-10 hematology analyzer with supervised cell image analysis: impact on quality parameters. Int J Lab Hematol 2019;41(5):601–6.

32. Eilertsen H, Sæther PC, Henriksson CE, et al. Evaluation of the detection of blasts by Sysmex hematology instruments, CellaVision DM96, and manual microscopy using flow cytometry as the confirmatory method. Int J Lab Hematol 2019;41(3): 338–44.

33. Henry S, Gérard D, Salignac S, et al. Optimizing the management of analytical interferences affecting red blood cells on XN-10 (Sysmex®). Int J Lab Hematol 2022;44(6):1068–77.

34. Zhang S, He Y, Wu W, et al. Comparison of the performance of two automatic cell morphology analyzers for peripheral-blood leukocyte morphology analysis: Mindray MC-100i and Sysmex DI-60. Int J Lab Hematol 2023. https://doi.org/10.1111/ijlh.14145.

35. Sacchetti S, Zanotti V, Giacomini L, et al. The role of infected red blood cells flag (InR) of Mindray BC 6800 plus in malaria diagnosis. Int J Lab Hematol 2024. https://doi.org/10.1111/ijlh.14172.

36. Katz B, Feldman MD, Tessema M, et al. Evaluation of Scopio Labs X100 Full Field PBS: the first high-resolution full field viewing of peripheral blood specimens combined with artificial intelligence-based morphological analysis. Int J Lab Hematol 2021;43(6):1408–16.

37. Katz BZ, Benisty D, Sayegh Y, et al. Remote digital microscopy improves hematology laboratory workflow by reducing peripheral blood smear analysis turnaround time. Appl Clin Inform 2022;13(05):1108–15.

38. Bachar N, Benbassat D, Brailovsky D, et al. An artificial intelligence-assisted diagnostic platform for rapid near-patient hematology. Am J Hematol 2021; 96(10):1264–74.

39. Atkins M, McGuire P, Balgobin B, et al. Point-of-care haematological monitoring during treatment with clozapine. J Lab Med 2022;46(3):187–93.

40. Jatoi A, Jaromin R, Jennings L, et al. Using the absolute neutrophil count as a stand-alone test in a hematology/oncology clinic: an abbreviated test can be preferable. Clin Lab Manag Rev Off Publ Clin Lab Manag Assoc. 1998;12(4): 256–60.

41. Bransky A, Larsson A, Aardal E, et al. A novel approach to hematology testing at the point of care. J Appl Lab Med 2021;6(2):532–42.

42. Larsson A, Carlsson L, Karlsson B, et al. Rapid testing of red blood cell parameters in primary care patients using HemoScreen™ point of care instrument. BMC Fam Pract 2019;20(1):1–7.

43. Kristian Kur D, Thøgersen D, Kjeldsen L, et al. The HemoScreen hematology point-of-care device is suitable for rapid evaluation of acute leukemia patients. Int J Lab Hematol 2021;43(1):52–60.

44. Linko-Parvinen AM, Keränen K, Kurvinen K, et al. HemoScreen hematology analyzer compared to Sysmex XN for complete blood count, white blood cell differential, and detection of leukocyte abnormalities. eJHaem 2022;3(4):1126–34.

45. Lindberg S, Jönsson I, Nilsson M, et al. A novel technology for 5-part differentiation of leukocytes point-of-care. Point Care J -Patient Test Technol 2014;13(2): 27–30.

46. Karawajczyk M, Haile S, Grabski M, et al. The HemoCue WBC DIFF system could be used for leucocyte and neutrophil counts but not for full differential counts. Acta Paediatr Oslo Nor 1992 2017;106(6):974–8.

47. Kur DK, Agersnap N, Holländer NH, et al. Evaluation of the HemoCue WBC DIFF in leukopenic patient samples. Int J Lab Hematol 2020;42(3):256–62.
48. Dale DC, Kelley ML, Navarro-De La Vega M, et al. A novel device suitable for home monitoring of white blood cell and neutrophil counts. Blood 2018; 132(Supplement 1):1103.
49. Sireci AN. Hematology testing in urgent care and resource-poor settings: an overview of point of care and satellite testing. Clin Lab Med 2015;35(1):197–207.
50. Merino A, Puigví L, Boldú L, et al. Optimizing morphology through blood cell image analysis. Int J Lab Hematol 2018;40(S1):54–61.
51. Khan S, Sajjad M, Hussain T, et al. A review on traditional machine learning and deep learning models for WBCs classification in blood smear images. IEEE Access 2021;9:10657–73.
52. Cheng JY, Abel JT, Balis UGJ, et al. Challenges in the development, deployment, and regulation of artificial intelligence in anatomic pathology. Am J Pathol 2021; 191(10):1684–92.
53. Lecompte TP, Bernimoulin MP. Novel parameters in blood cell counters. Clin Lab Med 2015;35(1):209–24.

Screening of Myelodysplastic Syndromes Using Research Parameters of Complete Blood Count
Automated Detection of Dysplasia

Eloísa Urrechaga, PhD

KEYWORDS

- Myelodysplastic syndromes • Cytopenia • Complete blood count
- Research use only parameters

KEY POINTS

- Myelodysplastic syndromes (MDS) are a heterogeneous group of clonal stem cell disorders yielding to an ineffective and dysplastic hematopoiesis which results in 1 or more cytopenias.
- The diagnosis of MDS is frequently challenging, especially in terms of the distinction from the other non-neoplastic causes of cytopenia.
- Peripheral blood smear review to assess dysplastic cellular morphology is helpful for the early screening. Nevertheless, manual review is time consuming and only a small fraction of blood smears is revised.
- Hematology analyzers perform the initial classification of blood cells. Due to technological progress, the number of parameters reported has increased, including the so called Research use only parameters (RUO).
- RUO might help to identify MDS in a routine clinical setting, triggering flag for blood smear examination, improving the Laboratory process, and the diagnosis of MDS.

BACKGROUND

Myelodysplastic syndromes (MDS) are a heterogeneous group of clonal stem cell disorders yielding to an ineffective and dysplastic hematopoiesis which result in 1 or more cytopenias (anemia in most cases, as well as thrombocytopenia and/or neutropenia).[1]

The progression to acute myeloid leukemia is observed in about 30% of MDS cases; until recently, MDS was treated with supportive therapy only, such as blood transfusions, but there have been advances in treatment of high-risk MDS. These facts make the early and correct diagnosis of the type of MDS crucial.[2]

Hematology Laboratory, Hospital Universitario Galdakao -Usansolo, Galdakao, Vizcaya, Spain
E-mail address: eloisamaria.urrechagaigartua@osakidetza.eus

Clin Lab Med 44 (2024) 387–396
https://doi.org/10.1016/j.cll.2024.05.001   labmed.theclinics.com
0272-2712/24/© 2024 Elsevier Inc. All rights reserved, including those for text and data mining, AI training, and similar technologies.

The diagnosis of MDS is frequently challenging, especially in terms of the distinction from the other non-neoplastic causes of cytopenia. The clinical presentation is typically insidious dependent on the depth and type of cytopenia, the signs and symptoms associated with anemia, thrombocytopenia, and neutropenia. The development of myelodysplastic syndrome (MDS) may be preceded by a few years by an unexplained macrocytic anemia with no evidence of megaloblastic anemia and a mild thrombocytopenia or neutropenia.[3]

MDS is suspected upon detection of cytopenia and morphologic changes of peripheral blood cells, and the diagnosis/prognosis must be comforted by bone marrow aspiration, flow cytometry, cytogenetic, and when needed, molecular analyses.[4] The recommended cytopenia thresholds for defining MDS are Hemoglobin (Hb) <100 g/L, absolute neutrophil count <1.8 × 10^9/L, and platelet count <100 × 10^9/L.[5]

However, blood counts above these thresholds do not exclude MDS and diagnosis may be made in patients with a milder degree of anemia or thrombocytopenia. Clinical symptoms that should prompt a workup for MDS are due to low peripheral blood counts, usually from the anemia but also from the thrombocytopenia or neutropenia.[6]

These syndromes can affect people of any age, but the risk of developing MDS increases with advancing age. The median age at onset is around 72 to 75 years old. Anemia is the most common feature of MDS which generally presents as a non-megaloblastic macrocytosis. Diagnosis when anemia is the only abnormality present can be complex, especially in older patients, but MDS must be considered a possible cause of unexplained anemia.[7]

Peripheral blood smear review to assess dysplastic cellular morphology, in particular neutrophil dysplasia, is helpful for the early screening and can guide to the diagnosis of MDS. Nevertheless, manual review is time consuming and only a small fraction of blood smears is revised; the review is only performed when quantitative or qualitative flags are present in a complete blood count (CBC). When cytopenia is moderate, as is frequently in asymptomatic patients, the absence of blood smear examination can delay diagnosis, which is crucial to initiate the diagnosis process by cytologic analysis of bone marrow aspiration[3]

Hematology analyzers perform complete blood counts and the initial classification of blood cells. Due to technological progress over past decades, the number of parameters reported has increased, the so-called Research use only parameters (RUO). In addition to the leukocyte differential counts, modern analyzers can also provide cell population data (CPD) parameters reflecting morphologic characteristics of the various cell populations. CPD provide quantitative information on the morphologic and functional characteristics of leukocytes: size, internal structure, and nucleic acid content. This added numerical information has been recognized as a new diagnostic tool that allows the automated detection of dysplasia, thus contributing to optimize the slide review, and improving the screening of MDS.[8] Multilineage dysplasia, including erythroid and megakaryocytic lineage, as well as dysgranulopoiesis can also be observed in MDS (**Fig. 1**).

RUO parameters give insights into morphology of blood cells which could be distinctively disrupted in MDS when compared with cytopenias of different etiology.

TECHNOLOGY: THE STATE OF THE ART
Red Blood Cell Extended Parameters

The flow-cytometric optical technology for red cells (RBC)-derived parameters measurement was first made available by the Technicon company in their H* series of instruments, later followed by the Advia analyzers (Bayer Diagnostics, presently Siemens Healthcare Diagnostics, Deerfield, IL, USA).

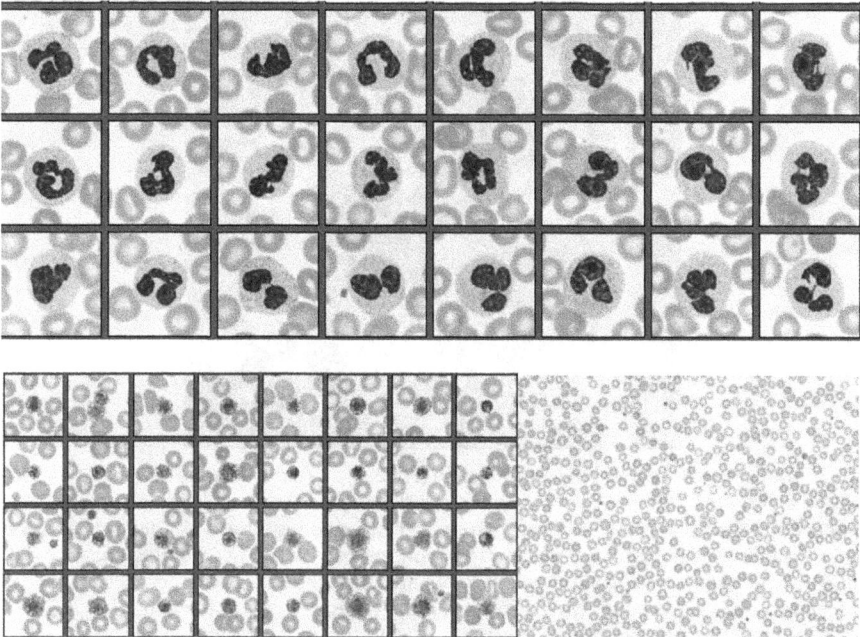

Fig. 1. Dysplasia in 3 lineages, including erythroid and megakaryocytic lineage, as well as neutrophils dysgranulopoiesis can be observed in myelodysplastic syndromes (MDS). Peripheral blood smear May-Grünwald-Giemsa stained in CellaVision DM96. (*With permission from* CellaVision.)

The technology is multi-angle laser light scattering by single cell, sphered RBC, and relies on the Mie optical theory. Mathematical models in the software use these scatter signals for calculating, for each individual cell, estimates of cellular volume (V) and cellular Hb concentration (CHC).

The whole RBC population can be classified considering the Hb concentration and cell volume: %HYPO is the percentage of hypochromic RBC with CHC <280 g/L, %HYPER the percentage the percentage of hyperchromic RBC, CHC >410 g/L. Red cells with a volume <60.0 fL are microcytic, while cells with a volume >120.0 fL are macrocytic.

In the same way, red cell distribution width reflects the anisocytosis; hemoglobin distribution width (HDW) is related with anisochromia of the RBC population.

Abbott Cell Dyn Saphire and BC 6800 Plus Mindray counters apply similar principles and reports, the Mie Map cytogram (**Fig. 2**).

Beckman Coulter (Beckman Coulter Inc. Miami, FL, USA) applies the Volume Conductivity Scatter technology to this field. Low hemoglobin density (LHD %) derives from the traditional mean cell hemoglobin concentration (MCHC), using a mathematical sigmoid transformation.

Leukocyte Cell Population Data

Automated hematology analyzers use various techniques for white blood cell counts and differential. The Coulter principle provided the basis for the first automated method for blood cell counting.

Beckman-Coulter (Brea, CA, USA) uses the VCS flow technology, based on a combination of 3 physical measurements: flow cell volume (V), conductivity (C), and light scatter (S) in their analyzers.

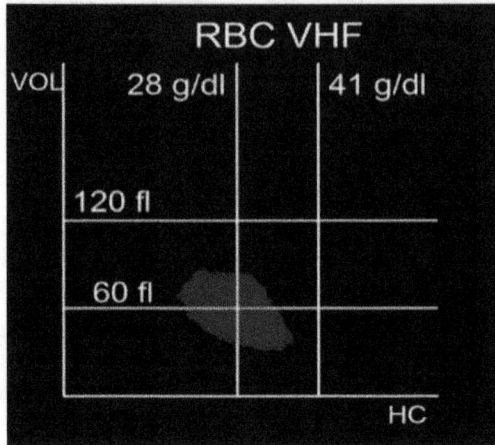

Fig. 2. The Volume/Hemoglobin concentration (V/HC) cytogram, Mie map, Hb concentration is plotted along the x axis and cell volume is plotted along the y axis. Only red blood cells (RBC) appear on this cytogram. Markers organize the cytogram into 9 distinct areas of RBC morphology. On the x axis, Hb concentration markers are set at 28.0 g/dL and 41.0 g/dL. RBC with an Hb concentration <28.0 g/dL are hypochromic, while cells with an Hb concentration >41.0 g/dL are hyperchromic. On the y axis, red cells volume markers are set at 60 fL and 120fL. Red cells with a volume <60.0 fL are microcytic, while cells with a volume >120.0 fL are macrocytic.

The CPD mean neutrophil volume (MNV), mean neutrophil conductivity (MNC), and mean neutrophil light scatter (MNS) (similar CPDs for monocytes and lymphocytes) were derived from this technology.

In addition to those CPD derived from volume and conductivity measurements, the Unicel DxH 800 analyzer generates an additional 5 angles of laser scatter, provides information regarding the granularity and membrane surface, in addition to optical signals related to cellular transparency and cellular complexity.

The optical flow cytometry technique has been combined with selective lysis and fluorescence flow cytometry in Mindray, Sysmex, and Abbott analyzers.

The Multi-Angle Polarized Scatter Separation (MAPSS) technology from Abbott uses 4 light scatter detectors to determine various cellular features. The recent Alinity-hq (Abbott, Santa Clara, CA), through 3 additional narrow-angle light scatter detectors, provides information on volume, hemoglobin content, and granularity, in a cell-by-cell count, of red cells and platelets.

In the BC-6800 Plus system (Mindray, Shenzhen, China), cells are counted and classified in diverse analytical channels, using various reagents; channel-specific light detectors at certain angles for each cell give information on cell size, cytoplasmic structures, and nuclear characteristics (S-Cube technology). The surfactant causes the hemolysis of erythrocytes and platelets, perforating the cell membranes of leukocytes. Next, the fluorescence reagent penetrates the leukocytes and labels the nucleic acids and the cytoplasmic organelles. After incubation, the sample is analyzed using the semiconductor laser and measuring the forward and side scatter fluorescent optical signals (**Fig. 3**).

Detailed information on blood cell morphology in terms of leukocyte volume, cytoplasmic and nuclear complexity, and nucleic acid content (DNA and RNA) is generated. This information is automatically converted into quantitative RUO parameters that describe the morphology of the cells: NeuX, NeuY, NeuZ for neutrophils; MonX, MonY, MonZ for monocytes; and LymX, LymY, LymZ for lymphocytes.

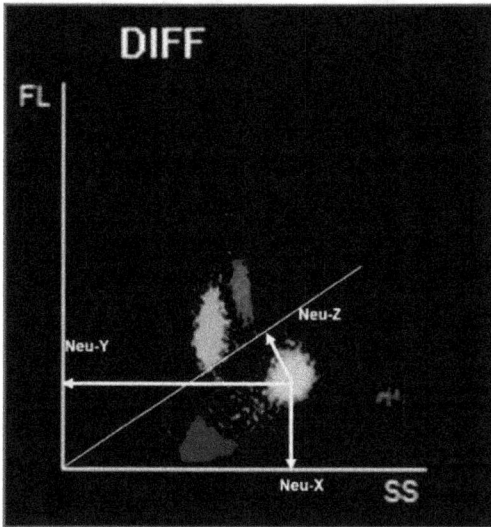

Fig. 3. Each leukocyte can be described by 3 optical signals appearing in the leukocyte differential (DIFF) scattergram: the coordinates to compose this scattergram are the morphometric parameters, so called Cell Population Data (CPD). CPD are related to the morphology and functional characteristics of leukocyte populations and report on the following: Internal cellular complexity: Neu X, Lym X, Mon X, Nucleic acid content: Neu Y, Lym Y, Mon Y, and Cell size: Neu Z, Lym Z, Mon Z.

Sysmex Corporation (Kobe Japan): The principles are similar to those described for Mindray counters. Using flow cytometry forward scatter (FSC), side scatter (SSC), and side fluorescence (SFL) optical signals are recorded. The intensities of the optical signals FSC and SSC reflect cell surface structure, shape and size, and internal granules of the leukocytes. SFL reflects the number of nucleic acids and cell organelles.

CPD is expressed as the mean (MN or M), standard deviation (SD), distribution width (W), distribution skewness (DS), or distribution kurtosis (DK) depending on the manufacturer.

Platelets

Reticulated platelets (RP) are immature, newly released platelets, which can be distinguished from mature platelets by their RNA content and their larger size.

The Abbott Cell-Dyn Sapphire (Abbott) measures RP as a part of reticulocyte analysis, which is based on the fluorescent dye CD4K530 that is excited by a 488-nm solid state laser. Scattered light (at a 7° angle) and fluorescence are recorded, which allows multi-dimensional separation of platelets and RP quantitation.

The Mindray analyzer performs immature platelets fraction (IPF%) detection together with the reticulocytes by means of proprietary asymmetric cyanine-based dye for staining RNA. IPF is derived from forward scatter versus sideward fluorescence scatterplot; results being expressed as a percentage. The IPF subpopulation is identified on the basis of size, cellular complexity, and nucleic acid content and then reported on the reticulocytes scattergram TRET (FS vs FL, **Fig. 4**).

The Sysmex XN analyzer has a dedicated channel for platelets based on fluorescence (PLT-F) channel which uses a new fluorescent dye (phenoxazine) for staining RNA. The stained cells are passed through a semiconductor diode laser

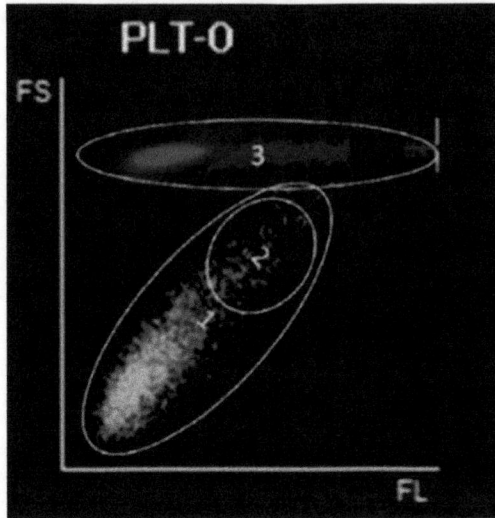

Fig. 4. Optical platelets (PLT-O) Scattergram (reticulocyte channel). X axis represents the fluorescence signal; Y axis forward scatters light. Immature platelets fraction is gated within a certain area showing stronger fluorescent signals. PLT-O optical platelets. 1 Platelets. 2 Immature platelets. 3 Optical red blood cells.

beam and the resulting forward scatter (cell volume) and fluorescence intensity (mainly due to RNA content) are measured. A computer algorithm discriminates between the mature and immature fraction (IPF) on the basis of the intensity of forward light and fluorescence. IPF is derived from the forward scatter (cell size) versus sideward fluorescence (RNA content) scatterplot.

AUTOMATIC DETECTION OF DYSPLASIA: A LITERATURE REVIEW

The diagnostic features of MDS are polymorphic and non-specific and the standard parameters reported by analyzers give little information to help in the detection of the disease. The diagnosis depends on the morphologic examination of the peripheral blood and bone marrow.[2]

Identification of MDS through CBC and RUO data has been explored over years. Among RUO parameters, the best attention has been paid to those related to the granulocyte dysplasia, typical feature of MDS. But those parameters are highly dependent on technology; due to the lack of standardization, these parameters cannot be used intercheangeably and instrument-specific clinical decision limits are required.

Different researchers have conducted studies using Sysmex analyzers[9–14] and have proposed predictive scoring systems utilizing these parameters for the diagnosis of MDS, also using advanced machine learning algorithms.[15,16] Few researchers have published data using Beckman Coulter counters.[17,18] Moreover, few articles include RUO parameters for RBC and platelets reported by Abbott or Coulter analyzers.[19,20]

Recently, using Coulter analyzers, Park and colleagues proposed a scoring system with 6 items: 2 routine CBC parameters and 4 RUO parameters (derived from red cells and leukocytes) showed satisfactory Area under curve (AUC) scores of >0.750 with high sensitivity in discriminating MDS patients from cytopenic patients without MDS.[21]

The dysplasia of neutrophils in MDS is defined by microscopic findings including nuclear hypolobulation, hypersegmentation, bizarre lobulation, clumping, cytoplasmic hypogranularity and pseudo-Chediak-Higashi granules, and small size.[22] Recent studies have found that CPD reflecting the cellular characteristics of neutrophils like cell internal complexity or granularity can be used to detect dysgranulopoiesis.[23]

Despite different technologies, Neu X provided by analyzers from different brands was correlated with the morphologic change of decreased neutrophil granules.

Granularity index can be derived from data of Sysmex, Abbott, Beckman Coulter, and Mindray analyzers.[24–27] Neu X, Neu Y, and Neu Z can reflect in numbers the severe alterations of the neutrophil morphology, internal complexity (Neu X), nucleic acid content (Neu Y), and cellular size (Neu Z). In our study, all of them presented significant lower values compared to the values seen in other maladies, macrocytic anemia and cytopenic non-MDS patients.

Le Roux and colleagues, using Sysmex XE-2100 counter, compared the values obtained for MDS patients with a group of patients with anemia and concluded that a low NEUT-X value in combination with anemia was strongly correlated with MDS.[24] Furundarena and colleagues with the same analyzer verified the value of NEUT-X and suggested the diagnostic value of NEUT-Y to detect neutrophil dysplasia arising from MDS.[9]

Sun and colleagues published the only report on the value of the CPD reported by Mindray analyzer to predict neutrophil dysplasia features of MDS combining Neu X and Neu Z.[27] In our set of patients, we also have found similar values.

Despite the technical matters, similar to those previously stated for RUO parameters, IPF has been considered a reliable marker for the differential diagnosis of thrombocytopenic disorders, and can contribute to distinguish peripheral thrombocytopenia with high diagnostic performance.[28,29]

Increased values have been found in patients with MDS, even in the absence of thrombocytopenia; in such cases, IPF would not be associated with an increase in megakaryopoiesis, but the underlying mechanism remains unknown. Moreover, a relationship between the increase in IPF and the poor prognosis in patients with MDS has been suggested.[30,31]

Macrocytic anemia, a hallmark of MDS, is due to ineffective erythropoiesis, with a high degree of apoptosis of marrow erythroid progenitors. Mean Cell Volume (MCV) is usually also increased in a large fraction of non-clonal anemias: liver diseases, endocrine diseases, vitamin deficiencies, etc. Diagnosis of MDS when anemia is the only abnormality can be complicated,[32] especially in the older population, in whom a certain degree of anemia is expected and considered normal by many clinicians. Early diagnosis enables optimal care of these diseases in aging MDS patients.

Several Articles Have Highlighted the Contribution of RBC Analysis to Myelodysplastic Syndromes Diagnosis

Using Sysmex-XN, Boutault and colleagues showed that MCV was significantly increased in MDS patients versus non-clonal cytopenias and included MCV in a score.[16] Ravalet and colleagues showed on DxH 800 that MCV, red cells distribution width (RDW), and the RUO Low Hemoglobin Density (derived from MCHC) were significantly higher in MDS patients compared to controls.[20] They also showed that diverse RBC-derived RUO, including the percentage of macrocytic hypochromic or hyperchromic RBCs, were higher in MDS patients compared to non-clonal cytopenia.

In microscopic examinations of RBCs from MDS patients, anisocytosis and poikilocytosis are also frequently observed, which can be quantified by means of RDW.

Certain hematology analyzers can report other distribution parameter similar to RBC distribution width, HDW, which reflects anisocytosis, or Hb distribution width, the distribution of Hb in the individual red cells, which reflects anisochromia. Both parameters could be useful in the screening in MDS among other anemias, as suggested by

Hwang and colleagues, using Abbott Alinity-hq analyzer. RDW, HDW, MCV, and MCH were higher in MDS patients than in non-clonal cytopenias.[21]

Neut X and Neut Y are the most potent diagnostic predictors for MDS, as was published for Sysmex analyzers[10] and by Sun and colleagues using Mindray counter.[27] These findings suggest that the dysplastic features of leukocytes, objectively measured by CPDs values, are strong predictors of MSD.

CBC is automatically obtained to detect hematological abnormalities; however, a manual examination of blood smear is essential to assess the morphologic changes in blood cells, but this procedure is labor intensive and time-consuming and requires experienced pathologists.

The use of Neu X and Neu Y in guiding the smear review could improve the sensitivity for the detection of MDS. These parameters are convenient and objective markers obtained from the automated analyzer along with the CBC. This could help to detect MDS rapidly without additional costs, improving the efficiency of the laboratory process, and contributing to make final diagnose of the patients in time.

SUMMARY

Myelodysplastic syndromes (MDS) are a heterogeneous group of clonal stem cell disorders yielding to an ineffective and dysplastic hematopoiesis which results in 1 or more cytopenias.

Until recently, MDS was treated with supportive therapy only, but advances in treatment make the early and correct diagnosis of MDS crucial.

The ultimate diagnosis depends on the morphologic examination of the peripheral blood and bone marrow. MDS is suspected upon detection of cytopenia and morphologic changes of peripheral blood cell.

Unfortunately, the MDS features are polymorphic and non-specific; moreover, manual review is time consuming and only a small fraction of peripheral blood samples is revised: blood smear review is only performed when quantitative or qualitative flags occur upon CBC.

Based on CB and RUO parameters, an automated and objective procedure, the generation of a flag for manual review, could be the initial trigger to screen for MDS among other cytopenias.

RUO reported during CBC might help to identify MDS in a routine clinical setting and could lead to a robust prediction of MDS in patients undergoing routine laboratory analysis.

DISCLOSURE

Author has nothing to disclosure.

REFERENCES

1. Sekeres MA, Taylor J. Diagnosis and treatment of myelodysplastic syndromes: a review. JAMA 2022;328(9):872–80.
2. Garcia-Manero G. Myelodysplastic syndromes: 2023 update on diagnosis, risk-stratification, and management. Am J Haematol 2023;98(8):1307–25.
3. Khan AM. Why are myelodysplastic syndromes unrecognized and underdiagnosed? A primary care perspective. Am J Med 2012;125:S15–7.
4. Bastida JM, López-Godino O, Vicente-Sánchez A, et al. Hidden myelodysplastic syndrome(MDS): a prospective study to confirm or exclude MDS inpatients with anemia of uncertain etiology. Int J Lab Hematol 2019;41:109–17.

5. Fenaux P, Haase D, Santini V, et al. Myelodysplastic syndromes: ESMO Clinical Practice Guidelines for diagnosis, treatment and follow-up. Ann Oncol 2021; 32(2):142–56.
6. Swerdlowm SH, Campo E, Harris NL, et al. World health organization classification of tumours of haematopoietic and lymphoid tissues. Lyon, France: IARC Press; 2008.
7. Greenberg PL, Tuechler H, Schanz J, et al. Revised international prognostic scoring system for myelodysplastic syndromes. Blood 2012;120:2454–65.
8. Zhu J, Clauser S, Freynet N, et al. Automated detection of dysplasia: data mining from our hematology analyzers. Diagnostics 2022;12:56.
9. Furundarena JR, Araiz M, Uranga M, et al. The utility of the Sysmex XE-2100 analyzer's NEUT-X and NEUT-Y parameters for detecting neutrophil dysplasia in myelodysplastic syndromes. Int J Lab Hem 2010;32:360–6.
10. Goel S, Sachdev R, Gajendra S, et al. Picking up myelodysplastic syndromes and megaloblastic anemias on peripheral blood: use of NEUT-X and NEUT-Y in guiding smear reviews. Int J Lab Hem 2015;37:e48–51.
11. Kim H, Han E, Lee HK, et al. Screening of myelodysplastic syndrome using cell population data obtained from an automatic hematology analyzer. Int J Lab Hematol 2021;43(2):e54–7.
12. Murphy PT, Bergin S, O'Brien M, et al. Cell population data from Sysmex XN analyzer and myelodysplastic syndrome. Int J Lab Hematol 2022;44:e138–9.
13. Di Luise D, Giannotta JA, Ammirabile M, et al. Cell Population Data NE-WX,NE-FSC, LY-Y of Sysmex XN-9000 can provide additional information to differentiate macrocytic anaemia from myelodysplastic syndrome: a preliminary study. Int J Lab Hematol 2022;44(1):e40–3.
14. Kwiecien I, Rutkowska E, Gawronski K, et al. Usefulness of new neutrophil-related hematologic parameters in patients with myelodysplastic syndrome. Cancers 2023;15:2488.
15. Boutault R, Peterlin P, Boubaya M, et al. A novel complete blood count-based score to screen for myelodysplastic syndrome in cytopenic patients. Br J Haematol 2018;183(5):736–46.
16. Pozdnyakova O, Niculescu RS, Kroll T, et al. Beyond the routine CBC: machine learning and statistical analyses identify research CBC parameter associations with myelodysplastic syndromes and specific underlying pathogenic variants. J Clin Pathol 2023;76(9):624–31.
17. Raess PW, van de Geijn GJM, Njo TL, et al. Automated screening for myelodysplastic syndromes through analysis of complete blood count and cell population data parameters. Am J Hematol 2014;89(4):369–74.
18. Kim SY, Park Y, Kim H, et al. Discriminating myelodysplastic syndrome and other myeloid malignancies from non-clonal disorders by multiparametric analysis of automated cell data. Clin Chim Acta 2018;480:56–64.
19. Ravalet N, Foucault A, Picou F, et al. Automated early detection of myelodysplastic syndrome within the general population using the research parameters of beckman–coulter DxH 800 hematology analyzer. Cancers 2021;13:389.
20. Hwang SM, Nam Y. Complete blood count and cell population data parameters from the Abbott Alinity hq analyzer are useful in differentiating myelodysplastic syndromes from other forms of cytopenia. Int J Lab Hematol 2022;44:468–76.
21. Park SH, Kim HK, Jeong J, et al. Research use only and cell population data items obtained from the Beckman Coulter DxH800 automated hematology analyzer are useful in discriminating MDS patients from those with cytopenia without MDS. J Hematop 2023;16:143–54.

22. Li H, Hu F, Gale R, et al. Myelodysplastic syndromes. Nat Rev Dis Primers 2022; 8:74.

23. Shekhar R, Srinivasan VK, Pai S. How I investigate dysgranulopoiesis. Int J Lab Hematol 2021;43(4):538–46.

24. Le R, Vlad A, Eclache V, et al. Routine diagnostic procedures of myelodysplastic syndromes: value of a structural blood cell parameter (NEUT-X) determined by the Sysmex XE-2100. Int J Lab Hem 2010;32:e237–43.

25. Inaba T, Yuki Y, Yuasa S, et al. Clinical utility of the neutrophil distribution pattern obtained using the CELL-DYN SAPPHIRE hematology analyzer for the diagnosis of myelodysplastic syndrome. Int J Hematol 2011;94:169–77.

26. Shestakova A, Nael A, Nora V, et al. Automated leukocyte parameters are useful in the assessment of myelodysplastic syndromes. Cytometry B Clin Cytom 2021; 100(3):299–311.

27. Sun P, Li N, Zhang S, et al. Combination of NeuX and NeuZ can predict neutrophil dysplasia features of myelodysplastic neoplasms in peripheral blood. Int J Lab Hematol 2023;45(4):522–7.

28. Dima F, Hoffmann JJML, Montolli V, et al. Assessment of reticulated platelets with automated hemocytometers: are we measuring the same thing? Diagnosis (Berl) 2016;3(2):91–3.

29. Briggs C, Kunka S, Hart D, et al. Assessment of an immature platelet fraction IPF in peripheral thrombocytopenia. Br J Haematol 2004;126:93–9.

30. Larruzea IA, Muñoz Marín L, Perea Durán G, et al. Evaluation of immature platelet fraction in patients with myelodysplastic syndromes. Association with poor prognosis factors. Clin Chem Lab Med 2019;57:e128–30.

31. Sugimori N, Kondo Y, Shibayama M, et al. Aberrant increase in the immature platelet fraction in patients with myelodysplastic syndrome: a marker of karyotypic abnormalities associated with poor prognosis. J Haematol 2019;82(1): 54–60.

32. Santini V. Anemia as the main manifestation of myelodysplastic syndromes. Semin Hematol 2015;52(4):348–56.

Digital Imaging and AI Pre-classification in Hematology

Kelly A. Bowers, DO, MPH, Megan O. Nakashima, MD*

KEYWORDS

- Digital imaging • Pre-classification • Neural networks • Differential count

KEY POINTS

- Digital imaging coupled with cellular pre-classification by artificial intelligence can provide a semi-automated morphology-based differential.
- These systems perform comparably to traditional manual optical microscopy when operated by a trained morphologist.
- These systems have several benefits including increased standardization, efficiency, and remote-review capabilities.

INTRODUCTION

The complete blood count with differential (CBCDIF) is one of the most commonly ordered routine laboratory tests. Advances in flow cytometry-based methods and automation have made automated analysis more accurate, precise, and efficient, as will be described elsewhere in this issue. However, a significant subset of cases still requires a morphology-based differential count (manual differential), especially in cases where there are abnormal cells (blasts and lymphoma cells) or abnormal morphology (eg, hypogranular neutrophils). This type of review is essential for clinical care but it is time-consuming and requires a skilled morphologist.[1]

In the past 2 decades, digital imaging (DI) coupled with artificial intelligence (AI) has provided a new tool for performing manual differentials. DI in this context includes detection of nucleated cells in the blood and capturing high resolution images of these cells, which can be automated. Larger fields of the slides may also be imaged in some systems. Then AI, typically an artificial neural network, is applied to pre-classify the image into a suggested cell type. The final determination of cell identity (eg, neutrophil, lymphocytes) is verified by the human operator and the results of the differential count can be released through the software into a laboratory information system, if interfaced.

Department of Pathology and Laboratory Medicine, Cleveland Clinic, 9500 Euclid Avenue L30, Cleveland, OH 44195, USA
* Corresponding author.
E-mail address: nakashm@ccf.org

Clin Lab Med 44 (2024) 397–408
https://doi.org/10.1016/j.cll.2024.04.002
0272-2712/24/© 2024 Elsevier Inc. All rights reserved.

The goal of this article is to review currently available options for digital imaging and AI pre-classification tools in the hematology laboratory and discuss the benefits of this technology, as well as potential obstacles to its use and implementation.

HISTORY AND BACKGROUND
Overview of Digital Imaging and Nucleated Cell Pre-classification Systems in the Hematology Laboratory

DI has been present in the hematology laboratory ever since digital cameras became available. The simplest method of capturing digital microscopy images is via an external camera system, which can be portable, such as a cell phone, or hard-mounted to the microscope; the image can be captured through the eye-piece or via a dedicated camera port. In this system, a human user must still manipulate the slide, find the cells, and choose which images to obtain. Because of the size of hematology cells, high-magnification (500–1000x) images, often using oil objectives, are typically required.

In 2001, Food and Drug Administration (FDA) approved the DiffMaster Octavia (CellaVision, Lund, Sweden) with an intended use of locating and imaging cells and providing suggested classification, with the caveat that the device be used by "skilled operators, trained in the use of the instrument and in recognition of leukocyte classes."[2] Several of the devices currently in use or development use this as a predicate device and methodology. These integrated systems incorporating robotics and AI can automate cell-finding and image acquisition, historically, by cell-finding using a low-power objective, then acquiring high-power cell "snapshot" images using a 1000x oil objective. An "overview image" corresponding to eight 1000x fields are also provided for platelet estimation and red blood cell (RBC) morphology assessment. This is the technology used by systems which use CellaVision software systems (CellaVision DM1200, DM9600, DC10, and Sysmex DI60, Kobe, Japan). A more recently employed technique instead uses computational photography to obtain a high-power image from multiple low-power images, allowing the system to capture a larger full-field of view corresponding to 1000 high-power fields. This is the technology used by the other currently FDA-approved systems from Scopio (X100, X100HT, Tel Aviv, Israel).

After capturing digital images, specialized image analysis software is used to process and analyze the data. This software can enhance image quality and perform quantitative measurements. This software also analyzes images using artificial neural networks (ANN), a form of AI, to recognize patterns and pre-classify each cell into a suggested type. The pre-classified cells are typically shown in a gallery view of all the images of each cell type, including artifacts and unclassified cells (**Figs. 1** and **2**). Because of the larger image ("Full Field") obtained by the Scopio system, users are able to see where each leukocyte is located within the peripheral smear (**Fig. 2**). The software may also provide the next most-likely classification. The human operator reviews the cells, reclassifies cell(s), if necessary, and releases the result wherein the software calculates the differential (%) count. These systems will be hereafter referred to as cell-locator/preclassification (CL/Pcell-locator/preclassification) and review using a traditional manual light microscope as optical microscopy (OM).

Classification of Leukocytes

Validations for these systems compare differential counts obtained from manual light microscopy to those from the final, operator re-classified differential counts. A subset of studies has addressed the accuracy of the pre-classification while the clinically-relevant result is the final, re-classified differential; accuracy of the pre-classification

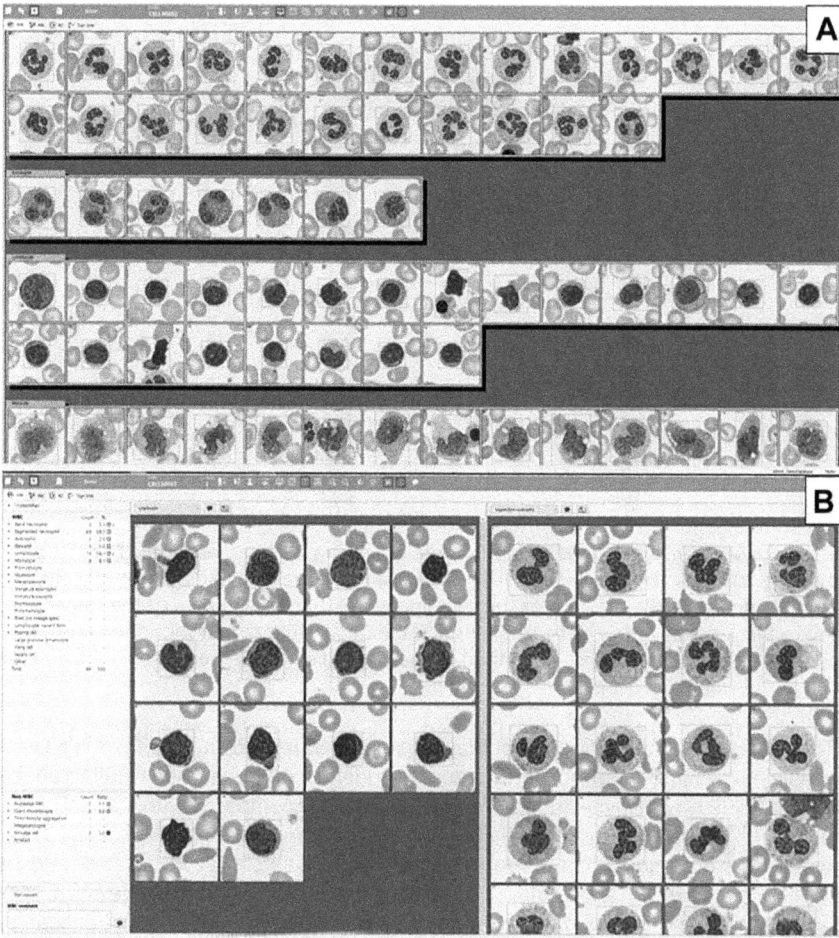

Fig. 1. Leukocyte images obtained by CellaVision systems. (*A*) gallery view of leukocyte images obtained by the CellaVision DC-1 instrument. (*B*) side-by-side view of two cell types (lymphocytes and segmented neutrophils) using images obtained by the DI-60 (Sysmex). The automatically calculated differential count is shown in the panel on the left. ([*A,B*] *With permission from* Scopio.)

can affect efficiency as a sample where many cells need to be reclassified will take the operator longer to result. The DM96 has several studies where the accuracy of the pre-classification was reported. Pre-classification of neutrophils and lymphocytes was generally excellent (>90% accuracy).[3–5] Monocytes and nucleated red blood cells (RBCs) were also pre-classified with greater than 80% accuracy. Accuracy was lower with less frequent cell types such as eosinophils, basophils, and various immature granulocytes. Stouten reported an R^2 of greater than 0.900 and slope 0.9 to 1.1 for neutrophils, lymphocytes, monocytes, eosinophils, and nucleated RBCs.[6] After re-classification, several of these cell types show excellent correlation to OM results with correlation slopes 0.9 to 1.1 for most cell types except rare events or cells with poor reproducibility on OM (eg, bands).[5,7,8] Similar, or even better performance has been reported for the more recently developed DI-60 and DC-1.[9,10] Published data regarding re-classified result on the Scopio system are similar.[11]

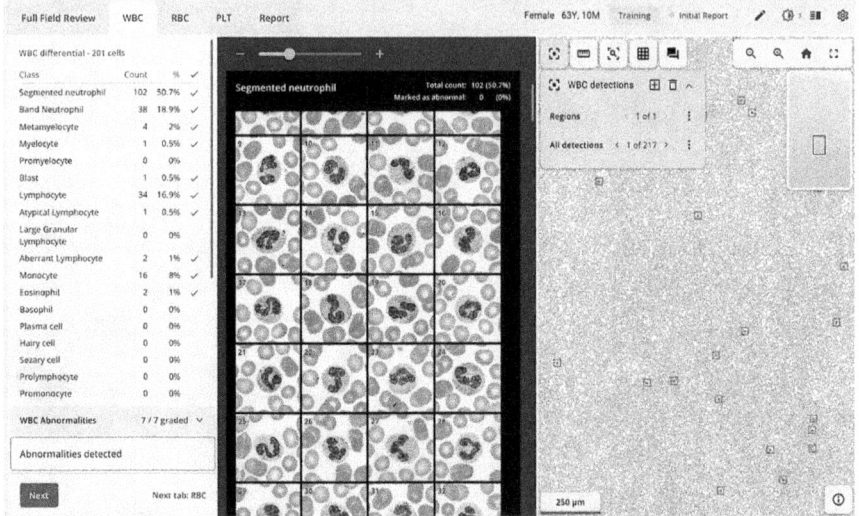

Fig. 2. Leukocyte images and differential obtained using a Scopio analyzer. The left panel shows the automatically calculated differential, center panel the gallery view of cells, and the right side shows the location of the cells imaged within a given area of the smear (indicated by black boxes with +). The small inset in the upper right corner shows the location of the current field of view (blue rectangle) in the context of the larger, "Full Field," image. (*With permission from* Scopio.)

The reported pre-classification of blasts has ranged from 65% to 83%.[3–5,12] Using re-classified results, reported performance for identification has been quite variable with 50% to 99% sensitivity and 91% to 99% specificity compared with manual microscopy.[3,7,13,14] Interestingly, sensitivity reportedly decreased in the Eilertsen study, however, the area under the curve to detect blasts was similar in the pre- and re-classified analyses. In a pediatric population, the DM96 performed better at pre-classifying myeloid blasts than lymphoid blasts, however, after re-classification, correlation between DM96 and OM was similar for total blast count.[15] Van der Vorm reported very good performance of the DC-1 to count blasts even on pre-classification, with a high clinical sensitivity and specificity for abnormal results.[10]

Other notable findings include that the absolute neutrophil counts are reportedly accurate even at low numbers on the DM96.[16] The DM96 also showed good sensitivity and specificity for left-shifted granulocytes, prolymphocytes, and plasma cells.[3,7] Also, variant morphology of lymphocytes can be detected and enumerated by the operator based on the images.[17]

Evaluation of Erythrocytes and Platelets

Digital images can also be used to assess RBCs and platelets with variable levels of sophistication. The Roche m511 system was unique in that; it performed all assessments of RBCs and platelets based on image analysis of specially created slides, including count, mean cell volumes, and hemoglobin or hematocrit measurements.[18] This instrument is no longer available in the United States.

The CellaVision systems provides the overview image for estimated platelet count; our laboratory also validated using these fields to perform RBC morphology assessment, which was also studied by Horn and colleagues[19,20] The CellaVision Peripheral Blood Application also pre-classifies anisocytosis, micro or macrocytosis, polychromatic cells, hypochromatic cells, and poikilocytosis. Their subsequently released Advanced Red Blood Cell Application (ARBCA) classifies RBCs into 21 categories including different shapes and inclusions (**Fig. 3**).[21–23] CellaVision, with or without ARBCA, performs well at identifying clinically-critical cell shapes such as sickle cells and schistocytes.[20,22] The system also detects intracellular inclusions such as Pappenheimer bodies and can identify parasites such as malaria, however, not at the clinically-required level of sensitivity.[24,25] The Scopio Peripheral Blood Smear application automates the platelet estimate and has similar erythrocyte pre-classification capabilities to ARBCA, although the performance of the latter has not been reported in detail.[11] Both of these systems also provide a semi-quantitative grade of the number of each poikilocyte present, which can be changed by the user if they disagree with the software.

One potential limitation of CL/P systems is an inability to completely visualize the edges of the smear, including the feathered edge, where abnormal cells and platelet clumps often localize. Previous studies reported CellaVision often failed to detect platelet clumps.[26] The company has recently released a "Feathered Edge" overview component to the software to address this issue, which allows visualization of the feathered edge (**Fig. 4**A). The "Full Field" view available on the Scopio system also visualizes the feathered edge and evaluates whether or not platelet clumps are present (**Fig. 4**B). However, there are yet no published data on the ability of these systems to identify platelet clumps or abnormal cells at the feathered edge that are not present on the other imaged areas of the slide.

Other Systems and Specimen Types

The digital imaging capabilities and pre-classification ANN are theoretically applicable to other Romanowsky-stained specimens with hematolymphoid cells. CellaVision has a Body Fluid Application, which provides a 5-part differential count on Romanowsky stained fluids. The pre-classification by DM96 showed reported high accuracy,

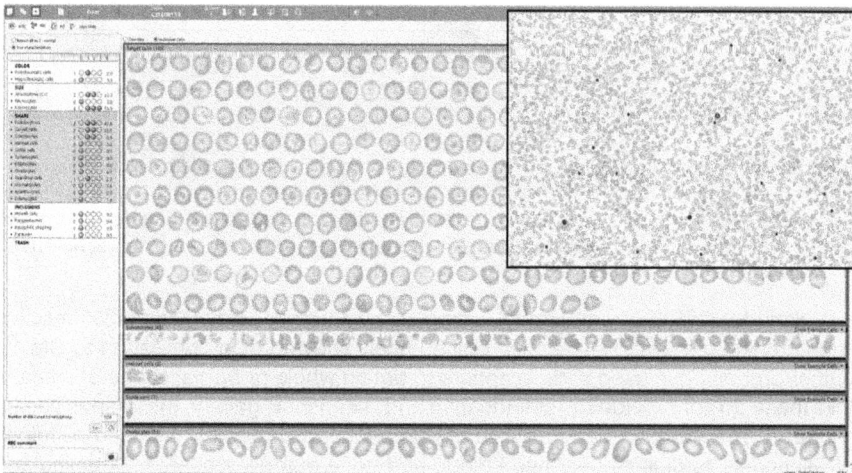

Fig. 3. CellaVision Advanced Red Blood Cell application. The main screen shows the gallery view of each poikilocyte while the left panel shows the automatically pre-assigned grading, which is programmed per laboratory cut-offs and manually changed by the user. The inset shows the "overview" image of the area of the slide from which the poikilocytes were imaged. (*With permission from* CellaVision.)

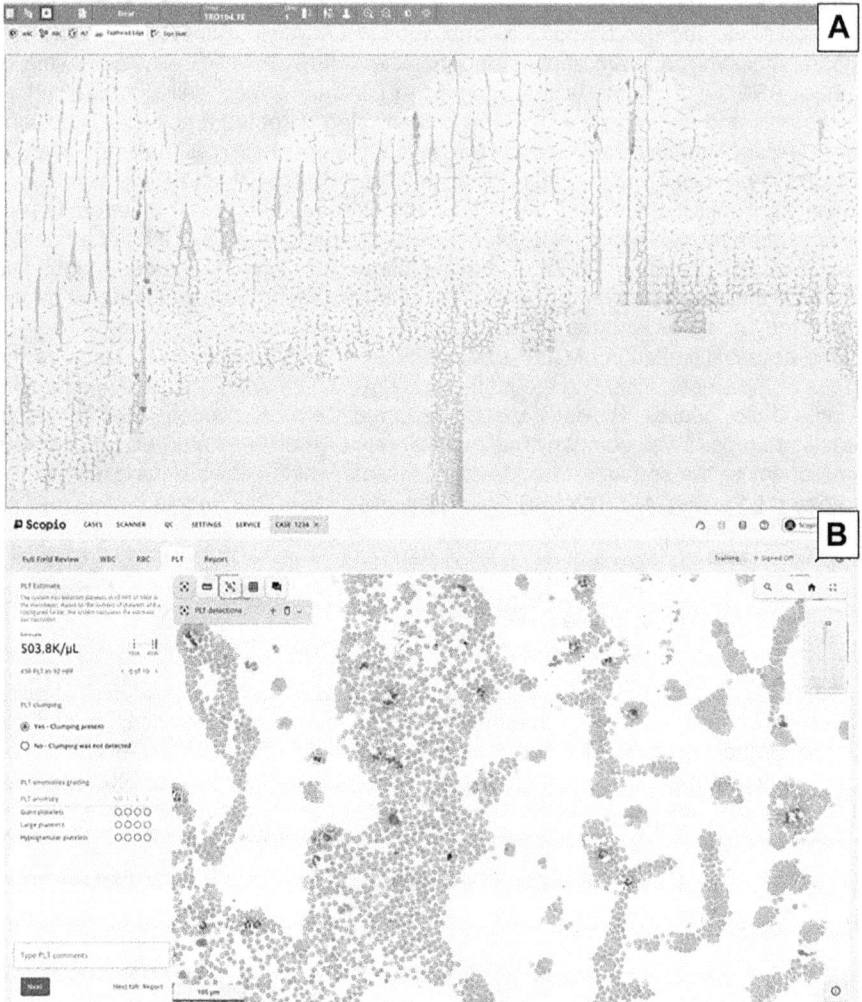

Fig. 4. Feathered edge visualization on the CellaVision and Scopio systems. (*A*) "feathered edge" application on CellaVision systems. The software flagged for "PLT clumps?" (not shown). (*B*) platelet tab of the Scopio software shows an estimated platelet count and whether or not the system detected platelet clumping. (*With permission from* Scopio.)

particularly for CSF (90% accuracy), compared with other body fluids (83%, ascites and peritoneal dialysis). Re-classified differentials showed high correlation to OM.[27]

Other groups have used slide scanners to obtain whole or partial scans of smears. While these do not provide the cell-locating and "snapshot" gallery, the images can be annotated. The Working Group WP10 of European LeukemiaNet has used histology slide-scanners to digitize peripheral blood and bone marrow smears for training and performance assessment of morphologists and reported an increased in intra-observer concordance using this technology from 62.5% to 83.0% They did note that an entire smear required 30 to 45 minutes to scan using a 40x oil-immersion objective, resulting in a 500 to 1000 MB file.[28] Whole slide images are also used in competency and proficiency testing programs.

Bone marrow aspirate smears are increasingly being evaluated using DI or AI. Several research groups have reported on using this technology to perform (*With permission from* Scopio.)automated differential counts, however, aspirate smears have other layers of complexity compared with peripheral blood smears. The smears are less uniform, requiring an extra step of finding the best areas of the slide for examination, and often nucleated cells are very near to each other. Recent advances in this research have been reviewed by Lewis and Pozdnyakova.[29] Commercial vendors are also actively working in this field, and Scopio and Morphogo (Zhiwei, Hangzhou, China) have bone marrow applications, which also image a smear and provide cell pre-classification, but are currently for research use-only[30] (See Joshua E. Lewis & Olga Pozdnyakova's article, "Advances in Bone Marrow Evaluation," in this issue).

DISCUSSION
Accuracy and Quality

As outlined earlier, the current CL/P systems have exhibited strong performance for routine differentials and for detecting abnormal cells, when operated by a trained morphologist. The pre-classification on DM96 has been shown to have less inter-laboratory variability than OM differentials.[31] The software also has a library of reference cells to aid the operator during re-classification. Depending on the storage capabilities or preferences, a patient's previous images may also be archived for comparison. The system also increased standardization because of a set area of the slide being examined. Nan and colleagues performed a failure mode and effect analysis and showed a 5-fold decrease in risk using DI-60 to count leukopenic slides compared with OM.[32]

Remote Review

Both of the currently FDA-approved systems have remote-review capabilities. This is particularly helpful at sites where OM cannot be performed because of space or equipment constraints or a lack of personnel trained to perform primary review. It is also helpful for cases which require secondary review by a more senior laboratory scientist or physician who may not work on-site, or after-hours.

Turnaround Time

Significant decreases in turnaround time can be achieved with these systems if remote-review replaces physically transporting slides to another location.[33,34] Within a site, results have been mixed, however, it is generally reported that it is faster to review a smear on the DM96 compared with OM.[3,15,31] In theory, review should be faster on CL/P, especially in low-cellularity samples because the operator does not have to spend time scanning the slide to find the cells. These authors found this to be the case and the technologists who were slower on OM, saved more time on using the DM96, similar to Kratz and colleagues finding that non-hematology specialists experienced more time-saving.[3,20] Nam and colleagues reported an overall longer turnaround time for leukopenic samples, however, their study design included time to scan the slides.[32] The time required to scan a slide is "hands-off," so it does not necessarily increase the amount of operator time required. The throughput for peripheral blood analysis of the 2 high-volume analyzers, Scopio X100HT and CellaVision DM9600, is 40 slides per hour and 30 slides per hour, respectively. If a very quick turnaround time is required, as in cancer centers where patients are waiting on differential results to receive treatment, then the time to scan may be prohibitive.

Automation

Analyzers designed for higher throughput laboratories allow a user to load slides (96 slides on DM9600, and 30 slides on X100HT) and then automatically retrieves and images each one before moving to the next. This allows the user to "walk away" and perform other laboratory tasks while leukocytes are located and the images are being obtained. Partnerships with cpmplete blood count analyzer manufacturers can facilitate end-to-end automation of CBCDIF. The Sysmex XN9000 automation line connects Sysmex XN10 or XN20 analyzers to automated slide-maker / stainers (SP-10) and a DI-60 module that utilizes CellaVision technology. The line will make and stain a peripheral blood smear when indicated, which is then automatically transferred to the DI-60 module and digitized without human intervention. Eventually, the slides and residual blood samples are archived. Scopio and Beckman Coulter (Brea, CA) have a similar system under development.

Other Benefits

Depending on file storage space, the images may be retained for several months to years, and selected images can be archived for longer. This is significantly longer than most laboratories can retain glass slides because of physical space constraints. Retained images can be used for teaching, as well as to compare abnormal cells in a current sample with a patient's previously diagnosed blasts or lymphoma cells. This repository of digital images also has potential to be used for training of future AI or machine learning algorithms, for detection of various disease states such as myelodysplasia, lymphoma, and sepsis.

Operators are able to sit upright and view the cells on the screen in a more ergonomically correct position compared with using OM. Users also reported less eye strain when using DM96 versus OM.[35] Respondees also indicated that results were more consistent and it was easier to train new employees using the DM96. The images can be used for competency assessment; unlike with a glass slide, using the captured digital images for the assessment assures that each assessee is reviewing the exact same cells during their assessment.

Operator Limitations

From anecdotal experience, some laboratory scientists are uncomfortable using the CL/P compared with OM. This may relate to the use of cell "snap-shots" on the CellaVision systems, leading to a lack of "context" in the overall slides. It remains to be seen whether innovations such as larger fields of view and the feathered edge scanning will decrease this hesitancy.

It should be noted that these systems are validated only for use by skilled operators, trained in identifying the cell types by morphology. CL/P systems do not replace proficient laboratory staff, and there is a theoretic risk of under-trained staff becoming over-reliant on the pre-classification.

Cost

The currently available systems require an outlay of capital for the digital imaging system and software. However, utilizing the technology may overall decrease costs because of the increased efficiency and remote-consultation capabilities. One study modeled using a point-of-care hematology paired with the DC-1 compared with a more sophisticated hematology analyzer and showed significant cost-savings.[36] Outside of the 2 currently FDA-approved systems, there is another system in development (Automated Blood Differential, Techcyte, Orem, UT) that uses a different model to achieve cell pre-classification; the laboratory can use their own slide-scanner and upload the images to the cloud, which could provide cost savings by utilizing technology already in the laboratory.[37] Other costs include maintaining the large volumes of digital data created, as well as cybersecurity, especially, if using a remote-review system, as well as laboratory resources needed for validation, inter-method comparisons, and operator competency assessment.

Validation

The International Council for Standardization in Hematology put forth recommended guidelines for validating digital cell-locator or pre-classification systems in 2014, which also references CLSI H20-A2.[38,39] Local regulations will vary as to what is required for validation. For analyzers with local approval, a validation emphasizing accuracy compared with the reference method, reproducibility, and reference range may be sufficient. Sensitivity and specificity analysis for clinically-significant findings, such as blasts, may also be prudent. For other non-approved or laboratory-developed systems, additional validation may be required. The College of American Pathologists has published a guideline on validating whole slide imaging for pathology.[40]

Future Possibilities

Several other companies are developing CL/P systems, but have not yet received FDA-approval. These include the Techcyte application and Mindray MC-80 (Shenzen, China).[41] The analytical software and algorithms including ANNs could be further optimized to include specific disease states. In addition to pre-classifying general cell types, some groups have applied other AI algorithms to try to differentiate between reactive lymphocytes and different types of lymphoma.[42,43] The number of cells imaged and analyzed could also be optimized to detect rare events such as for minimal or measurable residual disease detection. There are also possibilities to interface the results from a CL/P with the other data from hematology analyzers, other laboratory tests, and the electronic medical record to build larger diagnostic algorithms for detection of pathologies.[29]

SUMMARY

Automated cell-locators with DI, paired with AI, are capable of producing results comparable to optical manual microscopy. There are several benefits to these systems, including decreased turnaround time, especially in cases where remote-review replaces physically transporting slides. Use of these systems also increases standardization and reproducibility, and they can be used for training and competency of laboratory personnel. Some potential barriers to implementation include hesitancy of adopting the technology, cost of the system, data storage or cybersecurity, and resources to perform adequate validation. There are also applications for using this technology on other Romanowsky-stained specimens such as body fluids and bone marrow.

CLINICS CARE POINTS

- When operated by a trained morphologist, CL/P systems are accurate for both routine (normal 5-part differential) and abnormal white blood cell differential counting.

- CL/P systems can decrease turnaround time for peripheral blood smear review, especially when remote-review replaces physical transportation of slides.
- Performance at detecting blasts has been variable and this and other critical cell types may warrant a targeted validation study.

DISCLOSURE

The author has been a paid speaker for Sysmex, however, this was on a subject which is not related to this article. Dr K.A. Bowers has not disclosures.

REFERENCES

1. Bain BJ. Diagnosis from the blood smear. N Engl J Med 2005;353(5):498–507.
2. 510(k) summary for the DiffMaster OctaviaTM. U.S. Food & Drug Administration, Available at: https://www.accessdata.fda.gov/cdrh_docs/pdf/k003301.pdf, 2001. Accessed November 17, 2023.
3. Kratz A, Bengtsson HI, Casey JE, et al. Performance evaluation of the CellaVision DM96 system: WBC differentials by automated digital image analysis Supported by an artificial neural network. Am J Clin Pathol 2005;124(5):770–81.
4. Ceelie H, Dinkelaar RB, Van Gelder W. Examination of peripheral blood films using automated microscopy; evaluation of Diffmaster Octavia and Cellavision DM96. J Clin Pathol 2006;60(1):72–9.
5. Briggs C, Longair I, Slavik M, et al. Can automated blood film analysis replace the manual differential? An evaluation of the CellaVision DM96 automated image analysis system. Int J Lab Hematol 2009;31(1):48–60.
6. Stouten K, Riedl JA, Levin M-D, et al. Examination of peripheral blood smears: performance evaluation of a digital microscope system using a large-scale leukocyte database. Int J Lab Hematol 2015;37(5). https://doi.org/10.1111/ijlh.12391.
7. Park SH, Park C-J, Choi M-O, et al. Automated digital cell morphology identification system (CellaVision DM96) is very useful for leukocyte differentials in specimens with qualitative or quantitative abnormalities. Int J Lab Hematol 2013;35(5): 517–27.
8. Vergara-Lluri M, Kovach AE, Nakashima MO, et al. Significant variability in the identification and reporting of band neutrophils by Participants Enrolled in the College of American Pathologists proficiency testing program: time for a Change. Arch Pathol Lab Med 2023. https://doi.org/10.5858/arpa.2023-0015-CP.
9. Kweon OJ, Lim YK, Lee MK, et al. Red and white blood cell morphology characterization and hands-on time analysis by the digital cell imaging analyzer DI-60. PLoS One 2022;17(4):e0267638.
10. Van Der Vorm LN, Hendriks HA, Smits SM. Performance of the CellaVision DC-1 digital cell imaging analyser for differential counting and morphological classification of blood cells. J Clin Pathol 2023;76(3):194–201.
11. Katz B, Feldman MD, Tessema M, et al. Evaluation of Scopio Labs X100 Full Field PBS: the first high-resolution full field viewing of peripheral blood specimens combined with artificial intelligence-based morphological analysis. Int J Lab Hematol 2021;43(6):1408–16.
12. Eilertsen H, Sæther PC, Henriksson CE, et al. Evaluation of the detection of blasts by Sysmex hematology instruments, CellaVision DM96, and manual microscopy using flow cytometry as the confirmatory method. Int J Lab Hematol 2019;41(3): 338–44.

13. Eilertsen H, Henriksson CE, Hagve T-A. The use of CellaVision™ DM96 in the verification of the presence of blasts in samples flagged by the Sysmex XE-5000. Int J Lab Hematol 2017;39(4):423–8.

14. Rollins-Raval MA, Raval JS, Contis L. Experience with CellaVision DM96 for peripheral blood differentials in a large multi-center academic hospital system. J Pathol Inform 2012;3(1):29.

15. Billard M, Lainey E, Armoogum P, et al. Evaluation of the CellaVision™ DM automated microscope in pediatrics. Int J Lab Hematol 2010;32(5):530–8.

16. Amundsen EK, Urdal P, Hagve TA, et al. Absolute neutrophil counts from automated hematology instruments are accurate and precise even at very low levels. Am J Clin Pathol 2012;137(6):862–9.

17. Marionneaux S, Maslak P, Keohane EM. Morphologic identification of atypical chronic lymphocytic leukemia by digital microscopy. Int J Lab Hematol 2014; 36(4):459–64.

18. Bruegel M, George TI, Feng B, et al. Multicenter evaluation of the cobas m 511 integrated hematology analyzer. Int J Lab Hematol 2018;40(6):672–82.

19. Horn CL, Mansoor A, Wood B, et al. Performance of the CellaVision® DM96 system for detecting red blood cell morphologic abnormalities. J Pathol Inform 2015; 6(1):11.

20. Nakashima MO, Doyle TJ, Phelan-Lewin K, et al. Assessment of semi-quantitative grading of red blood cell abnormalities utilizing images from the CellaVision DM96 compared to manual light microscopy. Int J Lab Hematol 2017;39(5). https://doi.org/10.1111/ijlh.12673.

21. Egelé A, Stouten K, Van Der Heul-Nieuwenhuijsen L, et al. Classification of several morphological red blood cell abnormalities by DM96 digital imaging. Int J Lab Hematol 2016;38(5). https://doi.org/10.1111/ijlh.12530.

22. Criel M, Godefroid M, Deckers B, et al. Evaluation of the red blood cell advanced software application on the CellaVision DM96. Int J Lab Hematol 2016;38(4): 366–74.

23. Park SJ, Yoon J, Kwon JA, et al. Evaluation of the CellaVision advanced RBC application for detecting red blood cell morphological abnormalities. Ann Lab Med 2021;41(1):44–50.

24. Florin L, Maelegheer K, Muyldermans A, et al. Evaluation of the CellaVision DM96 advanced RBC application for screening and follow-up of malaria infection. Diagn Microbiol Infect Dis 2018;90(4):253–6.

25. Yoon J, Kwon JA, Yoon SY, et al. Diagnostic performance of CellaVision DM96 for Plasmodium vivax and Plasmodium falciparum screening in peripheral blood smears. Acta Trop 2019;193:7–11.

26. Gulati G, Uppal G, Florea AD, et al. Detection of platelet clumps on peripheral blood smears by CellaVision DM96 system and microscopic review. Lab Med 2014;45(4):368–71.

27. Riedl JA, Dinkelaar RB, Van Gelder W. Automated morphological analysis of cells in body fluids by the digital microscopy system DM96. J Clin Pathol 2010;63(6): 538–43.

28. Zini G, Barbagallo O, Scavone F, et al. Digital morphology in hematology diagnosis and education: the experience of the European LeukemiaNet WP10. Int J Lab Hematol 2022;44(S1):37–44.

29. Lewis JE, Pozdnyakova O. Digital assessment of peripheral blood and bone marrow aspirate smears. Int J Lab Hematol 2023;45(S2):50–8.

30. Fu X, Fu M, Li Q, et al. Morphogo: an automatic bone marrow cell classification system on digital images analyzed by artificial intelligence. Acta Cytol 2020; 64(6):588–96.

31. Riedl JA, Stouten K, Ceelie H, et al. Interlaboratory reproducibility of blood morphology using the digital microscope. SLAS Technol 2015;20(6):670–5.

32. Nam M, Yoon S, Hur M, et al. Digital morphology analyzer Sysmex DI-60 vs. Manual counting for white blood cell differentials in leukopenic samples: a Comparative assessment of risk and turnaround time. Ann Lab Med 2022;42(4):398–405.

33. Katz BZ, Benisty D, Sayegh Y, et al. Remote digital microscopy Improves hematology laboratory Workflow by Reducing peripheral blood smear analysis turnaround time. Appl Clin Inform 2022;13(05):1108–15.

34. Mayes C, Gwilliam T, Mahe ER. Improving turn-around times in low-throughput distributed hematology laboratory settings with the CellaVision® DC-1 instrument. J Lab Med 2023;0(0). https://doi.org/10.1515/labmed-2023-0073.

35. Vanvranken SJ, Patterson ES, Rudmann SV, et al. A Survey study of benefits and limitations of using CellaVisionTM DM96 for peripheral blood differentials. Clin Lab Sci 2014;27(1):32–9.

36. Stephens L, Bevins NJ, Bengtsson HI, et al. Comparison of different small clinical hematology laboratory Configurations with Focus on remote smear imaging. Arch Pathol Lab Med 2019;143(10):1234–45.

37. Makhija K, Lincz LF, Attalla K, et al. White blood cell evaluation in haematological malignancies using a web-based digital microscopy platform. Int J Lab Hematol 2021;43(6):1379–87.

38. Briggs C, Culp N, Davis B, et al. ICSH guidelines for the evalution of blood cell analysers including those used for differential leucocyte and reticulocyte counting. Int J Lab Hematol 2014;36(6):613–27.

39. Clinical and Laboratory Standards Institute (CLSI). Reference Leukocyte (WBC) Differential Count (Proportional) and Evaluation of Instrumental Methods - Approved Standard Second Edition. Published online January 18, 2017.

40. Evans AJ, Brown RW, Bui MM, et al. Validating whole slide imaging systems for diagnostic Purposes in pathology. Arch Pathol Lab Med 2022;146(4):440–50.

41. Merino A, Laguna J, Rodríguez-García M, et al. Performance of the new MC-80 automated digital cell morphology analyser in detection of normal and abnormal blood cells: Comparison with the CellaVision DM9600. Int J Lab Hematol 2023;14178. https://doi.org/10.1111/ijlh.14178.

42. Alférez S, Merino A, Mujica LE, et al. Automatic classification of atypical lymphoid B cells using digital blood image processing. Int J Lab Hematol 2014;36(4): 472–80.

43. Puigví L, Merino A, Alférez S, et al. Quantitative Cytologic Descriptors to differentiate CLL, Sézary, granular, and Villous lymphocytes through image analysis. Am J Clin Pathol 2019;152(1):74–85.

Advances and Progress in Automated Urine Analyzers

Nicholas E. Larkey, PhD[a], Ifeyinwa E. Obiorah, MD, PhD[b],*

KEYWORDS

- Urinalysis • Microscopy • Flow cytometry • Analyzer • Automated

KEY POINTS

- Recent advances have cleared the pathway to significant progress in automated urinalysis that may alter the pathologic detection of abnormal urinary elements.
- The automation and standardization of urinalysis improve efficacy, save labor costs, and reduce preanalytical variables due to sample processing.
- Automated flow cytometers serve as an efficient screening method in urinary tract infection and may reduce and eliminate unnecessary urine cultures in the laboratory.
- Fully automated instrumentation with automated strip and urine sediment analyzers streamline workflow to decrease the need for manual review.

INTRODUCTION

Urinalysis is the one of the most frequently used screening tests in the clinical laboratory. In general, urinalysis consists of 3 major components; physical, chemical, and microscopic examination.[1] Physical evaluation of a urine specimen includes description of color, odor, clarity, volume, and specific gravity. Chemical examination entails detection of protein, blood cells, glucose, pH, bilirubin, urobilinogen, ketone bodies, nitrites, and leukocyte esterase.[1] In addition, microscopic examination involves formed elements including identification of crystals, epithelial and blood cells, casts, and microorganisms. Testing is commonly performed using traditional methods such as test strip tests, urine microscopy, and cultures. However, these methods can be time consuming and more labor intensive. Interpretation of the tests can be subjective due to variations in reaction time for test strips, and interobserver/intraobserver variation, which can both lead to analytical errors.[2,3] Technological advances have revealed a variety of instrumentations that standardize sample processing, analysis of the test strips, and microscopy analysis.[4] In addition to performing a complete

[a] Department of Pathology, Division of Clinical Chemistry, University of Virginia Health, 1215 Lee Street, Charlottesville, VA 22903, USA; [b] Department of Pathology, Division of Hematopathology, University of Virginia Health, 1215 Lee street, Charlottesville, VA 22903, USA
* Corresponding author
E-mail address: jnp5qm@uvahealth.org

Clin Lab Med 44 (2024) 409–421
https://doi.org/10.1016/j.cll.2024.04.003
0272-2712/24/© 2024 Elsevier Inc. All rights reserved.

labmed.theclinics.com

analysis, these automated urine systems can incorporate result reporting. Over the years, automated urinalysis has undergone extensive advancement. For examination of the physical and chemical components, semiautomated biochemical analyzers have evolved to fully automated systems. Urine sediment evaluation has utilized manual techniques such as counting in a standardized or non-standardized method under a coverslip or counting of centrifuged or uncentrifuged urine specimens in a chamber.[5] Subsequently, automated microscopy and flow cytometry are now established for urine sediment examination in modern clinical laboratories. Digitized urine microscopy analyzers provide efficient standardized results with a quick turnaround time using artificial intelligence (AI) techniques.[5] Flow cytometry utilizes forward light scatter, fluorescence, and impedance detection to identify stained urine sediment particles presented in scattergrams.[6] In this review, the progress and major developments in automated urinalysis will be discussed.

SEMIAUTOMATED AND FULLY AUTOMATED URINE ANALYZERS

Urine test strips typically detect either all or a portion of the following 10 routine urine components: specific gravity, pH, protein, glucose, ketones, blood, bilirubin, urobilinogen, nitrite, and leukocyte esterase. In conjunction, these analytes can screen for numerous glomerular abnormalities. Additional components that can be evaluated, sometimes on a separate strip, are albumin, creatinine, and human chorionic gonadotropin. Test strips that are designed for only albumin and creatinine are used to determine the albumin/creatinine ratio (urine ACR) which is useful in the evaluation of kidney disease.[7] Each individual pad on the test strip contains unique reagents for a color-changing chemical reaction for the analyte of interest, where the degree of color change can be correlated to the concentration of the analyte. Test strips are dipped into a urine sample and are then interpreted manually by a user by comparing the color of each pad to a reference color chart that correlates the color to a specific concentration or the presence/absence of the analyte. Parameters such as color and clarity/turbidity are not interpreted by the urine test strips and must be recorded by the user manually. Notably, urine color can be affected by certain foods, drugs, as well as systemic medical diseases.[8]

Semiautomated analyzers allow for more accurate measurement of the urine test strips by using reflectometry. The test strip must be dipped manually into the urine specimen before inserting into the analyzer. Upon placement into the analyzer, light is shone on the reagent pad for a given analyte. The reflectance from the light is measured and correlated to provide qualitative or semiquantitative results. The results can be reported as negative/trace/positive or small/moderate/large or have numerical results reported over specified ranges. Similar to manual urine test strip methods, color and clarity of the urine is manually recorded by the user. An advantage of the semiautomated analyzers over manual test strip methods is that the analyzers can be interfaced to laboratory middleware and results are uploaded to the medical record. Thus, this decreases the error associated with the manual transcription of results.

Semiautomated analyzers obtain either Food and Drug Administration (FDA) 510k approval or seek class I device exemptions, and their complexity is typically considered waived. This allows the devices to be used by the maximum amount of people with minimal training or required qualifications. There are numerous different brands of semiautomated analyzers with approval in the United States, and select examples are included in **Table 1**. These brands include a semiautomated analyzer that work with their proprietary test strips. Popular brands and platforms include the Clinitek

Table 1
Semiautomated and automated urine analyzers

Manufacturer	Platform	Reagent Strips or Cartridges	Automation Level
Siemens	Clinitek Status+ Clinitek Advantus	Uristix, Multistix, Multistix PRO, Hema-Combistix, CLINITEK Microalbumin 2,	Semiautomated
	Clinitek Novus	CLINITEK Novus	Automated
ARKRAY	AUTION Elevent AE-4022 AUTION MAX AX-4280 AUTION MAX AX-4030	AUTION sticks	Automated
Roche	Urisys 1010 Cobas u 411 Cobas u 601	Chemstrip Combur-Test	Semiautomated Automated
ACON Labs	Mission U120 Mission U500	Mission urinalysis reagent strips	Semiautomated
AccuBioTech	Accu-Tell Urine Analyzer	Accu-Tell urine reagent strips	Semiautomated
BTNX	Rapid Response Urine Analyzer U120	Rapid Response urinalysis reagent strips	Semiautomated
Cardinal Health	Cardinal Health Urinalysis Analyzer	ACR urinalysis test strips SGL urinalysis test strips	Semiautomated
Clarity Diagnostics	Platinum Urocheck 120c	Clarity Urocheck Clarity Platinum	Semiautomated
EKF Diagnostics	Uri-Trak 120	Stanbio Uri-Chek 10 SG	Semiautomated
Germaine Laboratories	AimStrip Urine Analyzer 2	Aimstick urine reagent strips	Semiautomated
Jant Pharmacal	Accustrip URS Reader	Accustrip URS 10	Semiautomated
Macherey-Nagel	URYXXON Relax URYXXON 200 URYXXON 500	URYXXON Stick 10	Semiautomated
McKesson	Consult 120	Consult urine reagent strips	Semiautomated
NDC	Pro Advantage Urine Analyzer	Pro Advantage urine reagent strips	Semiautomated
Teco Diagnostics	TC-201	URS-10	Semiautomated
YD Diagnostics	URiSCAN Optima	URiSCAN 10ACR urine strips	Semiautomated

Status+ (Siemens Healthineers, Erlangen, Germany), Aution Eleven AE-4022 (Arkray Inc., Kyoto, Japan), and the Roche Urisys (Roche Diagnostics, Rotkreuz, Switzerland).

Fully automated urine strip analyzers have integrated specimen handlers which automatically pipette samples onto the test strip, thus decreasing labor and inter-operator variability in the reaction time. Popular manufacturers and platforms can be found in **Table 1** and include the Siemens Novus (Siemens Healthineers, Erlangen, Germany), Arkray Aution Max series (Arkray Inc., Kyoto, Japan), and Roche Cobas u series (Roche Diagnostics, Rotkreuz, Switzerland). The automated urinalysis analyzers utilize the same chemical components used by the conventional test strips with the capacity to include additional parameters. The fully automated systems can evaluate for the different parameters using reflectance photometry and specific gravity using refractometry. Some automated urine strip analyzers, such as the Arkray Aution

Max series, can determine urine color and turbidity/clarity, which is an advancement over most semiautomated analyzers. Certain analyzers may allow for quantitative results to be determined on the urine test strips.[9] Additionally, automated urinalysis analyzers can be combined with automated urine microscopy analyzers to become a more complete system.[10] The Arkray Aution series has been combined with the DxU Iris system, an automated microscopy analyzer.

Smartphone cameras are capable of performing image analysis for the detection of various types of chemical reactions for devices at the point-of-care.[11,12] For over a decade, researchers have developed proof-of-concept models and devices to use smartphones to read urine test strips.[13,14] Some platforms have been developed into commercial products, including the uChek system from Biosense (Biosense Technologies, Bhiwandi, India) and the Minuteful in-Home Urine Analysis Test System from Healthy.io. These products are regarded as in vitro diagnostics and require FDA clearance. Machine learning and AI have been used to interpret urine test strip results using training sets and machine learning workflows.[15,16] Other potential advancements for test strip design come from the development of more advanced paper-based microfluidics, which may decrease manufacturing costs of these tests in the future.[17]

MANUAL URINE MICROSCOPY

Manual urine microscopy remains one of the few manual procedures performed in clinical laboratories. Bright-field microscopy (BFM) was initially the technique of choice used for routine microscopic urine analysis.[18] It is now well known that this method allows for poor visualization of particles with low refractive index such as hyaline casts and "ghost" erythrocytes (red blood cells [RBCs] with low hemoglobin).[19] Phase-contrast microscopy (PCM) has superseded BFM and enables better identification of elements with low refractive indices. PCM demonstrates superior enhancement of the morphologic details of dysmorphic RBCs, renal tubular epithelial cells (ECs), and atypical/neoplastic urothelial cells.[19,20] BFM can be utilized when PCM is unavailable. Strategies including lowering the condenser[21] and the use of supravital stains[22] may enhance the sensitivity of BFM. The one advantage that BFM has over PCM is for crystals, whose tridimensional morphology is best examined by BFM.[19] In addition, hemocytometer slides for more accurate counting and centrifugation to concentrate the sediment for less frequent bodies, such as casts, has been attempted to improve efficacy. However, the loss of particles and interobserver variability remain problematic challenges. Polarized light microscopy aids in the identification of cholesterol in oval fat bodies, fatty casts, including characteristic Maltese cross patterns, and various crystals. Polarized microscopy may be helpful in the differentiation of morphologically similar urine sediment components such as erythrocytes and monohydrate calcium oxalate crystals.[23] Interference contrast microscopy provides 3-dimensional microscopy images and layer-by-layer imaging of cellular elements. Differential interference contrast microscopy possesses higher contrast and resolution compared with BFM or dark-field microscopy.[24,25] With experience, the microscopic techniques are easy to use and less time consuming than BFM due to the enhanced imaging. However, high costs and technical expertise are the major deterrents to routine use in clinical practice.

AUTOMATED URINE MICROSCOPY

The manual urine microscopy of urine sediment is labor intensive, time consuming, and imprecise (**Table 2**) when compared to automated methods. Wallace Coulter

Table 2
Comparison of manual urine examination and automated urinalysis

Variable	Manual	Automated
Sample processing	Vigorous sample processing	Limited or no processing
Bias	Interobserver variability	None
Sample volume	Up to 12 mL	Up to 4 mL
Standardization	limited	Excellent
Throughput (samples/hour)	Very low	high
Crystal and cast classification	Excellent	Limited
Microbial subclassification	Excellent	Possible but limited
Lipid	Excellent	Poor
Quantification of particles	Estimate	Exact numbers
Automatic resulting	Not possible	Present
Turnaround time	Slow	Fast
Transcription errors	Increased	Markedly reduced with barcode option
Cost	Inexpensive	Expensive

developed a method for counting particles in electrolyte solutions known as the Coulter principle.[26] Subsequently, the Coulter counter model enabled the rapid and accurate enumeration of cells in blood. Machines based on the Coulter principle became the mainstream equipment in clinical hematology laboratories. The Coulter method could not be easily applied in urinalysis until the late 1990s, due to the broad spectrum of urinary particles including crystals and cells that do not exist in blood.[4] Automated urine microscopy utilizes computerized analysis of digitized monochrome images of urinary particles. Two major types of analyzers using digitized microscopy in the laboratory are identified. The first is based on automated intelligent or automated particle recognition microscopy and the second utilizes cuvette-based image microscopy. The iQ200 (Iris Diagnostics, Chatsworth, USA.) uses a digital flow morphology technology through the incorporation of an auto-particle recognition (APR) software, that identifies and characterizes urine particles on the screen.[27] The laminar flow allows the specimen particles to be observed with their largest projection facing the direction of the lens. The particles can be seen through the objective lens of a microscope coupled to a charged coupled device video camera.[28] Five hundred images are created for each particle and are then analyzed by a neural network which contains up to 26,000 reference images. Subsequently, the particle is isolated within 1 image and is inserted in the 1-particle category. Digital images of flagged particles are visually examined and reclassified, by the operator. A strong correlation has been reported between iQ200 output and manual cell counts for RBCs, white blood cells (WBCs), and ECs.[29,30] The analyzer can recognize 12 particles (**Fig. 1**) with up to 27 categories and eliminates manual sample preparation, but requires a well-trained technologist for reclassification of findings. The FUS100 (Dirui Industrial Co. Ltd., China) is another digital image–based APR system. Similar to the IQ200, FUS100 uses uncentrifuged urine for digital imaging to capture and analyze photos from each sample to auto-classify and report them quantitatively.[31]

The cuvette-based microscopy includes the sediMAX (77 Elektronika, Budapest, Hungary) analyzer, also known as UriSed in certain countries. These instruments differ

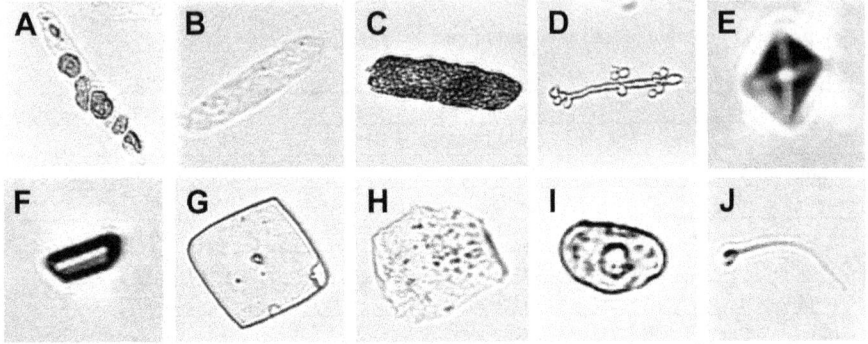

Fig. 1. Demonstration of images of select particles analyzed in the iQ200 analyzer. The analyzer displays images of (*A*) white blood cell casts (*B*) hyaline casts (*C*) granular casts (*D*) yeast (*E*) calcium oxalate crystals (*F*) triple phosphate crystals (*G*) uric acid crystals (*H*) squamous cell (*I*) transitional cell (*J*) sperm.

from the APR method by producing a monolayer of urine sediment by centrifugation in a special cuvette.[32] The sediment is analyzed by a BFM and digital camera to capture particle images using image-processing software. For each sample, 15 images are captured and the identification and quantification of particles is carried out by a complex neural network structure specifically developed for the model. The most significant advantage of the iQ200 over the sediMAX is the ability to individually display the sediment images by categorizing them (RBCs, WBCs, and casts). On the other hand, the cuvette-based system displays the entire field image, similar to microscopic fields seen with manual microscopy.[33] The operator may detect particles present in the whole field of view not identified by the analyzer. Comparisons with manual urinary microscopy between the various automated devices show good concordance on detection of RBCs, WBCs, bacteria, and squamous ECs.[33,34] However, more complex particles such as non-squamous ECs, non-hyaline casts, lipids, and less-common crystals may require additional manual review.[35,36]

Technical advances have led to improved versions of both types of instrumentation. More recently, a newer model of the iQ200 was launched in 2021, now known as the DxU Microscopy Series (Beckman, Brea, USA). The improved model analyses higher sample numbers, and streamlines urinalysis workflow to achieve manual review rates of 4%.[37] A newer version of the FUS-100, namely, FUS-200, handled a higher specimen load but showed unsatisfactory analytical sensitivity for bacteria recognition and quantification.[38] Notably, the latest SediMax (CONTRUST) analyzer incorporates both PCM and BFM to capture high-quality images in 1 optical system, leading to improved accurate results including certain crystals[35] and parasites.[39] The automated analyzers Cobas u 701 (Roche Diagnostics, Mannheim, Germany) and Atellica UAS 800 (Siemens Healthineers, Eschborn, Germany) are cuvette-based analyzers, more recently introduced in the market.[40,41] The sensitivities of Cobas u 701 and Atellica UAS 800 for pathologic casts (73.6% and 81.1%, respectively) and crystals (62.2% and 49.5%, respectively) were high, along with high image review rates (24.6% and 25.2%, respectively).[42] Similar to the sediMAX and IQ200, these automated urine microscopy analyzers are capable of interfacing with automated physiochemical strip analyzers in a single efficient device,[10] and may also be coupled to a laboratory information system software for electronic transmission and enable consultation with experts for unusual cases.

AUTOMATED FLOW CYTOMETRY

Models of automated urine flow cytometers (FCs) are quite limited in comparison to the image-based analyzers (**Table 3**). The first urine FC, the UF-100 (Sysmex, Kobe, Japan) classifies uncentrifuged urine particles labeled with fluorophores.[43] Measurement is obtained by an array of detectors as the stained cells flow in a fluid stream through a laser beam. The methodology employs argon laser technology and produces scatter-grams rather than images that are viewed or saved by the operator. For each urinary particle, forward and side scatters and fluorescence intensities are detected and then converted to optoelectronic signals for the easy identification and quantification of particles.[44] A new generation UF-1000i superseded the UF-100 in 2007. While precision was satisfactory for RBCs, WBCs, and ECs when compared to manual micro-scopy and automated image-based analyzers, microscopic observation was required for more complex particles such as casts.[45,46] These laser-based FCs are particularly useful in the screening of pyuria, bacteriuria, and hematuria, thus reducing the need for microscopy or culture.[47] Although urine culture remains the gold standard for the detection of urinary tract infection (UTI), the high percentage of negative results (~60%) necessitates the requirement for an efficient screening method.[48] Gessoni and colleagues[49] utilized bacteria forward scatter (B_FSC) and fluorescent light scatter to distinguish UTIs caused by gram-positive or gram-negative bacteria. The resultant data suggest that B_FSC could be useful in presumptive exclusion of UTI caused by gram-positive bacteria. The argon-laser–based FCs have been replaced by semicon-ductor lasers, which are more economical due to a longer life span.[50] The semicon-ductor lasers operate at another blue wavelength, thus forcing manufacturers to completely redesign the system and adapt the dyes. The newer UF-5000 and UF-4000 (Sysmex, Kobe, Japan) models recognize, count, and classify cells by analyzing forward scatter light, side scatter light, side fluorescent light, and depolarized side scat-tered light (DSS). DSS was incorporated to improve sensitivity of crystals and better differentiate RBCs and crystals.[51] UF-5000 showed a better diagnostic agreement for most clinical parameters with manual PCM in comparison to the u 701 image-based module[52] However, when compared to the microscopy-based analyzers, the dif-ferentiation of crystals is still challenging.[42,52,53] In addition, automated FCs and strip analyzers have been combined into fully automated workstations.[54]

MASS SPECTROMETRY–BASED MODELS

Despite advancements made with the automated examination of urine sediments, some particle detection involving certain micro-organisms need improvement. Matrix-associated laser desorption ionization time-of-flight (MALDI-TOF) mass spectrometry (MS) is now used in routine clinical microbiology laboratories for bacteria identification. Several studies have explored using MALDI-TOF-MS to eliminate the time delay due to conventional culture methods. Direct identification of bacteria by combining MALDI-TOF-MS with automated urine sediment analyzers were comparable to bacteria detec-tion from positive cultures.[55,56] The disadvantage of this method is the requirement of sample preparation and the hampering of results by polymicrobial samples. The devel-opment of an automated MALDI-TOF-MS-based method for the direct detection of carbapenemase-producing enterobacteriaceae rapidly improved turnaround time.[57] The samples were initially evaluated with a urine FC and processed directly by MALDI-TOF-MS for bacterial identification and detection of carbapenemase produc-tion. The results were interpreted using a MALDI-TOF software module that automati-cally calculates the imipenem logRQ value (which indicates the rate of hydrolysis).[58] The automated interpretation spectra revealed 100% sensitivity and specificity with a

Table 3
Current automated urine microscopy analyzers and flow cytometers

Features	Automated Urine Microscopy	Automated Flow Cytometry
Centrifugation	iQ200, DxU series, FUS-100/200 (not required) SediMAX, Atellica UAS 800, Cobas u701 (required)	Not required
Minimum sample volume	3 mL (iQ200) 2 mL DxU series 3 mL (FUS-100/FUS-200) 2 mL (SediMAX series) 2 mL (Atellica UAS 800) 2 mL (Cobas u701)	4 mL (UF-100) 4 mL (UF-1000) 2 mL (UF-5000)
Analytical volume	2 mL (iQ200) 1.3 mL DxU series 1 mL (FUS-100/FUS-200) 0.2 mL (SediMAX series) mL (Atellica UAS 800) 0.17 mL (Cobas u701)	0.8 mL (UF-100) 1.2 mL (UF-1000) 0.45 mL (UF-5000)
Throughput (maximum samples/hour)	101 (iQ200 and DxU series) 60 (FUS-100) 120 (FUS-200) 130 (SediMAX series) 106 (Atellica UAS 800) 116 (Cobas u701)	100 (UF-100) 100 (UF-1000) 105 (UF-5000)
Result output	500 images/sample (iQ200 and DxU series) 850 images/sample (FUS-200) 15 images/sample using WFM (SediMAX series) 15 images/sample using WFM (Cobas u701)	Scattergrams,; no particle images
Crystal differentiation	Certain crystals	Rarely
Number of particles recognized and counted	12 (iQ200 and DxU series) 12 (FUS-100/FUS-200) 12 (SediMAX series) 11 (Atellica UAS 800) 11 (Cobas u701)	12 (UF-100) 11 (UF-1000) 17 (UF-5000)
Bacteria classification	No bacteria classification	Classifies bacteria with improved bacteria counting
Data storage (number of patient results)	10,000 (iQ200 and DxU series) >10,000 (FUS-100/FUS-200) 10,000 (SediMAX/UridSed) 10,000 (Atellica UAS 800) None (Cobas u701). Uses a database	1000 (UF-4000/5000)
Integrated systems with urine strip reader (and automated urine sediment analyzers)	DxU Iris Workcell (DxU series) iRICELL 3000 (iQ200) FUS-2000 Urinalysis Hybrid (FUS-100/FUS-200) Atellica 1500 (Atellica UAS 800) Cobas 6500 (Cobas u701)	UN series (UF-4000/5000)

Abbreviation: WFM, whole-field microscopy.

rapid turnaround time of 90 minutes after sample reception. Roux-Dalvai and colleagues[59] developed a rapid and accurate method of bacterial species detection in urine samples using liquid chromatography tandem MS and AI. In the first training step, libraries of peptides are obtained on pure bacterial colonies, their identification in urine is then verified, followed by the use of machine learning classifiers to define a peptidic signature that differentiates each bacterial species from the others. The second stage involves monitoring of this signature in unknown urine specimens using targeted proteomics. Within 4 hours and without bacterial culture, the predominant bacteria infecting a sample were detected in 97% of cases and 100% above the standard threshold. Perhaps this machine learning–based method could be extended in the future to other biological specimens which are not readily detected by the automated analyzers.

DISCUSSION AND SUMMARY

Remarkable technical advances have occurred in automated urinalysis over the past 3 decades. Each automated urinary system uses a different technology to classify and quantify urine particles. This offers an improvement in standardization over manual examination by eliminating potential interobserver variability during slide or dipstick/urine test strip interpretation. Improved quality of results is obtained due to more efficient sample processing since samples are analyzed closer to their collection time. Subsequently, there is decreased likelihood of cell lysis, microbial contamination, or precipitation from prolonged storage. The automated analyzers handle large numbers, eliminate or reduce sample processing, and can interface with laboratory information systems for transmission, storage, and data analysis. Furthermore, newer applications show promising results for early detection of urothelial cancer.[60] To streamline workflows, manufacturers have combined their microscopic analyzers with automated strip analyzers to form a single workstation device which has marked decreased the need for manual review.[54] In certain instances, confirmation of results by manual methods may be required. Combination of the automated urine analyzers with MS improve specific bacterial classification and possibly other complicated particles, but this requires further validation studies. Importantly, urinalysis testing may vary among laboratories due to laboratory size and frequently used tests. For instance, various departments such as urology, oncology, and emergency (ED) departments have different requirements for what to examine in a urine sample. It may be reasonable to have portable semiautomated point-of-care instruments in the ED or a more sophisticated fully automated instrument that includes detection of neoplastic urothelial cells in a urologic cancer center. Therefore, a reflex-based system using solution software to customize rules based on testing and define when to reflex to microscopy may be necessary. The urinary system a laboratory chooses is likely dependent on the technology, cost, technical expertise, and various needs of the user.

CLINICS CARE POINTS

- Automated urinalysis methods show an improvement over manual examination through elimination of sample processing and result bias.
- The major disadvantage of the automated analyzers lies in the detection of non-hyaline casts, lipids, certain bacteria, and crystals, which reflex to a manual review.
- Improved automated detection of more complex urine particles may benefit from combining fully automated urine analyzers with other instruments such as MS.

ACKNOWLEDGMENTS

The authors are grateful to Chris Powell for proving the images from the instrument and staff members of the Clinical Core Laboratory of the University of Virginia Health System.

DISCLOSURE

The authors have nothing to disclose.

REFERENCES

1. Echeverry G, Hortin GL, Rai AJ. Introduction to urinalysis: Historical Perspectives and clinical application. In: Rai AJ, editor. The urinary Proteome. Methods in Molecular Biology. 1st edition. New Jersey: Humana Totowa; 2010. p. 1–12.
2. Chien TI, Kao JT, Liu HL, et al. Urine sediment examination: a comparison of automated urinalysis systems and manual microscopy. Clinica chimica acta; international journal of clinical chemistry 2007;384(1–2):28–34.
3. Young PE, Diaz GJ, Kalariya RN, et al. Comparison of the time required for manual (visually read) and semi-automated POCT urinalysis and pregnancy testing with associated electronic medical record (EMR) transcription errors. Clinica chimica acta; international journal of clinical chemistry 2020;504:60–3.
4. Cho SY, Hur M. Advances in automated urinalysis systems, flow cytometry and digitized microscopy. Annals of laboratory medicine 2019;39(1):1–2.
5. İnce FD, Ellidağ HY, Koseoğlu M, et al. The comparison of automated urine analyzers with manual microscopic examination for urinalysis automated urine analyzers and manual urinalysis. Practical laboratory medicine 2016;5:14–20.
6. Manoni F, Fornasiero L, Ercolin M, et al. Cutoff values for bacteria and leukocytes for urine flow cytometer Sysmex UF-1000i in urinary tract infections. Diagn Microbiol Infect Dis 2009;65(2):103–7.
7. Gässler NS,H, Luppa PB. In: Luppa PBJR, editor. Urine and stool analyses. 1st edition. Germany: Springer; 2018. p. 181–92.
8. Fan S-L, Bai S. Chapter 38 - urinalysis. In: Clarke W, Marzinke MA, editors. Contemporary practice in clinical Chemistry. 4h edition. Academic Press; 2020. p. 665–80.
9. Delanghe JR, Himpe J, DeCock N, et al. Sensitive albuminuria analysis using dye-binding based test strips. Clinica chimica acta; international journal of clinical chemistry 2017;471:107–12.
10. Cobbaert CM, Arslan F, Caballé Martín I, et al. Automated urinalysis combining physicochemical analysis, on-board centrifugation, and digital imaging in one system: a multicenter performance evaluation of the cobas 6500 urine work area. Practical laboratory medicine 2019;17:e00139.
11. Vashist SK, Mudanyali O, Schneider EM, et al. Cellphone-based devices for bioanalytical sciences. Anal Bioanal Chem 2014;406(14):3263–77.
12. Wang P, Kricka LJ. Current and emerging Trends in point-of-care technology and Strategies for clinical validation and Implementation. Clinical chemistry 2018;64(10):1439–52.
13. Lee DS, Jeon BG, Ihm C, et al. A simple and smart telemedicine device for developing regions: a pocket-sized colorimetric reader. Lab Chip 2011;11(1):120–6.
14. Smith GT, Dwork N, Khan SA, et al. Robust dipstick urinalysis using a low-cost, micro-volume slipping manifold and mobile phone platform. Lab Chip 2016;16(11):2069–78.

15. Cao Y, Cheng M, Hu C. UrineCART, a machine learning method for establishment of review rules based on UF-1000i flow cytometry and dipstick or reflectance photometer. Clin Chem Lab Med 2012;50(12):2155–61.

16. De Bruyne S, De Kesel P, Oyaert M. Applications of artificial intelligence in urinalysis: is the future Already Here? Clinical chemistry 2023;69(12):1348–60.

17. Mohammadi S, Maeki M, Mohamadi RM, et al. An instrument-free, screen-printed paper microfluidic device that enables bio and chemical sensing. The Analyst 2015;140(19):6493–9.

18. Sharda N, Bakhtar O, Thajudeen B, et al. Manual urine microscopy versus automated urine analyzer microscopy in Patients with Acute kidney Injury. Lab Med 2014;45(4):e152–5.

19. Fogazzi GB, Delanghe J. Microscopic examination of urine sediment: phase contrast versus bright field. Clinica chimica acta; international journal of clinical chemistry 2018;487:168–73.

20. Fogazzi GB, Pallotti F, Garigali G. Atypical/malignant urothelial cells in routine urinary sediment: Worth knowing and reporting. Clin Chim Acta 2015;439:107–11.

21. Barros Silva GE, Costa RS, Ravinal RC, et al. Evaluation of erythrocyte dysmorphism by light microscopy with lowering of the condenser lens: a simple and efficient method. Nephrology 2010;15(2):171–7.

22. Chu-Su Y, Shukuya K, Yokoyama T, et al. Enhancing the detection of dysmorphic red blood cells and renal tubular epithelial cells with a modified urinalysis protocol. Sci Rep 2017;7(1):1–10.

23. Frochot V, Daudon M. Clinical value of crystalluria and quantitative morphoconstitutional analysis of urinary calculi. Int J Surg 2016;36(Pt D):624–32.

24. Tsunoda M, Isailovic D, Yeung ES. Real-time three-dimensional imaging of cell division by differential interference contrast microscopy. Journal of microscopy 2008;232(2):207–11.

25. Chen J, Xu Y, Lv X, et al. Super-resolution differential interference contrast microscopy by structured illumination. Opt Express 2013;21(1):112–21.

26. Becker GJ, Garigali G, Fogazzi GB. Advances in urine microscopy. Am J Kidney Dis : the official journal of the National Kidney Foundation 2016;67(6):954–64.

27. Altekin E, Kadiçesme O, Akan P, et al. New generation IQ-200 automated urine microscopy analyzer compared with KOVA cell chamber. J Clin Lab Anal 2010; 24(2):67–71.

28. Linko S, Kouri TT, Toivonen E, et al. Analytical performance of the Iris iQ200 automated urine microscopy analyzer. Clin Chim Acta 2006;372(1):54–64.

29. Budak YU, Huysal K. Comparison of three automated systems for urine chemistry and sediment analysis in routine laboratory practice. Clin Lab 2011;57(1–2): 47–52.

30. Park J, Kim J. [Evaluation of iQ200 automated urine microscopy analyzer]. The Korean journal of laboratory medicine 2008;28(4):267–73.

31. Yüksel H, Kiliç E, Ekinci A, et al. Comparison of fully automated urine sediment analyzers H800-FUS100 and Labumat-Urised with manual microscopy. J Clin Lab Anal 2013;27(4):312–6.

32. Block D.R., Lieske J.C., Automated urinalysis in the clinical lab. *MLO Med Lab Obs.* 2012;44(10):8-10, 12; quiz 14.

33. Akin OK, Serdar MA, Cizmeci Z, et al. Comparison of LabUMat-with-UriSed and iQ200 fully automatic urine sediment analysers with manual urine analysis. Biotechnol Appl Biochem 2009;53(Pt 2):139–44.

34. Ma J, Wang C, Yue J, et al. Clinical laboratory urine analysis: comparison of the UriSed automated microscopic analyzer and the manual microscopy. Clin Lab 2013;59(11–12):1297–303.

35. Castiglione V, Cavalier E, Diop C, et al. Distinction between urine crystals by auto-mated urine analyzer SediMAX conTRUST is specific but lacks sensitivity. Clin Chem Lab Med 2017;55(12):e288–90.

36. Bottini PV, Martinez MH, Garlipp CR. Urinalysis: comparison between micro-scopic analysis and a new automated microscopy image-based urine sediment instrument. Clin Lab 2014;60(4):693–7.

37. Aller R. Urinalysis Instrumentation. Cap Today. 2023;48-50.

38. Kocer D, Sarıguzel FM, Karakukcu C. Cutoff values for bacteria and leukocytes for urine sediment analyzer FUS200 in culture-positive urinary-tract infections. Scand J Clin Lab Invest 2014;74(5):414–7.

39. Intra J, Sala MR, Falbo R, et al. Improvement in the detection of enteric protozoa from clinical stool samples using the automated urine sediment analyzer sed-iMAX(®) 2 compared to sediMAX(®) 1. Eur J Clin Microbiol Infect Dis 2017; 36(1):147–51.

40. Wesarachkitti B, Khejonnit V, Pratumvinit B, et al. Performance evaluation and comparison of the fully automated urinalysis analyzers UX-2000 and cobas 6500. Lab Med 2016;47(2):124–33.

41. Aper SJA, Gijzen K, Luimstra JJ, et al. Evaluation of the Atellica® UAS 800: a new member of the automated urine sediment analyzer family. Scand J Clin Lab In-vestig 2021;81(7):585–92.

42. Cho J, Oh KJ, Jeon BC, et al. Comparison of five automated urine sediment an-alyzers with manual microscopy for accurate identification of urine sediment. Clin Chem Lab Med 2019;57(11):1744–53.

43. Kouri TT, Kähkönen U, Malminiemi K, et al. Evaluation of Sysmex UF-100 urine flow cytometer vs chamber counting of supravitally stained specimens and con-ventional bacterial cultures. Am J Clin Pathol 1999;112(1):25–35.

44. Mejuto P, Luengo M, Díaz-Gigante J. Automated flow cytometry: an Alternative to urine culture in a routine clinical microbiology laboratory? International Journal of Microbiology 2017;2017:8532736.

45. Manoni F, Tinello A, Fornasiero L, et al. Urine particle evaluation: a comparison between the UF-1000i and quantitative microscopy. Clin Chem Lab Med 2010; 48(8):1107–11.

46. Lee W, Ha JS, Ryoo NH. Comparison of the automated cobas u 701 urine micro-scopy and UF-1000i flow cytometry systems and manual microscopy in the ex-amination of urine sediments. J Clin Lab Anal 2016;30(5):663–71.

47. Millán-Lou MI, García-Lechuz JM, Ruiz-Andrés MA, et al. Validation and Search of the ideal Cut-Off of the Sysmex UF-1000i(®) flow cytometer for the diagnosis of urinary tract infection in a Tertiary hospital in Spain. Front Med 2018;5:92.

48. Jolkkonen S, Paattiniemi EL, Kärpänoja P, et al. Screening of urine samples by flow cytometry reduces the need for culture. J Clin Microbiol 2010;48(9):3117–21.

49. Gessoni G, Saccani G, Valverde S, et al. Does flow cytometry have a role in pre-liminary differentiation between urinary tract infections sustained by gram posi-tive and gram negative bacteria? An Italian polycentric study. Clinica chimica acta; international journal of clinical chemistry 2015;440:152–6.

50. Oyaert M, Delanghe J. Progress in automated urinalysis. Annals of laboratory medicine 2019;39(1):15–22.

51. Previtali G, Ravasio R, Seghezzi M, et al. Performance evaluation of the new fully automated urine particle analyser UF-5000 compared to the reference method of

the Fuchs-Rosenthal chamber. Clinica chimica acta; international journal of clinical chemistry 2017;472:123–30.

52. Enko D, Stelzer I, Böckl M, et al. Comparison of the diagnostic performance of two automated urine sediment analyzers with manual phase-contrast microscopy. Clin Chem Lab Med 2020;58(2):268–73.

53. Liu H, Li Q, Zhang Y, et al. Consistency analysis of the Sysmex UF-5000 and Atellica UAS 800 urine sedimentation analyzers. J Clin Lab Anal 2022;36(9):e24659.

54. Tantisaranon P, Dumkengkhachornwong K, Aiadsakun P, et al. A comparison of automated urine analyzers cobas 6500, UN 3000-111b and iRICELL 3000 with manual microscopic urinalysis. Practical laboratory medicine 2021;24:e00203.

55. Íñigo M, Coello A, Fernández-Rivas G, et al. Direct identification of urinary tract Pathogens from urine samples, combining urine screening methods and matrix-assisted laser desorption ionization-time of flight mass spectrometry. J Clin Microbiol 2016;54(4):988–93.

56. Wang XH, Zhang G, Fan YY, et al. Direct identification of bacteria causing urinary tract infections by combining matrix-assisted laser desorption ionization-time of flight mass spectrometry with UF-1000i urine flow cytometry. J Microbiol Methods 2013;92(3):231–5.

57. Oviaño M, Ramírez CL, Barbeyto LP, et al. Rapid direct detection of carbapenemase-producing Enterobacteriaceae in clinical urine samples by MALDI-TOF MS analysis. The Journal of antimicrobial chemotherapy 2017;72(5):1350–4.

58. Oviaño M, Sparbier K, Barba MJ, et al. Universal protocol for the rapid automated detection of carbapenem-resistant Gram-negative bacilli directly from blood cultures by matrix-assisted laser desorption/ionisation time-of-flight mass spectrometry (MALDI-TOF/MS). Int J Antimicrob Agents 2016;48(6):655–60.

59. Roux-Dalvai F, Gotti C, Leclercq M, et al. Fast and accurate bacterial species identification in urine specimens using LC-MS/MS mass spectrometry and machine learning. Molecular & cellular proteomics : MCP. 2019;18(12):2492–505.

60. Anderlini R, Manieri G, Lucchi C, et al. Automated urinalysis with expert review for incidental identification of atypical urothelial cells: an anticipated bladder carcinoma diagnosis. Clinica chimica acta; international journal of clinical chemistry 2015;451(Pt B):252–6.

Opportunities and Drawbacks of Digitalized Morphologic Analysis of Body Fluids

Giuseppe Lippi, MD[a,b,*], Brandon M. Henry, MD[c],
Sabrina Buoro, PhD[d]

KEYWORDS

• Digitalization • Body fluid • Analysis • Robotics

KEY POINTS

- Body fluid analysis is a cornerstone of diagnostic and clinical decision-making for a wide spectrum of human pathologies.
- Digitalized morphologic analysis of body fluids is an emerging and appealing alternative to optical microscopy.
- Implementation and validation of new software programs are necessary before digitalized morphology of body fluids will be ready for prime time.

INTRODUCTION

The usual activity of medical laboratory services focuses primarily on the analysis of "conventional body fluids," which includes whole blood or its major derivatives (eg, serum and plasma) and urine. However, the human body contains a variety of other fluids, both physiologic and pathologic, the analysis of which has gradually become a cornerstone of diagnosis and clinical decision-making for a wide range of pathologic conditions.[1]

Tears, saliva, cerebrospinal, nasal, pericardial, pleural, peritoneal, pancreatic, gastric, synovial, amniotic and seminal fluids, breast milk, and other fluids contained in cysts and other lesions that develop almost anywhere in the human body are the

[a] Section of Clinical Biochemistry and School of Medicine, University of Verona, Verona, Italy; [b] Section of Clinical Biochemistry, University Hospital of Verona, Piazzale L.A. Scuro, 10, Verona 37134, Italy; [c] Clinical Laboratory, Division of Nephrology and Hypertension, Cincinnati Children's Hospital Medical Center, Cincinnati, OH, USA; [d] Centro Regionale di Coordinamento della Medicina di Laboratorio, Milan, Italy
* Corresponding author. Section of Clinical Biochemistry, University Hospital of Verona, Piazzale L.A. Scuro, 10, Verona 37134, Italy.
E-mail address: giuseppe.lippi@univr.it

Clin Lab Med 44 (2024) 423–429
https://doi.org/10.1016/j.cll.2024.04.004
0272-2712/24/© 2024 Elsevier Inc. All rights reserved.

most commonly studied para-physiologic fluids.[2] Morphologic examination of these fluids, as well as measurement of a number of laboratory biomarkers, is an excellent aid in the diagnosis, monitoring, and follow-up of a kaleidoscope of human diseases.[3]

The ability to qualitatively or quantitatively analyze nontraditional body fluids has gained popularity in the last 2 to 3 decades. This is the result of new biological discoveries that have helped to illuminate new pathologic pathways, as well as of remarkable analytical breakthroughs that have made it possible to partially or even completely automate the analysis of body fluids. The development of a new generation of laboratory instruments equipped with small volume aspiration modules and specialized software versions that allow the visualization, identification, and potential classification of numerous human cells, including those not normally found in blood or urine, has led to the most significant advances in the field.[4] The remainder of this article is, therefore, devoted to providing an up-to-date overview of the advantages and limitations of digital morphologic analysis of body fluids.

CLINICAL APPLICATIONS OF BODY FLUIDS ANALYZERS

Automation of body fluid analysis has significant advantages over conventional methods based on counting chambers, since sample pretreatment and preparation can be avoided, allowing faster and more standardized analysis and virtually eliminating the influence of subjective operator skill.[5] These new "modules," whose commercialization began at the turn of the century, have gradually gained acceptance in laboratory medicine with the increasing number of validation studies, although their use has remained largely limited to routine hematology.[4]

In general, automated morphologic analysis of body fluids may consist of 2 (sequential) steps, the first involving enumeration of blood cells and other elements in the biological fluid using the same techniques used for routine hematologic testing (ie, "flow cytometers"), and the second (additional) step may involve morphologic analysis using cell imaging techniques (ie, "digital morphology analyzers"). Digital analyzers typically consist of an automated microscope, a high-quality digital camera, and a software designed to identify and classify cells and other elements in smears stained with Romanowsky-type reagents (eg, May Grünwald-Giemsa, Wright Giemsa, and Wright).

The software of digital morphology analyzers has been developed for automatic recognition of specific cellular features in digital images, with an initial "preclassification" based on artificial neural network technology, which should always be followed by subsequent review and verification (ie, postclassification) by a trained and knowledgeable laboratory expert to confirm or modify the initial sorting. The CellaVision series (DM96, DM1200, and DM9600) and Sysmex DI-60 (which use identical software to the CellaVision DM1200 in conjunction with a different camera lens system) digital analyzers, which have now been released with a specific "body fluid application," produce a "white blood cell (WBC) preclassification" of cells into neutrophils, lymphocytes, macrophages (which include monocytes), eosinophils, "other cells" (which may include basophils, atypical lymphocytes, blasts, and other cancer cells), and unidentified elements. With the "non-WBC preclassification" option, the analyzer can also detect artifacts and smear cells, allowing the user to improve the classification process by adding additional cell categories during revision. Therefore, these integrated systems are capable of reclassifying and renaming a variety of normal or pathologic cells that may be present in various biological fluids. Other similar analyzers are now commercially available (eg, Mindray MC-80, West Medica Vision Hema, Medica Corporation EasyCell, Nextslide Imaging LLC Nextslide, and Roche Cobas m511 automated digital cell morphology analyzers), but no validation studies involving body fluids have appeared in PubMed or Scopus so far, as a recent digital search using the keywords "instrument name" and "body fluid(s)" revealed.

In the following section of this article, we will briefly outline some published experiences with digital morphologic instruments for body fluid analysis.

Narrative Review of Some Validation Studies

The analysis of the cerebrospinal fluid (CSF) is an integral part of the diagnostic process of a multitude of human pathology that may primarily or secondarily affect the central nervous system, especially encompassing infectious, autoimmune, neoplastic, traumatic, and neurodegenerative diseases.[6] A preliminary study was published by Riedl and colleagues with the CellaVision DM96 digital cell morphology system.[7] The authors assayed 177 body fluids (CSF: n = 100, abdominal fluids: n = 62, continuous ambulant peritoneal dialysis fluid: n = 15), the measurement of which were compared between manual review and digital microscopy system. Compared to manual review, the study showed a cumulative 90% classification accuracy of elements contained in CSF samples. Specifically, the preclassification and postclassification agreement with manual review were 96.1% and 95.0% for neutrophils, 94.6% and 93.5% for lymphocytes, 80.1% and 87.5% for macrophages, 56.7% and 73.1% for eosinophils, 41.7% and 32.5% for other cells, 89.7% and 76.0% for smudge cells, and 89.2% and 96.9% for artifacts, respectively. The correlation coefficients (r) between manual revision and CellaVision DM96 were comprised between 0.92 and 0.99 for CSF samples. Compared to manual review, the study also showed a cumulative 83% classification accuracy of elements contained in non-CSF samples. The preclassification and postclassification agreement with manual review were 95.2% and 92.6% for neutrophils, 87.7% and 93.6% for lymphocytes, 84.9% and 83.9% for macrophages, 91.9% and 55.0% for eosinophils, 64.1% and 27.8% for other cells, 73.7% and 42.5% for smudge cells, and 55.4% and 96.3% for artifacts, respectively. The correlation coefficients (r) between manual revision and CellaVision DM96 were comprised between 0.83 and 0.98 for non-CSF samples. Interestingly, manual revision displayed a 2.2 minute average hands-on time, while the postclassification on DM96 took an average of 2.7 minutes. Finally, the intra-assay imprecision was found to be less than 6% for all categories of cells.

In a subsequent study, Takemura and colleagues assessed the performance of the Sysmex DI-60 compared to manual microscopic analysis.[8] Compared to microscopic examination of 34 CSF samples, the digital analyzer displayed acceptable performance, with correlation coefficients (r) of 0.743 for neutrophils, 0.819 for lymphocytes, 0.778 for monocytes, and 0.770 for eosinophils, respectively. The same authors investigated the performance of DI-60 in 60 ascites and pleural effusion samples.[8] Compared to microscopic examination, the correlation coefficients (r) with the digital analyzer were 0.973 for neutrophils, 0.939 for lymphocytes, 0.638 for monocytes, and 0.803 for eosinophils, respectively.

More recently, Ivady and colleagues conducted a comparative assessment of morphologic analysis of 40 CSF and 40 ascitic samples with manual microscopy and digital cell morphology, using a CellaVision DM1200.[9] The correlation coefficients (r) of both polymorphonuclear and mononuclear cells between these 2 techniques were as high as 0.969 in CSF samples and 0.984 in ascites samples, respectively.

An interesting analysis was published by Yamatani and colleagues.[10] In brief, the authors used the Sysmex DI-60 integrated cell image analyzer for assaying 68 body fluids samples (CSF: n = 9, pleural effusion: n = 56, ascitic fluid: n = 3), 21 of which were positive and 47 were negative for the presence of malignant cells previously identified with cytologic testing. The simple postclassification diagnostic performance of DI-60 for tumor cell detection displayed 50.0% sensitivity and 95.7% specificity, which considerably increased to 81.0% and 97.9%, respectively, using the overview analysis, that is, a tool designed to optimize the area of interest, enabling the generation of clear images with 10× to 50× magnification and thus ultimately allowing better detection and reclassification of cancer cells by the operator.

Yoon and colleagues examined 213 body fluid samples (47 CSF, 80 pleural effusion samples, and 86 ascites samples) with DI-60 and compared the analytical performance of the analyzer with manual counting.[11] In total samples, the diagnostic sensitivity of DI-60 was 95.9% for neutrophils, 83.1% for lymphocytes, 69.4% for eosinophils, 99.4% for macrophages, and 33.7% for other cells, respectively. The corresponding values of diagnostic specificity for neutrophils, lymphocytes, eosinophils, macrophages, and other cells were 99.7%, 99.6%, 99.5%, 96.5%, and 95.3%, respectively. Overall, the calculated diagnostic accuracy resulted to be 98.7% for neutrophils, 94.3% for lymphocytes, 99.3% for eosinophils, 97.7% for macrophages, and 94.6% for other cells. In CSF, pleural effusion samples, and ascites, the sensitivity varied between 69.0% and 99.6%, 33.3% and 99.0% and 30.5% and 99.7%, respectively.

The iQ200 is another laboratory instrument that has been used for morphologic analysis of body fluids. This is basically an automated urine microscopy analyzer, encompassing a specific trained neural network (called "Auto-Particle Recognition") for classifying and enumerating several formed elements (ie, leukocytes, leukocyte clumps, squamous and nonsquamous epithelial cells, hyaline and unclassified casts, crystals, yeast, bacteria, sperm, and mucus). The results could be self-reported according to user-defined criteria and captured images could be seen on-demand at the workstation monitor, thus reducing the need for manual analysis of urine by microscopy. In a recent study, Goubard and colleagues assessed red blood cells and nucleated elements in 247 body fluid samples (CSF: n = 96, ascitic and pleural fluids: n = 151) and compared the performance of this analyzer with the manual microscopic method.[12] The concordance (correlation coefficient) between automated analysis and microscopy was 0.82 to 0.91 for nucleated elements and 0.96 to 0.98 for erythrocytes in CSF samples, and 0.82 to 0.85 for nucleated elements and 0.92 to 0.94 for erythrocytes in non-CSF fluids. Overall, the authors failed to find significant difference in the time needed for classification of cells between the 2 methods.

ADVANTAGES AND DRAWBACKS OF DIGITALIZED MORPHOLOGIC ANALYSIS OF BODY FLUIDS

As previously stated, digitalization analysis is now widely used in routine hematology, where these analyzers provide a reliable and rapid alternative to manual blood smear inspection. Nonetheless, the desire to provide speedy and accurate detection of nonhematological disorders by morphologic study of cells found in various body fluids represents a paradigm change in body fluid analysis. While this possible breakthrough has undeniable benefits, it may also have some potential drawbacks, as summarized in **Box 1**.

One of the major advantages of these techniques is represented by the partial automation of the preanalytical phase of cytospin slide evaluation, since the elimination of this manually intensive process enables to obtain standardized and reproducible body fluid smears within the same local system, saving precious human and economic resources (ie, always using the necessary amount of reagent).[8] It is noteworthy, however, that the methodologic limitations of cytospin preparation may have an impact on

---

Box 1
Advantages and limitations of digitalized morphologic analysis of body fluids

Advantages
- Highly standardized and reproducible generation of body fluid smears
- Saving of human and economic resources
- Improving operator's health and wellness
- Preclassification
- Better visualization of cell classes and specific cell features
- Creating a reference library of images
- Use of the images for remote analysis, future revision, and educational purposes
- Digitalized images may become an integral part of the electronic health record

Drawbacks
- Impact of the quality of cytospin preparation
- Initial cost
- Space
- Impossibility to focus
- Different approach for cell recognition and classification
- Some cells and elements cannot be preclassified
- Time needed for reclassification

---

the quality of tests results. For example, morphologic alteration of cells during the centrifugation procedure used for preparing the cytospin, the staining method, and the type of slide maker used may lead to misclassify the cells in wrong categories, thus reducing the correlation with manual microscopic examination.

The digitization of vast sample areas, possibly tagging specific regions of interest, and its reproduction within a monitor then enables to avoid using a manual microscope, an activity that is frequently associated with the development of stress, visual, and musculoskeletal problems (mostly in neck and back).[13] The analyzer provides already a preclassification of the major cell types, specifically depending on the digitalized microscopy system in use. The possibility to rapidly adjust magnification of cell images allows to better visualize cell classes side-by-side and specific cell features, which will considerably facilitate the process of cell recognition and classification. The customable cell sorting enables to add new categories of reference cells and create a reference library that can be stored in the form of digital image(s) for remote analysis (eg, body fluid samples can be analyzed in remote networked laboratories and the captured images could then digitally transferred to the core laboratory for review), future revision (eg, for patient monitoring), and even for educational purposes (training, presentations, and so forth). The digitalized images could then become an integral part of the patient's medical history, permanently stored in the electronic health record. Understandably, these last aspects would only be possible using the last generation of hematology image analysis systems, since those designed for urinalysis are still plagued by a very limited menu of cells for enabling a useful preclassification in the morphologic analysis of body fluids.

On the other hand, there may also be some drawbacks linked to the use of these innovative means of body fluid analysis, beside cytospin preparation (as previously highlighted): available literature is relatively scarce, no direct comparison aimed at evaluating the potential bias among the different methods has been conducted, the clinical impact has not been thoughtfully assessed, and no quality control materials (either internal or external) have become available so far. Additional limitations include the initial cost of the instrumentation and the space needed for its installation. Digital analyzers should be typically connected to hematological and/or urinalysis instrumentation, in a physical continuum that may occupy a large space (as

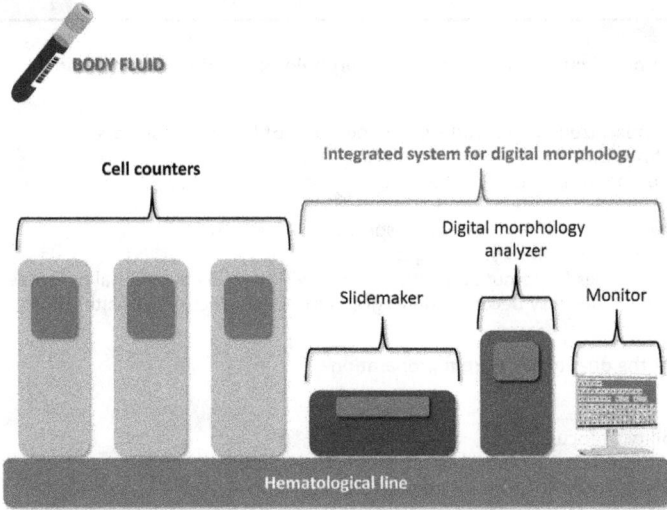

Fig. 1. Digital analyzers connected to hematological and/or urinalysis instrumentation.

shown in **Fig. 1**), which may even be unavailable in some medical laboratories. The frequent impossibility to manually focusing into the digital images, with the purpose of better appreciating some detailed cellular features, is another potential drawback. Laboratory professionals may then develop a different approach to that typically used with manual microscopy for cell recognition and classification. The appearance of cells and other elements is somehow different from that seen with traditional microscopy, and this may require a period of adaptation to the new appearance. To this end, the current hematological and/or urinalysis digital analyzer allow the preclassification of a limited number of elements (typically normal and abnormal leukocytes), while body fluids may contain a vast array of additional cells (either physiologic or pathologic) and other elements that need to be interpreted and recognized by a skilled operator, who will reclassify them into an appropriate category. Unlike routine hematological testing where the use of these techniques has become widespread in many modern laboratories, the opportunity to use digital morphology for body fluids analysis is still in embryo. As shown by Yamatani and colleagues in their recent work,[10] the accurate identification and classification of cancer cells still requires an overview analysis by an expert laboratory professional, whose reclassification process may contribute to enhance the diagnostic sensitivity from 50% to over 80%.[11] Yet, additional studies would be needed to confirm this promising performance in detecting cancer cells, as well other elements. To this end, the software versions that are currently used by CellaVision and Sysmex analyzers for preclassification of cells would need to be improved, to become capable of recognizing a wider array of physiologic and pathologic elements that are not commonly observed in whole blood samples.

With respect to the time needed to perform the morphologic analysis of body fluids, the use of digital analyzers is conventionally believed to be faster than optical revision by conventional microscopy. Nonetheless, preliminary evidence suggests that this claim may not always be true, as the time needed for reclassifying cells and other elements potentially present in body fluids may take time. Thus, irrespective of future technological improvements in preclassification, the activity of an expert morphologist, who will need to be accurately trained to the use of digital cytology, will remain for long crucial for reclassification and diagnostic interpretation.

DISCLOSURE

None of the authors have any potential conflict of interest that might constitute an embarrassment.

REFERENCES

1. Lippi G, Plebani M. Opportunities and drawbacks of nonstandard body fluid analysis. Clin Chem Lab Med 2017;55:907–9.
2. Brinkman JE, Dorius B, Sharma S. Physiology, body fluids. In: StatPearls [Internet]. Treasure Island (FL). StatPearls Publishing; 2023.
3. Block DR, Algeciras-Schimnich A. Body fluid analysis: clinical utility and applicability of published studies to guide interpretation of today's laboratory testing in serous fluids. Crit Rev Clin Lab Sci 2013;50:107–24.
4. Kratz A, Lee SH, Zini G, et al. Digital morphology analyzers in hematology: ICSH review and recommendations. Int J Lab Hematol 2019;41:437–47.
5. Alcaide Martín MJ, Altimira Queral L, Sahuquillo Frías L, et al. Automated cell count in body fluids: a review. Adv Lab Med 2021;2:149–77.
6. Hrishi AP, Sethuraman M. Cerebrospinal fluid (CSF) analysis and interpretation in neurocritical care for acute neurological conditions. Indian J Crit Care Med 2019; 23:S115–9.
7. Riedl JA, Dinkelaar RB, van Gelder W. Automated morphological analysis of cells in body fluids by the digital microscopy system DM96. J Clin Pathol 2010;63: 538–43.
8. Takemura H, Ai T, Kimura K, et al. Evaluation of cell count and classification capabilities in body fluids using a fully automated Sysmex XN equipped with high-sensitive Analysis (hsA) mode and DI-60 hematology analyzer system. PLoS One 2018;13:e0195923.
9. Ivady G, Barath S, Szaraz-Szeles M, et al. Comparative evaluation of body fluid analysis by Sysmex XN hematology analyzers, cellavision, manual microscopy and multicolor flow cytometry. Ann Clin Lab Sci 2022;52:314–22.
10. Yamatani K, Tabe Y, Ai T, et al. Performance evaluation of the Sysmex DI-60 overview application for tumor cell detection in body fluid samples. Int J Lab Hematol 2019;41:e134–8.
11. Goubard A, Marzouk M, Canoui-Poitrine F, et al. Performance of the Iris iQ(R)200 Elite analyser in the cell counting of serous effusion fluids and cerebrospinal drainage fluids. J Clin Pathol 2011;64:1123–7.
12. Yoon S, Kim HR. Analytical performance of the digital morphology analyzer Sysmex DI-60 for body fluid cell differential counts. PLoS One 2023;18:e0288551.
13. Jain G, Shetty P. Occupational concerns associated with regular use of microscope. Int J Occup Med Environ Health 2014;27:591–8.

Advances in Bone Marrow Evaluation

Joshua E. Lewis, MD, PhD[a], Olga Pozdnyakova, MD, PhD[b],*

KEYWORDS

- Bone marrow • Aspirate • Trephine biopsy • Artificial intelligence • Machine learning

KEY POINTS

- Manual microscopy has remained the standard for bone marrow aspirate and biopsy evaluation due to barriers in instrumentation, software, and workflow optimization necessary for digital evaluation.
- Recent research has demonstrated the feasibility of applying artificial intelligence toward assisted bone marrow evaluation, including automated differential cell counts on aspirate smears, biopsy image segmentation for cell lineage enumeration, and identification of novel features predictive of hematologic neoplasms.
- Many potential models exist for implementation of digital bone marrow evaluation into the hematopathology workflow, with the ultimate implementation likely being a mixture of multiple approaches.

INTRODUCTION TO THE CURRENT STATE OF DIGITAL EVALUATION OF BONE MARROW SPECIMENS

Manual microscopic evaluation of bone marrow aspirate and trephine biopsy specimens remains the standard of clinical practice for the pathologic diagnosis of hematologic conditions.[1] In the case of bone marrow aspirate smears, a critical barrier to digital analysis remains the lack of viable slide scanners. Microscopic assessment of bone marrow aspirate smears is typically performed with a 100x objective (1000x magnification) with oil immersion to obtain sufficient cytomorphologic detail.[1] Scanners currently used clinically can reach magnifications of only 400x and do not allow for oil immersion due to difficulties in dispensation and containment which can contaminate imaging systems and increase maintenance requirements. Machine learning-based studies have suggested that bone marrow aspirate differentials obtained from digital assessment at 400x magnification correlate well with manual differentials obtained from 1000x microscopic assessment.[2] However, a comprehensive

[a] Department of Pathology, Brigham and Women's Hospital, 75 Francis Street, Boston, MA 02215, USA; [b] The Hospital of the University of Pennsylvania, 3400 Spruce Street, Philadelphia, PA 19104, USA
* Corresponding author.
E-mail address: olga.pozdnyakova@pennmedicine.upenn.edu

Clin Lab Med 44 (2024) 431–440
https://doi.org/10.1016/j.cll.2024.04.005   labmed.theclinics.com
0272-2712/24/© 2024 Elsevier Inc. All rights reserved, including those for text and data mining, AI training, and similar technologies.

comparison of bone marrow aspirate smear analysis between 400x and 1000x magnifications has yet to be performed. Additionally, the identification of subtle morphologic details of atypical cell populations, such as in the assessment of atypical blast and plasma cell populations for the diagnosis of leukemia and plasma cell neoplasms, respectively, often requires 1000x microscopic assessment.[3,4] These limitations restrict the use of conventional anatomic pathology slide scanners for clinical assessment of bone marrow aspirate smears.

To address these limitations, a handful of solutions including high-resolution digital slide scanners tailored for analysis of bone marrow aspirate smears have been developed. Jin and colleagues and Fu and colleagues coupled a digital microscope with 100x objective, oil-dropping unit, digital camera, and autofocusing software to obtain 1000x images of bone marrow aspirate smears as part of the Morphogo system for automated bone marrow aspirate assessment.[5,6] Similar commercial solutions are available including the Leica Biosystems Aperio VERSA, which utilizes an automated oiler, 63x objective, and automated tissue detection software for high-resolution image acquisition. While this coupling of digital microscope and high-resolution camera for image acquisition could avoid the need for stand-alone slide scanning instrumentation, significant commercial interest in developing digital slide scanners for this purpose has been raised. Scopio Labs X100 and X100HT instruments, previously developed for digital assessment of peripheral blood smears, are currently in a multicenter trial for full-field morphologic evaluation of whole-slide bone marrow aspirate smears.[7] By coupling a series of low-resolution images of slide regions at different illumination conditions with a physical reconstruction model, these instruments are capable of obtaining 100x resolution images of peripheral blood and bone marrow aspirate smears, overcoming technical challenges met by previously developed digital slide scanners.[8] The X100HT instrument has a throughput comparable to conventional digital slide scanners (40 slides per hour). CellaVision is currently developing software to tailor their peripheral blood smear scanners and digital analysis software for bone marrow aspirate analysis as well. These dedicated high-resolution bone marrow aspirate slide scanners and automated analysis software solutions are likely to become commercially available within the next few years.

Conventional anatomic pathology slide scanners with a 40x objective would allow for optimal digital analysis of bone marrow trephine biopsies, given that these specimens are often microscopically assessed at a maximum of 400x resolution. However, scanning of whole-slide bone marrow biopsy slides is currently not commonplace in clinical practice. There have been few studies critically analyzing the improvement in clinical workflow by digital scanning of hematopathology slides including bone marrow trephine biopsies and aspirate smears. Chen and colleagues found that digital review of lymph nodes, bone marrow core biopsies and aspirate smears, and peripheral blood smears resulted in improved outcomes at a hematopathology tumor board, including presentation efficiency, clinical decision-making, and overall satisfaction.[9] Further studies have demonstrated improved hematology laboratory workflow by implementation of remote digital peripheral blood smear analysis,[10] but analogous studies for digital bone marrow aspirate and trephine biopsy analysis have yet to be performed. Nonetheless, numerous institutions have begun implementing digital pathology into their case workup and sign-out workflows for other anatomic pathology services, with overall strong concordance between digital and glass diagnoses, as well as variable improvements in pathologist efficiency and satisfaction[11–14]; similar outcomes are expected for hematopathology services, but validation studies would need to be performed.

ARTIFICIAL INTELLIGENCE FOR BONE MARROW ASPIRATE ASSESSMENT

Numerous research studies have explored the use of artificial intelligence to recapitulate or improve upon aspects of bone marrow aspirate assessment which are currently performed manually (**Table 1**). Early studies utilized convolutional neural networks (CNNs) and machine learning models tailored to learning of image-based data, to perform automated classification of cell types from scanned bone marrow aspirate smears. These included Choi and colleagues, who trained CNNs to classify cells into 10 different classes along the myeloid and erythroid maturation series,[15] and Matek and colleagues, who trained CNNs to classify 21 different bone marrow cell types from slides across a range of hematologic conditions.[16] The models from both of these studies reached hematopathologist-level performance and also demonstrated fair agreement between each other,[16] suggesting interinstitution applicability of these models. Jin and colleagues and Fu and colleagues performed cell classification studies with the Morphogo system as described earlier, allowing for 1000x magnification and associated performance improvements.[5,6] Other studies including Chandradevan and colleagues combined CNNs with other machine learning models called Faster region-based convolutional neural network (R-CNNs), tailored for object detection applications, to sequentially perform bone marrow cell detection and classification from scanned slides.[17] These early studies provided significant promise toward automated bone marrow aspirate cell preclassification similar to that already applied to peripheral blood smears, but nonetheless fell short of performing fully automated aspirate cell differentials.

Later studies implemented CNN-based region classification models to identify cellular and spicular areas on bone marrow aspirate smears for downstream analysis; when coupled with cell detection and classification models, these provided end-to-end pipelines for digital bone marrow aspirate assessment. Wang and colleagues and Tayebi and colleagues implemented this approach on whole-slide bone marrow aspirate smears to obtain slide-level cell distributions while also demonstrating strong cell type classification accuracy.[18,19] Lewis and colleagues developed a similar end-to-end pipeline with further validation studies, including the direct comparison of automated pipeline-derived differential cell counts to manual hematopathologist-derived cell counts with

Table 1		
Highlighted research on the implementation of artificial intelligence toward evaluation of bone marrow aspirate smears		
References	**Summary**	
Cell detection and classification		
Choi et al,[15] 2011	10 class cell classification along myeloid and erythroid series	
Matek et al,[16] 2017	21 class cell classification across range of hematologic conditions	
Jin et al,[5] 2020	Integrated hardware and software for cell classification	
Fu et al,[6] 2020	Cell classification and 500 cell differential cell counts	
Chandradevan et al,[17] 2020	Coupled cell detection and classification models	
Automated differential cell counts on whole-slide images		
Wang et al,[18] 2022	Coupled region of interest (ROI) detection with cell detection/classification on WSI	
Tayebi et al,[19] 2022	Automated pipeline for developing histogram of cell types	
Lewis et al,[2] 2023	Automated pipeline for automated differential cell counts	
Slide-level classification		
Manescu et al,[20] 2023	Weakly supervised classification of acute promyelocytic leukemia	

strong correlations.[2] This study also demonstrated the ability of these automated pipelines to identify and classify many more than the typical 500 cells used in manual bone marrow aspirate analysis, greatly decreasing the associated variance in differential cell counts. Thus, these artificial intellignece (AI)-based approaches can not only recapitulate manual bone marrow aspirate analysis but additionally improve upon manual analysis in ways which can ultimately impact pathologic diagnoses.

While the abovementioned approaches to digital bone marrow aspirate analysis have shown strong performance compared to manual analysis, they require the generation of large training datasets through manual slide annotation to train neural network models. Weakly supervised learning provides an alternative approach, whereby only a slide-level class is given (eg, the marrow diagnosis), and a machine learning model is trained to associate differences in cellular morphology with the given class. Manescu and colleagues applied this approach to differentiate bone marrow aspirate slides from cases of acute promyelocytic leukemia from those of acute myeloid leukemia, showing strong performance without requiring cellular-level annotations.[20] This approach could be applied to use cases where the pathologic diagnosis is of greater importance than the quantitative marrow differential cell count.

Based on the promising results of these research studies, significant interest in the development of commercially available instrumentation and AI-based software for automated bone marrow aspirate smear analysis has been garnered. Scopio Labs have developed software for automated bone marrow aspirate region and cell classification, including differential cell count calculation, from slides scanned on their X100 and X100HT instruments.[7] A multicenter trial is evaluating the software's accuracy of cell classifications, consistency of automated cell differentials with manual analysis, and repeatability and reproducibility of results. Other companies including CellaVision are developing similar software applications for their existing instrumentation. While current commercial focus is software development for accurate quantification of differential cell counts, other applications including the identification of rare cell subsets or integration with bone marrow trephine biopsy findings may be explored as adoption of AI-based assistance tools increases.

ARTIFICIAL INTELLIGENCE FOR BONE MARROW TREPHINE BIOPSY ASSESSMENT

Research studies applying artificial intelligence to the analysis of bone marrow trephine biopsies can be categorized into 2 major groups: (1) the implementation of focused models for an individual component of biopsy assessment and (2) the implementation of more generalizable models for end-to-end biopsy assessment, such as in automated diagnosis or prognostic assessment (**Table 2**). The former includes the development of CNN-based models for identification and quantification of specific cell types. Baranova and colleagues analyzed CD138 immunohistochemical stain (CD138 IHC) stains for accurate quantification of plasma cells across a wide range of bone marrow plasma cell percentages.[21] Van Eekelen and colleagues used CNN models for automated segmentation of bone marrow biopsy regions, including bone, fat, and nucleated cells[22]; this allowed for accurate quantification of bone marrow cellularity as well as quantification of myeloid, erythroid, and megakaryocytic lineages. Song and colleagues utilized an autoencoder neural network architecture to combine cell detection and classification steps, allowing for accurate identification of myeloid and erythroid elements.[23] These focused models demonstrate similarly strong performance as their counterparts in bone marrow aspirate analysis. When combined, these models allow for characterization of individual aspects bone marrow biopsy assessment that can directly contribute to case diagnosis.

Table 2
Highlighted research on the implementation of artificial intelligence toward evaluation of bone marrow trephine biopsies

Reference	Summary
Models for individual components of biopsy evaluation	
Baranova et al,[21] 2021	Plasma cell quantification from CD138 IHC
Van Eekelen et al,[22] 2022	Biopsy segmentation for cellularity and lineage quantification
Song et al,[23] 2018	Cell detection and classification for lineage quantification
Automated case diagnosis and prognosis prediction	
Irshaid et al,[24] 2022	Prediction of large cell transformation of B-cell lymphomas
Brück et al,[25] 2021	Prediction of molecular aberrancies and prognosis in myelodysplastic syndrome (MDS)

Other approaches to digital bone marrow trephine biopsy analysis include automated case diagnosis and patient prognosis based on AI-identified histologic features. Irshaid and colleagues used CNN models to identify novel histologic features in bone marrow biopsies that correlated with large cell transformation of follicular lymphoma and chronic lymphocytic leukemia as well as traditionally used morphologic features, including large lymphoma cells, chromatin pattern, nucleoli, and proliferation index.[24] Brück and colleagues used a similar approach to identify novel features that are collectively predictive for genetic/cytogenetic aberrations and prognosis for patients with myelodysplastic syndrome.[25] While newly identified AI-based features have primarily been explored in the context of automated diagnosis and prognostication, these features could be further explored for improved biologic understanding of hematologic conditions as well as AI-based diagnostic assistance tools for hematopathologists.

ADVANTAGES AND BARRIERS FOR ARTIFICIAL INTELLIGENCE-ASSISTED BONE MARROW EVALUATION

The digitization of bone marrow aspirate smear and trephine biopsy slides affords the opportunity to apply AI-based models for automated and assisted sample analysis, as described earlier. The incorporation of artificial intelligence into the hematopathology workflow for bone marrow evaluation provides many advantages compared to the current state of hematopathology. Perhaps the largest and most immediate advantage is that whereas humans are limited to the number of cells/slide areas they can fully analyze within a timely manner, machine learning models are capable of analyzing the thousands to hundreds-of-thousands of marrow nucleated cells on bone marrow aspirate smears and trephine biopsies within minutes.[2,23] This allows for automated enumeration of cell types (differential cell count on bone marrow aspirate smears, cell types, and immunohistochemistry results on trephine biopsies), assisting hematopathologists by providing this highly useful information in an objective manner. In addition, whereas manual bone marrow evaluation is subject to interobserver variability in slide areas examined, cell classification, and case diagnosis, machine learning models provide consistent outputs based on all slide areas, as well as interpretation mechanisms to understand which histologic features contributed to model predictions.[26] By providing more complete and objective cell differentials and other diagnostically relevant morphologic features, AI-based models will become an invaluable tool for assisting hematopathologists in making timely pathologic diagnoses.

Artificial intelligence also allows for the performance of hematopathology-related tasks that are impossible for humans regardless of time constraints. In the prior section, we highlighted studies using machine learning models to identify novel histologic features which predict disease presence and molecular/cytogenetic subtypes of hematologic neoplasms more accurately than manually identified features. While humans are limited to analyzing a finite number of image-based patterns to correlate with patient diagnosis and outcomes, machine learning models can efficiently identify predictive and prognostic histologic patterns over a much wider search space.[27] Additionally, methods for interpreting CNN-based model predictions have become widely adopted to improve human understanding of these novel features, providing insight into the "black box" of machine learning models.[28] Thus, artificial intelligence can help eliminate much of the bias and subjectivity in bone marrow assessment, relying less on antiquated histologic features which may only have minimal diagnostic utility, and more on unbiased features optimized by machine learning algorithms.

While the promise of artificial intelligence for assisting bone marrow evaluation is strong, there remain many barriers to its successful adoption. Foremost, digital slide scanning must be adopted for training and execution of machine learning models, ideally at 400x magnification for bone marrow trephine biopsies and 1000x magnification for aspirate smears. As mentioned earlier, this adoption has yet to become widespread, owing in part to the current lack of 1000x magnification oil objective slide scanners for bone marrow aspirates. In addition to slide scanning, investment must be placed on digital slide storage and computational resources for execution of machine learning models, training of laboratory personnel and pathologists, and incorporation of digital bone marrow evaluation into existing hematopathology workflows. These raises yet unanswered questions regarding digital slide storage and security, quality improvement/quality assurance in digital slide scanning, minimum thresholds for machine learning model performance accuracy, and regulation/oversight across institutions.

Finally, the approach to which AI-based bone marrow evaluation will be implemented has yet to be determined. Two potential avenues include (1) a centralized approach, where companies or institutions develop models trained on interinstitutional data and deliver their models as a "digital send out test" to be applied to cases at individual institutions and (2) a decentralized approach, where individual institutions develop their own models as a "digital laboratory-developed test" and train/execute these models independently of other institutions (**Fig. 1**). Benefits to the former include having models trained on larger and diverse datasets, thus improving interinstitution model generalizability, as well as making AI-based assistance tools more accessible without the need for costly computational resources and skilled informaticists at each institution. Benefits to the later include focusing model training on data from an individual institution, likely yielding improved model performance on local data as a trade-off for model generalizability, and the potential to develop highly specialized models based on the needs and patient population of an individual institution. The optimal solution may be a mixed approach, where an institution relies on outside models for more streamlined applications (eg, quantification of bone marrow aspirate differential cell counts) and develops in-house models for specific applications related to their patient population (eg, for institutions with a large population of patients with lymphoplasmacytic lymphoma, developing models that integrate IHC data from B-lymphocyte and plasma cell markers). Nonetheless, the cost-effectiveness and marginal utility of each approach will need to be determined at the individual institution level.

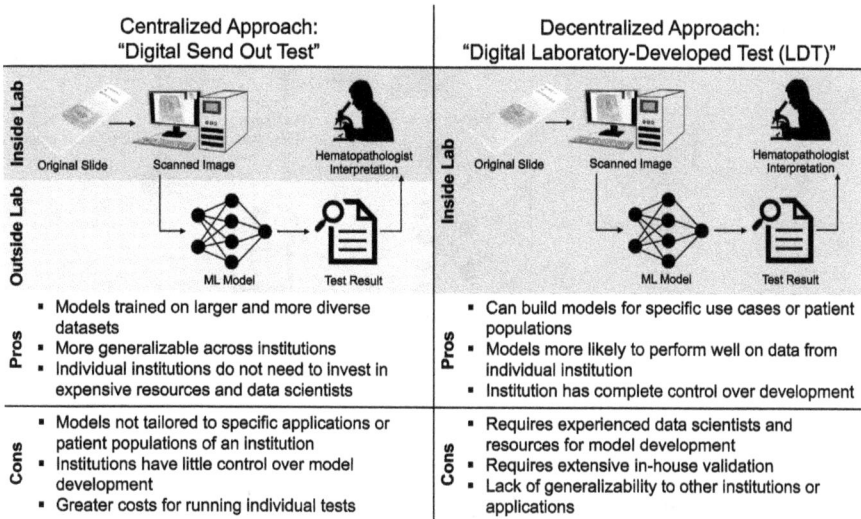

Fig. 1. Potential approaches to implementation of AI-based bone marrow evaluation. (*Left*) Centralized approach or "digital send out test," where the institution sends scanned whole-slide images of bone marrow aspirates and/or biopsies to an outside laboratory, which runs a machine learning model on the images and obtains a corresponding test result that is sent back to the original institution. (*Right*) Decentralized approach or "digital laboratory-developed test," where each individual institution implements machine learning models on their own scanned slides for use in hematopathology diagnosis. Pros and cons of the 2 approaches are outlined.

FUTURE VISION FOR ARTIFICIAL INTELLIGENCE-ASSISTED BONE MARROW EVALUATION

Once the abovementioned barriers to AI-assisted bone marrow evaluation are addressed, integration of AI into the hematopathology workflow can be initiated and will likely become commonplace. This integration can occur in 2 different forms (**Fig. 2**). First, AI-based models can be used in an assistance role to aid the hematopathologist in organizing relevant data and performing time-consuming tasks. These tasks include enumeration of bone marrow aspirate differential cell counts and trephine biopsy cell lineages, detection of rare cell subsets (eg, dysplastic cells, mast cells), quantification of IHC results (eg, blast and plasma cell percentages), and formatting of bone marrow biopsy findings with ancillary data into integrated and easily interpretable reports. This method of AI integration would not replace the hematopathologist at any level, but rather aid them in making more accurate, objective, and timely diagnoses.

AI-based models may also be used in a triaging role, performing automated bone marrow evaluation and categorizing cases as those that have a straightforward diagnosis versus those that require manual review. In light of the increasing workload of most hematopathologists, this approach would allow one to focus their efforts on more complex cases. While the potential for this type of approach is significant, it would require sophisticated machine learning models that integrate bone marrow aspirate and trephine biopsy findings with ancillary data including flow cytometry, cytogenetics, and molecular diagnostics, which have yet to be developed. Additionally, this approach would require considerable performance evaluation to ensure accurate

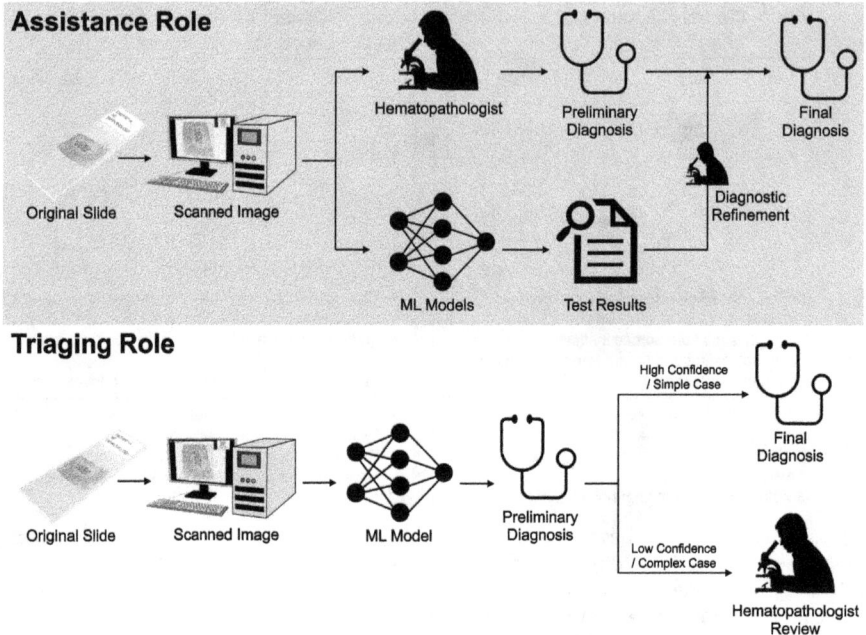

Fig. 2. Methods of integrating AI-based bone marrow evaluation into the hematopathology workflow. (*Top*) Use of AI in an "assistance role," where machine learning models analyze scanned whole-slide images of bone marrow aspirates and/or biopsies in parallel with the hematopathologist, who then analyzes the results of these models toward making a final diagnosis. (*Bottom*) Use of AI in a "triaging role," where a machine learning model makes a preliminary diagnosis from scanned slides; based on the relative confidence of the model and/or the complexity of the case, this preliminary diagnosis is accepted as the final diagnosis, or the case is routed to the hematopathologist for manual review.

diagnosis is being made, as well as a low threshold for considering cases as "complex" and routing to manual hematopathologist review.

Regardless of the method of implementation, artificial intelligence will significantly affect the clinical workflow for bone marrow evaluation. Nonetheless, the current role of the hematopathologist will largely remain the same that being the integration and synthesis of data sources toward making a conclusive diagnosis for the patient. Up until now, these data sources have been raw data in the form of histologic, immunophenotypic, and molecular genetic information, which the hematopathologist must fully assess on their own. With the assistance of artificial intelligence, these raw data sources can be made more easily and objectively analyzed, integrated, and utilized by the hematopathologist to make more accurate and timely diagnoses. Thus, this current role will be improved upon but not replaced by artificial intelligence. Hematopathologist will play a new role in overseeing AI-based model design, application, and refinement to ensure these models address the correct clinicopathologic questions, perform at a high enough standard for clinical use, and keep up with the inevitable evolution of the field of hematopathology. This new role will require collaboration with data scientists, software engineers, and clinicians who are able to effectively communicate across disciplines toward a common goal of improving patient care. While this new role may appear daunting, it will undoubtedly bring upon significant improvements to bone marrow evaluation and the field of hematopathology as a whole.

CLINICS CARE POINTS

- Artificial intelligence has the potential to revolutionize evaluation of bone marrow aspirate and biopsy specimens through implementation of automated computational models analyzing scanned aspirate and biopsy slides.

- Multiple barriers to this implementation need to be addressed, including a lack of instrumentation for scanning bone marrow aspirate smears, unclear quality and regulatory standards for AI-based models, and unanswered questions regarding how AI will be integrated into the hematopathology workflow.

DISCLOSURE

O. Pozdnyakova is a consultant for Scopio and serves as a speaker for Sysmex.

REFERENCES

1. Lee SH, Erber W, Porwit A, et al. ICSH guidelines for the standardization of bone marrow specimens and reports. Int J Lit Humanit 2008;30(5):349–64.
2. Lewis JE, Shebelut CW, Drumheller BR, et al. An automated pipeline for differential cell counts on whole-slide bone marrow aspirate smears. Mod Pathol 2023;100003.
3. Bain BJ, Béné MC. Morphological and immunophenotypic clues to the WHO categories of acute myeloid leukaemia. Acta Haematol 2019;141(4):232–44.
4. Ribourtout B, Zandecki M. Plasma cell morphology in multiple myeloma and related disorders. Morphologie 2015;99(325):38–62.
5. Jin H, Fu X, Cao X, et al. Developing and preliminary validating an automatic cell classification system for bone marrow smears: a pilot study. J Med Syst 2020; 44:1–10.
6. Fu X, Fu M, Li Q, et al. Morphogo: an automatic bone marrow cell classification system on digital images analyzed by artificial intelligence. Acta Cytol 2020; 64(6):588–96.
7. Ragg A, Raess P, Rund D, et al. Performance evaluation study of a novel digital microscopy system for the quantitative analysis of bone marrow aspirates. Blood 2021;138:4000.
8. Katz BZ, Feldman MD, Tessema M, et al. Evaluation of Scopio Labs X100 Full Field PBS: the first high-resolution full field viewing of peripheral blood specimens combined with artificial intelligence-based morphological analysis. Int J Lit Humanit 2021;43(6):1408–16.
9. Chen ZW, Kohan J, Perkins SL, et al. Web-based oil immersion whole slide imaging increases efficiency and clinical team satisfaction in hematopathology tumor board. J Pathol Inf 2014;5(1):41.
10. Katz BZ, Benisty D, Sayegh Y, et al. Remote digital microscopy improves hematology laboratory workflow by Reducing peripheral blood smear analysis turnaround time. Appl Clin Inf 2022;13(5):1108–15.
11. Hanna MG, Reuter VE, Hameed MR, et al. Whole slide imaging equivalency and efficiency study: experience at a large academic center. Mod Pathol 2019;32(7): 916–28.
12. Wilbur DC, Madi K, Colvin RB, et al. Whole-slide imaging digital pathology as a platform for teleconsultation: a pilot study using paired subspecialist correlations. Arch Pathol Lab Med 2009;133(12):1949–53.

13. Graham AR, Bhattacharyya AK, Scott KM, et al. Virtual slide telepathology for an academic teaching hospital surgical pathology quality assurance program. Hum Pathol 2009;40(8):1129–36.
14. Jukić DM, Drogowski LM, Martina J, et al. Clinical examination and validation of primary diagnosis in anatomic pathology using whole slide digital images. Arch Pathol Lab Med 2011;135(3):372–8.
15. Choi JW, Ku Y, Yoo BW, et al. White blood cell differential count of maturation stages in bone marrow smear using dual-stage convolutional neural networks. PLoS One 2017;12(12):e0189259.
16. Matek C, Krappe S, Münzenmayer C, et al. Highly accurate differentiation of bone marrow cell morphologies using deep neural networks on a large image data set. Blood 2021;138(20):1917–27.
17. Chandradevan R, Aljudi AA, Drumheller BR, et al. Machine-based detection and classification for bone marrow aspirate differential counts: initial development focusing on nonneoplastic cells. Lab Invest 2020;100(1):98–109.
18. Wang C-W, Huang S-C, Lee Y-C, et al. Deep learning for bone marrow cell detection and classification on whole-slide images. Med Image Anal 2022;75:102270.
19. Tayebi RM, Mu Y, Dehkharghanian T, et al. Automated bone marrow cytology using deep learning to generate a histogram of cell types. Commun Med 2022;2:45.
20. Manescu P, Narayanan P, Bendkowski C, et al. Detection of acute promyelocytic leukemia in peripheral blood and bone marrow with annotation-free deep learning. Sci Rep 2023;13(1):2562.
21. Baranova K, Tran C, Plantinga P, et al. Evaluation of an open-source machine-learning tool to quantify bone marrow plasma cells. J Clin Pathol 2021;74(7):462–8.
22. van Eekelen L, Pinckaers H, van den Brand M, et al. Using deep learning for quantification of cellularity and cell lineages in bone marrow biopsies and comparison to normal age-related variation. Pathology 2022;54(3):318–27.
23. Song T-H, Sanchez V, Daly HE, et al. Simultaneous cell detection and classification in bone marrow histology images. IEEE journal of biomedical and health informatics 2018;23(4):1469–76.
24. Irshaid L, Bleiberg J, Weinberger E, et al. Histopathologic and machine deep learning criteria to predict lymphoma transformation in bone marrow biopsies. Arch Pathol Lab Med 2022;146(2):182–93.
25. Brück O, Lallukka-Brück S, Hohtari H, et al. Machine learning of bone marrow histopathology identifies genetic and clinical determinants in patients with MDS. Blood Cancer Discov 2021;2:238–49 [Europe PMC free article][Abstract][CrossRef][Google Scholar];2021.
26. Saleem R, Yuan B, Kurugollu F, et al. Explaining deep neural networks: a survey on the global interpretation methods. Neurocomputing 2022;513:165–80.
27. Alzubaidi L, Zhang J, Humaidi AJ, et al. Review of deep learning: concepts, CNN architectures, challenges, applications, future directions. Journal of big Data 2021;8:1–74.
28. Haar LV, Elvira T, Ochoa O. An analysis of explainability methods for convolutional neural networks. Eng Appl Artif Intell 2023;117:105606.

Advances in Hemoglobinopathies and Thalassemia Evaluation

Archana M. Agarwal, MD*, Anton V. Rets, MD, PhD[1]

KEYWORDS

- Hemoglobinopathy • Thalassemia • Sequencing • Capillary electrophoresis
- High-performance liquid chromatography • Next-generation sequencing

KEY POINTS

- Hemoglobin disorders are one of the most common genetic disorders worldwide with broad clinical presentations.
- Diagnostic modalities vary from widely available complete blood count to advanced molecular techniques.
- Newer diagnostic modalities, for example, next-generation sequencing and third-generation sequencing are promising for future.

INTRODUCTION

Hemoglobin (Hb), a tetrameric protein containing 4 prosthetic heme moieties, plays a crucial role in the physiologic transport of oxygen.[1] In broader sense, thalassemias result from the quantitative decrease in the globin chain (eg, due to decrease in globin expression) and hemoglobinopathies are due to structural alterations in the globin chains.[2–4] The diagnosis of Hb disorders heavily relies on clinical laboratory assessments, employing a combination of biophysical, biochemical, and molecular assays to substantiate and confirm the diagnosis.

The fully assembled Hb molecule consists of 4 globin subunits formed through the pairing of α (alpha)-globin or α-like globin chains with β (beta)-globin or β-like globin chains.[1] The predominant Hb in adults, Hb A, comprises 2 α and 2 β subunits. Hb composition undergoes switching in the early years of life due to the changes in gene expression.

Department of Pathology, University of Utah Health and ARUP Laboratories, 500 Chipeta Way, Salt Lake City, UT 84108, USA
[1] Present address: 4313 S Zarahemla Drive, Salt Lake City, UT, 84124.
* Corresponding author. 500 Chipeta Way, Salt Lake City, UT 94108.
E-mail address: archana.agarwal@hsc.utah.edu

Clin Lab Med 44 (2024) 441–453
https://doi.org/10.1016/j.cll.2024.04.006
0272-2712/24/© 2024 Elsevier Inc. All rights reserved.

The α-globin gene cluster resides on chromosome 16, featuring 2 copies of α gene (*HBA2* and *HBA1*) per chromosome. The α-like protein, ζ, is expressed in the embryo but becomes virtually absent after the first trimester.[4] The β-globin gene cluster is located on chromosome 11 and includes β-globin (*HBB*) and multiple flanking β-like genes. The embryonic β-like globin, ε, is expressed solely in the first trimester, followed by the production of the fetal β-like globin, γ.[2] Hb F is a tetramer of γ-globin and α-globin. The expression of γ-globin gene peaks in mid-gestation, gradually declining approximately 6 months after birth, with small residual expression persisting throughout life.[2,3] Hb A_2 is a tetramer of δ-globin and α-globin chains. The expression of δ-globin gene (*HBD*), another β-like subunit, commences shortly before birth and continues throughout life. Although produced in small quantity, Hb A_2 is crucial for β-thalassemia screening. Hb disorders are recognized by disruptions in the ratios of normal Hb tetramers or the presence of structurally abnormal Hbs.

PATHOPHYSIOLOGY OF HEMOGLOBINOPATHY AND THALASSEMIA

Genes encoding for globin chains and those regulating their expression can undergo spontaneous mutations. The incidence of these aberrations is so frequent, that inherited Hb disorders are the most prevalent inherited diseases in the world. Chiefly, genetic alterations can affect (1) the amino acid sequence of a globin chain, thus changing the chain's structure, or (2) the rate of globin chain expression. The former group is referred to as "variant Hbs" or hemoglobinopathies and the latter as "thalassemias." This is a very basic approach as some mutations can affect both the globin chain structure and its expression rate, for example, Hb E or Hb constant spring among others. It is estimated that approximately 5.2% of the world population are carriers of an Hb disorder.[5] About 330,000 affected infants are born annually, 83% of them having sickle cell disorders and 17% with thalassemias.[5] The increasing rates of international migration have introduced Hb disorders to the parts of the world where they were previously rare.

The classification system for thalassemias encompasses molecular/pathogenetic and clinical aspects. Considering the affected gene/globin chain, they are subdivided into α-, β-, δβ-, γδβ-thalassemias, and so forth, with β-thalassemia and α-thalassemia being the most clinically relevant. Clinical classification, based on the severity of symptomatology and transfusion dependence, divides thalassemia into "major," "intermedia," and "minor."[3]

The presentation and the clinical course of thalassemias depend on 2 main pathogenetic mechanisms: decreased production and imbalance between the globin chains. The diminished production of Hb results in microcytic hypochromic red blood cells (RBCs) and oftentimes anemia, wherein an imbalance between different globin chains may lead to a relative excess of a non-affected chain. For example, in some forms of α-thalassemia, β-globin chains (adults) or γ-globin chains (neonates and infants) form homotetramers, Hb H and Hb Bart's, respectively.[4] In β-thalassemia, α-chain homotetramers are insoluble and precipitate in maturing RBCs causing their destruction introducing a hemolytic component. Anemia and tissue hypoxia stimulate RBC production in the bone marrow. As a result, a "classic" thalassemic presentation includes complete blood count (CBC) abnormalities, particularly microcytic hypochromic anemia with compensatory increase in RBCs, and often some degree of hemolysis.[2]

The clinical significance of α-thalassemias and β-thalassemias is largely determined by the genotype. Because there are 4 α-globin genes as opposed to only 2 β-globin genes, genotypic spectrum of α-thalassemia is much broader than that in β-thalassemia. The most severe form of α-thalassemia is Hb Bart's hydrops fetalis, occurs when there is a complete absence of α-globin chains. Patients with β-thalassemia major (Cooley's anemia), the most severe form of β-thalassemia, are dependent on blood transfusions throughout their life.[2]

Variant Hbs occur due to mostly point mutations of the globin genes resulting in altered amino acid sequence. Over 1400 variant Hbs are currently described.[6] The majority of these are of no clinical significance, but some are associated with important functional alterations such as Hb polymerization (Hb S), crystallization (Hb C), decreased stability (unstable Hbs), increased or decreased oxygen affinity, or propensity to form methemoglobin. Of variant Hbs, conditions associated with Hb S are by far the most impactful health problems worldwide.[6] Prevalence of Hb S can be as high as 40% in some populations (Eti Turks) and is around 4% to 10% in African Americans. Whereas Hb S trait is usually asymptomatic, Hb S disease is a severe debilitating condition. Sickling syndromes, in addition to homozygous Hb S, also develops in compound heterozygosity of Hb S with Hb C (Hb SC disease), β-thalassemia, Hb D-Los Angeles, and so forth.[7]

WHY IS CORRECT AND TIMELY DIAGNOSIS OF A HB DISORDER IMPORTANT?

Hb disorders pose a significant disease burden on the world population. Although many forms of thalassemias/Hb variants are clinically asymptomatic, their detection is necessary for the following reasons:

- Prevention of clinically severe forms of disease and management of the overall disease burden.
- Affected individuals and couples must receive genetic counseling and offering appropriate pre-conception or post-conception measures to avoid birth or appropriately manage an affected child.
- Distinction of the patient's condition from iron deficiency anemia (IDA). Both IDA and thalassemia present with microcytic hypochromic anemia. Although both conditions may coexist, their treatments are different as iron supplementation that resolves IDA can further advance iron overload with severe clinical sequelae in a patient with thalassemia.
- In addition, management of thalassemia may encompass prevention or mitigation of growth retardation, osteoporosis, and endocrine dysfunction.

Current Diagnostic Workup

Diagnosis of Hb disorders requires the knowledge of clinical presentation, family history, and laboratory tests. The laboratory workup is performed in a stepwise manner. Although currently available molecular testing is essential for a definitive diagnosis, it is prudent and cost-effective to utilize other tests to effectively identify individuals with a high probability of an Hb disorder who would need molecular testing specially in resource limited situation.

The common clinical settings triggering an investigation for a Hb disorder include preconceptional or postconceptional screening, abnormal neonatal screening results, abnormal CBC indices, and family history of Hb disorder. The laboratory workup should begin with routine tests invariably including CBC and morphologic review of the blood smear. In addition, laboratory assessment of hemolysis (including Coombs test) and iron metabolism are strongly recommended. The second step is Hb fractionation followed by more specialized tests targeting certain major groups of Hb disorders, if appropriate. Ultimately, molecular tests are strongly recommended as a definitive and final step of the investigation.

Routine Tests

CBC, being the most ordered and performed laboratory test, provides crucial information.[8] Microcytosis (reflected by decreased mean corpuscular volume [MCV]) and hypochromia (represented by low mean corpuscular Hb [MCH] concentration and MCH) are commonly seen in α- and β-thalassemias. Microcytosis and hypochromia are also associated with IDA, therefore, concurrent iron studies must be performed. Increased RBC count and normal RBC distribution width favor thalassemia over IDA, but these features are neither sensitive nor specific. The utility of RBC indices and their combination (variable calculated indexes) have been shown to have some reliability to distinguish between IDA and thalassemias, but their application is setting-dependent.[9–11] If the iron studies suggest IDA, it may be prudent to provide iron supplementation and re-evaluate for persistence of anemia before proceeding with the workup. Many carriers of thalassemia and variant Hbs may have normal RBC parameters, therefore CBC results must be interpreted in the context of clinical and family history.

Morphologic review of blood can provide valuable information to guide further workup in certain scenarios.[12] For example, it provides correlation between the CBC indices and morphology (microcytosis with low MCV, etc.), detection of dimorphic RBC population, assessment of the regeneration (polychromasia and nucleated RBCs), and identification of morphologic clues associated with certain Hb conditions (eg, sickle-shaped RBCs in sickle cell anemia, Hb C crystals, "boat cells" in Hb SC disease, target cells in thalassemia and IDA, "bite cells" in unstable Hbs). Morphologic findings may also expand the differential diagnosis, for example, "bite cells" which can be seen in unstable Hbs also raise a possibility of enzyme deficiency (G6PD) and exposure to certain toxins.

Hemoglobin Fractionation Tests

These tests allow to separate and detect/visualize Hb fractions, normal and abnormal, if present. The separation is achieved by various methodologies (**Table 1**). Hb fractionation serves 2 main purposes: (1) quantification of normal Hbs (Hb A, Hb A_2, Hb F) and (2) detection of variant Hbs. Quantification of Hb A_2 plays a critical role in screening for β-thalassemia as almost all β-thalassemia patients have increased Hb A_2.[13–15] This phenomenon is likely due to excess of α-globin chains and an increase in δ-chain synthesis in at least a subset of cases. One should be mindful of common caveats. For example, high-performance liquid chromatography (HPLC), a widely used methodology, cannot separate Hb A_2 from Hb E (a relatively common β-chain variant with thalassemic features) or Hb Lepore.[14] Products of Hb S degradation also co-elute with Hb A_2 on HPLC falsely increasing the Hb A_2 percentage.[14] Therefore, an alternative technique such as capillary electrophoresis (CE) must be applied. A methodology-independent underestimation of Hb A_2 happens in δ-chain variant or δ-thalassemia.[16] Neonates with β-thalassemia may have normal Hb A_2 level up to 3 to 4 months after birth because of physiologic γ-chain to β-chain switching. Being a very useful testing modality to screen for β-thalassemia, Hb fractionation has little to offer for screening of α-thalassemia carriers.[4] Because all 3 normal Hb fractions contain α-globin chains, the decreased α-globin chain production will result in a proportionate decrease of all fractions preserving the pattern and percentage of Hbs.

Variant Hbs are easier to identify, they usually present as an abnormal peak/band. Its location helps to narrow the list of possible variants, but definitive conclusion can be made without molecular confirmation. For Hb S, acceptable diagnostic certainty can

Table 1
Summary of tests used for Hb fractionation profiling[13,15,17]

Test/Methodology	Hb Separation Principle	Advantages	Disadvantages
Gel electrophoresis	Migration of Hb depending on the charge	Rapid Low cost Separates major clinically relevant Hbs (Hb A$_2$, Hb S, and Hb C)	Low throughput Labor intensive Low resolution Imprecise quantification Cannot separate many Hb variants
Isoelectric focusing	Migration of the Hb fraction within a pH gradient (isoelectric point)	Low cost Separation of Hb fractions superior to gel electrophoresis Higher definition of the Hb fractions	High resolution for minor insignificant fractions (eg, Hb degradation products)
High-performance liquid chromatography	Interaction between staticnary phase (negatively charged silica) and mobile phase (buffer)	Rapid Good quantification Good resolution Low specimen volume	Cannot quantify Hbs with retention time <1 min (Hb H, Hb Bart's) Cannot separate Hb A$_2$ from Hb E and Hb Lepore Cannot separate some other Hb variants Highly skilled laboratory personnel
Capillary electrophoresis	Electroosmotic flow created between negatively charged capillary wall and positively charged buffer with electric field	Rapid Good resolution Good quantitation Separates Hb A$_2$ from Hb E Quantifies Hb H and Hb Bart's Low specimen volume	Cannot separate some Hb variants Highly skilled laboratory personnel

be achieved by using 2 independent techniques if molecular testing is not available. The pattern of tracing by HPLC and/or CE as well as their percentage can help to distinguish α-chain from β-chain variants as well as favor γ or δ variants. Accurate measurements of the variant Hb are important to identify cases with concurrent thalassemias (eg, in sickle cell trait, Hb S <35% is often indicative of concurrent α-thalassemia).[13–15] Unstable variant Hbs show lower-than-expected percentages of the abnormal peaks/bands to the point of being not detectable by these techniques (eg, hyper-unstable Hbs). β-chain variants including Hb S and Hb C may not be apparent in neonates and repeat testing after 6 months of age may be strongly advised. Similarities of physical/chemical properties of some Hb variants do not allow them to be separated for normal Hbs using certain methodologies.

Other screening laboratory tests

An additional arsenal of screening tests for abnormal Hbs can be performed when appropriate (**Table 2**). These tests aim to demonstrate abnormal functional properties of Hbs and should be considered in the diagnostic workup for additional information.

MOLECULAR DIAGNOSTICS TECHNIQUES: CURRENT STATE

Molecular testing, becoming more available and affordable world-wide, has demonstrated its diagnostic value to definitively confirm a Hb disorder (**Table 3**). Technological advances have been continuously expanding a menu of clinically validated molecular tests. Understanding of advantages and pitfalls of these tests is key to accurate, timely, and cost-effective workup.

Detection of Large Deletions

Large deletions in the *HBA* and *HBB* gene clusters, responsible for 90% of α-thalassemias and approximately 5% of β-thalassemias can be detected using Gap-PCR and multiplex ligation-dependent probe assay (MLPA) or comparative genomic hybridization array (CGH).

Gap-PCR: PCR primers are designed to flank a potentially deleted region. In the wild type allele (no deletion), the primers are located too far apart to yield a product. In contrast, the presence of a deletion shortens the distance between the forward and reverse primers allowing the DNA amplification.[21] A gap-PCR method is used by many laboratories to detect the 7 common α-thalassemia deletions (−α3.7, −α4.2, −α20.5, −−SEA, −−MED, −−FIL, and −−THAI).[22] The downside of this technology is that it will only detect the known targeted deletions.

MLPA is employed for the multiplex detection of gene-specific deletions and/or duplications. It is a high-throughput and relatively cost-effective method for detecting copy number variations. It uses a set of short oligonucleotide probes designed to anneal to an area of interest. The MLPA reaction begins with the denaturation of patient's DNA, followed by hybridization with the probes and then amplification using universal primer sequences. The PCR products are then analyzed by CE. The peak height of the amplified probe is compared to the corresponding peak height of a reference sample to generate a ratio. Wild type alleles produce a ratio of 1.0 (2 alleles) while a deletion produces a ratio of 0.5 (1 allele) while a duplication produces a ratio of 1.5 (3 alleles) or more. MLPA does not require exact knowledge of the breakpoints, however, it cannot detect the precise deletion points.[15,23]

CGH array: Comprehensive and precise characterization of the breakpoints can be achieved CGH. Although not routinely used, this can be useful in detecting unusual or novel large deletions or duplications.[24]

Table 2
Summary of other screening tests used in workup for Hb disorders [18–20]

Test	Principle	Test Description	Clinical Utility	Caveats
Sickle solubility test	Polymerization and precipitation of certain Hbs (sickling Hbs) in deoxygenated environment.	Addition of deoxygenating agent (dithionate) to the hemolysate causes precipitation of abnormal Hb visually detected by increased turbidity.	Alternative/additional test for sickling disorders mostly Hb S.	False-negative results at low concentration of the sickling Hb (severe anemia or infant younger than 6 mo). Positive results in Hbs other than Hb S: Hb I, Hb Bart's, Hb C-Harlem, etc.
Hb stability test	Precipitation of unstable Hb in harsh environment.	Exposure of the hemolysate to heat (heat stability test) or isopropanol (isopropanol stability test) causes enhanced precipitation of unstable Hbs visually detected as flocculation.	Demonstration of altered Hb stability.	False-negative results in super-unstable Hbs (low concentration of the Hb variant in the hemolysate). Hb F, being less stable than Hb A, may show positive results in conditions with increased Hb F. Avoid testing infants younger than 6 mo.
Heinz body detection	Visualization of precipitated Hb using supravital stains.	The blood sample is incubated with supravital stain. Heinz bodies (stained intraerythrocytic inclusions) are assessed in smears under the microscope. Crystal violet stain detects pre-existing Heinz bodies. Brilliant cresyl blue, being an oxidizer, induces formation Heinz bodies during incubation, increasing the robustness if the test.	Detection of decreased Hb stability. Brilliant cresyl blue stain can also be used to detect Hb H inclusions.	Decreased Hb stability can be due to a variant Hb with decreased stability, enzyme deficiency (eg, G6PD), and acquired conditions (oxidizing medication, toxins, etc.). Interpretation requires morphologic skills.

(continued on next page)

Table 2
(continued)

Test	Principle	Test Description	Clinical Utility	Caveats
Hb F distribution	Patterns of distribution of Hb F between RBCs: • Keilhauer–Betke test • Flow cytometry-based assay.	Keilhauer–Betke test is based on the increased resistance of RBCs with high Hb F to acid detected morphologically. Hb F can be labeled by fluorochrome-conjugated antibody and detected by flow cytometry.	Hb F distribution pattern (pancellular vs heterocelluar) helps to distinguish many forms of HPFH from δβ-thalassemia trait, respectively. Detection of fetal–maternal hemorrhage.	Keilhauer–Betke is rarely used in Hb disorder workup due to low sensitivity and poor reproducibility.
Osmotic fragility	RBCs with decreased volume/surface area ratio show increased resistance to osmotic lysis (decreased fragility).	Incubation of patient's RBCs in progressively hypotonic solutions to determine their resistance to lysis.	The test is frequently used for screening for hereditary membrane disorders (increased fragility in HS), decreased fragility is seen in thalassemias.	Limited specificity: any condition with decreased volume/surface area ratio (eg, IDA) can have decreased osmotic fragility.
P50 determination	p50 value as measurement of Hb affinity to oxygen.	Measurement of oxygenated and deoxygenated Hb at different oxygen tension points.	Demonstration of abnormal (increased or decreased) oxygen affinity of Hb.	Technically complex and challenging. Very strict specimen requirements. Not sensitive and specific.

Abbreviations: G6PD, glucose-6-phosphate dehydrogenase; Hb, hemoglobin; HS, hereditary spherocytosis; IDA, iron deficiency anemia; RBC, red blood cell.

Table 3
Comparison of the molecular technologies used for hemoglobin analysis

Methodology	Application	Limitations
Gap-PCR	Detection of common deletions in α-globin and/or β-globin genes	Detects only the deletions specifically targeted by the assay
MLPA	Detection of both common and uncommon deletions and duplications in α-globin and/or β-globin genes	Does not detect exact breakpoints; similar variants may be indistinguishable
Dot blot/allele-specific oligonucleotide	Detection of targeted point mutations	Detects only the targeted variants
Allele-specific PCR/ARMS	Detection of targeted point mutations	Detects only the targeted variants
Sanger sequencing	Detection of point mutations and small insertions/deletions, including novel variants	Not suitable for large deletions/duplications and complex rearrangements
Next-generation sequencing	Detection of point mutations, small insertions/deletions	Not suitable for large deletions/duplications yet, need sophisticated bioinformatics pipeline
Third-generation sequencing	Can detect large deletions/duplications and complex rearrangement	High cost, sophisticated analysis, lack of expertise

Abbreviation: ARMS, amplification refractory mutation system.

Detection of Point Mutations

This approach is frequently taken in investigation of β-thalassemia (since the majority [>90% cases] are due to point mutations, small insertion/deletions) and variant Hbs. Non-deletional α-thalassemia that represents approximately 5% to 10% of α-thalassemias can also be investigated with this approach.

The detection of characterized point mutations can be accomplished by dot blot or reverse dot blot with allele-specific oligonucleotide probes. It is an inexpensive test employed by many laboratories. Hybridization between the probe and the amplified patient DNA reveals a particular point mutation. In dot blot, the patient's amplified DNA is fixed to a nylon membrane strip.[15] In reverse dot blot, probes are fixed to a nylon membrane strip and the patient's genomic DNA is amplified, labeled, and hybridized to the filter. Here, multiple mutations, rather than multiple patients, can be tested in one hybridization reaction. Similarly, allele-specific PCR, known as amplification refractory mutation system, can be used to detect predefined point mutations. The PCR products are analyzed by electrophoresis.

Methodologies such as high-resolution melting, denaturing gradient gel electrophoresis, denaturing HPLC, and single-strand conformation polymorphism can also be employed to detect point mutations; these methods are also suitable for the detection of small insertions and deletions.[15]

Sanger sequencing can detect point mutations and small insertions/deletions in both α-globin and β-globin genes. These genes are small and have been very well characterized. However, Sanger sequencing should not be used as a first-line detection method for α-thalassemia as it is not suited for large deletions/duplications. It works great for β-thalassemia due to point mutation, small insertion/deletion.[15,23]

ADVANCED/EVOLVING TECHNOLOGIES: FROM PRESENT TO FUTURE

Next-generation sequencing (NGS), also known as "second-generation sequencing," has been established as a diagnostic tool for many genetic disorders including thalassemia.[25–27] Several modalities are available: whole-genome sequencing, exome sequencing, and targeted gene panels. However, because of the short-read lengths and long fragments of homologous regions in the *HBA* gene cluster, an accurate evaluation of α-globin genes by NGS is challenging. Until now, NGS has mainly been useful to evaluate β-globin genes, modifier genes that is, *KLF1, BCL11, HBS1L,* and *MYB* and non-deletional α-thalassemias.[26,28]

Third-generation sequencing (TGS) employs single molecule sequencing of either DNA or RNA. It differs from NGS in that it omits the amplification step and can generate data on large DNA fragments. TGS is gaining popularity for initial diagnosis as well as for preimplantation and noninvasive prenatal diagnosis specially in China where α-thalassemia is prevalent.[29,30] Earlier version of these technologies had a sequencing error rate of 5% to 25%, however, since 2018, with newer bioinformatics and algorithms, the accuracy has been improved.[31]

Single molecule real-time (SMRT) sequencing, nanopore sequencing, and synthetic long-read sequencing are some of the techniques within this category. SMRT, pioneered by Pacific Biosciences (PacBio) in 2010[31] uses a SMRTbell library format wherein a double stranded DNA fragments are capped at both ends by ligated hairpin adapter and converted to a single stranded circular DNA. Each circular DNA also contain sequencing primer and polymerase. Single DNA molecules are immobilized on to the SMRT cell chip unit with millions of microwells called "zero-mode wavelengths."[29] As the polymerase incorporates each nucleotide during replication, a fluorescent pulse is generated and read in real time. The same DNA sequence is sequenced multiple times generating highly accurate long reads (from 250 to >25000 base pairs) also known as HiFi reads.

Oxford nanopore technology introduced in 2014 uses a nanopore/nanoscale protein pore as a biosensor. This protein pore is embedded in an electrically resistant polymer membrane. DNA or RNA molecule passes through these nanopore and the sequencers measure changes in ionic current.[26,30] This methodology provides long reads and can detect complex rearrangements and copy number variants.

Synthetic long read sequencing developed by Illumina utilizes the long DNA fragments that are enzymatically "land marked" with unique patterns than amplified and sequenced.

Mass spectrometry (MS) offers a rapid and accurate detection of many Hb variants, but can be technologically complex, and expensive. MS is extensively used for the detection of protein. Tandem MS also known as MS/MS is the reference technique classically combining 2 mass analyzers in a single instrument, that is, electrospray ionization and matrix-assisted laser desorption ionization. These analyzers utilize 2 strategic approaches: top-down and bottom-up. In top-down approach, direct sample infusion happens in mass spectrometer without enzyme digestion. In bottom-up approach, the protein is digested into corresponding peptides and then analyzed.[17,32,33] There have been a lot of technological advancements in recent past. However, most of the laboratories still lack the technical expertise to use MS for the evaluation of hemoglobinopathies and thalassemia.

SUMMARY

The laboratory diagnosis of Hb disorders has been gradually transforming to reflect changes in the incidence of these conditions and embracing technological advances. This necessitates adjustments of our clinical and diagnostic practices. Among these are (1) increased awareness of Hb disorders among general practitioners, as well as specialists in obstetrics/gynecology, pediatrics, hematology, and so forth; (2) understanding the diagnostic utility of routine tests, and recognition of the benefits of current and upcoming molecular methodologies; and (3) development of workup models to ensure accurate, timely, and cost-effective result. To summarize, no single test is adequate for the definitive diagnosis. Combining several modalities (eg, HPLC and CE along with molecular technologies) helps to alleviate some of the methodology-dependent drawbacks and improve diagnostic utility.

CLINICS CARE POINTS

- High index of suspicion is necessary to make a diagnosis of hemoglobinopathy/thalassemia as these disorders are becoming common due to migration and population intermingling.
- Careful evaluation of CBC, especially MCV, MCH, and RBC count is essential for diagnosis.
- Elevated Hb A2 levels by HPLC or CE can be used as a surrogate marker for β-thalassemia trait; however, α-thalassemia trait often requires molecular techniques, for example, deletion/duplication analysis for diagnosis.
- Advanced molecular techniques, for example, NGS or third-generation sequencing, still have limitations due to cost and complex nature of the involved genes.

DISCLOSURE

The authors have nothing to disclose.

REFERENCES

1. Schechter AN. Hemoglobin research and the origins of molecular medicine. Blood 2008;112(10):3927–38.
2. Taher AT, Musallam KM, Cappellini MD. β-Thalassemias. N Engl J Med 2021; 384(8):727–43.
3. Taher AT, Weatherall DJ, Cappellini MD. Thalassaemia. Lancet Lond Engl 2018; 391(10116):155–67.
4. Piel FB, Weatherall DJ. The α-thalassemias. N Engl J Med 2014;371(20):1908–16.
5. Modell B, Darlison M. Global epidemiology of haemoglobin disorders and derived service indicators. Bull World Health Organ 2008;86(6):480–7.
6. Giardine B, Borg J, Viennas E, et al. Updates of the HbVar database of human hemoglobin variants and thalassemia mutations. Nucleic Acids Res 2014; 42(Database issue):D1063–9.
7. Steinberg MH. Treating sickle cell anemia: a new era dawns. Am J Hematol 2020; 95(4):338–42.
8. Ma I, Guo M, Lau CK, et al. Test volume data for 51 most commonly ordered laboratory tests in Calgary, Alberta, Canada. Data Brief 2019;23:103748.
9. Matos JF, Dusse LMS, Borges KBG, et al. A new index to discriminate between iron deficiency anemia and thalassemia trait. Rev Bras Hematol Hemoter 2016; 38(3):214–9.
10. Jameel T, Baig M, Ahmed I, et al. Differentiation of beta thalassemia trait from iron deficiency anemia by hematological indices. Pakistan J Med Sci 2017;33(3): 665–9.
11. Sari DP, Wahidiyat PA, Setianingsih I, et al. Hematological parameters in individuals with beta thalassemia trait in South Sumatra, Indonesia. Anemia 2022;2022: 3572986.
12. Beckman AK, Ng VL, Jaye DL, et al. Clinician-ordered peripheral blood smears have low reimbursement and variable clinical value: a three-institution study, with suggestions for operational efficiency. Diagn Pathol 2020;15(1):112.
13. Munkongdee T, Chen P, Winichagoon P, et al. Update in laboratory diagnosis of thalassemia. Front Mol Biosci 2020;7:74.
14. Joutovsky A, Hadzi-Nesic J, Nardi MA. HPLC retention time as a diagnostic tool for hemoglobin variants and hemoglobinopathies: a study of 60000 samples in a clinical diagnostic laboratory. Clin Chem 2004;50(10):1736–47.
15. Greene DN, Vaughn CP, Crews BO, et al. Advances in detection of hemoglobinopathies. Clin Chim Acta Int J Clin Chem 2015;439:50–7.
16. Rets AV, Reading NS, Agarwal AM. δ-Globin chain variants associated with decreased Hb A2 levels: a national reference laboratory experience. Hemoglobin 2020;44(6):438–41.
17. Xu M, Wang Y, Xu A. A Comparative evaluation of capillary electrophoresis, cation-exchange high-performance liquid chromatography, and matrix-assisted laser desorption/ionization time-of-flight mass spectrometry for the screening of hemoglobin variants. Am J Clin Pathol 2021;156(3):445–54.
18. Huntsman RG, Barclay GP, Canning DM, et al. A rapid whole blood solubility test to differentiate the sickle-cell trait from sickle-cell anaemia. J Clin Pathol 1970; 23(9):781–3.
19. Kaushansky K. Hematology. 9th edition. McGraw-Hill; 2016.
20. Kjeldsberg CR. Practical diagnosis of hematologic disorders. 4th edition. ASCP Press; 2006.

21. Sabath DE. Molecular diagnosis of thalassemias and hemoglobinopathies: an ACLPS critical review. Am J Clin Pathol 2017;148(1):6–15.
22. Tan AS, Quah TC, Low PS, et al. A rapid and reliable 7-deletion multiplex polymerase chain reaction assay for alpha-thalassemia. Blood 2001;98(1):250–1.
23. Sabath DE. The role of molecular diagnostic testing for hemoglobinopathies and thalassemias. Int J Lab Hematol 2023;45(Suppl 2):71–8.
24. Blattner A, Brunner-Agten S, Ludin K, et al. Detection of germline rearrangements in patients with α- and β-thalassemia using high resolution array CGH. Blood Cells Mol Dis 2013;51(1):39–47.
25. Agarwal AM, McMurty V, Clayton AL, et al. Clinical utility of targeted next-generation sequencing panel in routine diagnosis of hereditary hemolytic anemia: a national reference laboratory experience. Eur J Haematol 2023;110(6):688–95.
26. Hassan S, Bahar R, Johan MF, et al. Next-generation sequencing (NGS) and third-generation sequencing (TGS) for the diagnosis of thalassemia. Diagn Basel Switz 2023;13(3):373.
27. He J, Song W, Yang J, et al. Next-generation sequencing improves thalassemia carrier screening among premarital adults in a high prevalence population: the Dai nationality, China. Genet Med 2017;19(9):1022–31.
28. Rizzuto V, Koopmann TT, Blanco-Álvarez A, et al. Usefulness of NGS for diagnosis of dominant beta-thalassemia and unstable hemoglobinopathies in five clinical cases. Front Physiol 2021;12:628236.
29. Lou J, Sun M, Mao A, et al. Molecular spectrum and prevalence of thalassemia investigated by third-generation sequencing in the Dongguan region of Guangdong Province, Southern China. Clin Chim Acta Int J Clin Chem 2023;551:117622.
30. Wu J, Xie D, Wang L, et al. Application of third-generation sequencing for genetic testing of thalassemia in Guizhou Province, Southwest China. Hematol Amst Neth 2022;27(1):1305–11.
31. Ling X, Wang C, Li L, et al. Third-generation sequencing for genetic disease. Clin Chim Acta Int J Clin Chem 2023;551:117624.
32. Dasauni P, Chhabra V, Kumar G, et al. Advances in mass spectrometric methods for detection of hemoglobin disorders. Anal Biochem 2021;629:114314.
33. Lin Y, Agarwal AM, Anderson LC, et al. Discovery of a biomarker for β-thalassemia by HPLC-MS and improvement from proton transfer reaction - parallel ion parking. J Mass Spectrom Adv Clin Lab 2023;28:20–6.

Automation in Flow Cytometry

Giovanni Insuasti-Beltran, MD[a],*, Ahmad Al-Attar, PhD, ASCP(SCYM)[b]

KEYWORDS

- Automation • Flow cytometry • Artificial intelligence • Sample handling
- Throughput • Turnaround time

KEY POINTS

- Workforce shortage and increased workload necessitate the application of automation in clinical flow cytometry laboratories.
- Automation in flow cytometry has largely been limited to distinct workflow tasks.
- Current automation solutions offer walkaway (or near-walkaway) solutions.
- Machine learning and artificial intelligence are being tested and deployed in an effort to automate data analysis.

INTRODUCTION

Automation in the clinical laboratory has emerged as a pivotal force, reshaping the landscape of diagnostic processes and the way health care is delivered. Flow cytometry, once a manual and labor-intensive process, has also benefited from and has the potential to undergo a revolutionary transformation with the advent of automation. With many advances in hardware and software, come possibilities of a better-streamlined workflows as well as enhanced accuracy, reproducibility, and efficiency of the entire diagnostic process.

Clinical laboratory automation has been available for many years, with clinical chemistry automated analyzers making their debut in 1956.[1] Laboratory information systems (LISs) began to rise in the 1970s; this, together with analytical automation, has made a connection between electronic data management and laboratory instrumentation.[2,3]

In general, one of the primary advantages of automation lies in its ability to improve workflow efficiency. Traditional manual laboratory processes are often time-consuming and prone to human errors. With automation, routine and repetitive tasks

[a] Wake Forest University, 1 Medical Center Boulevard, Winston-Salem, NC 27157, USA; [b] Flow Cytometry Laboratory, University of Louisville Health, 529 S Jackson Street, Louisville, KY 40202, USA
* Corresponding author.
E-mail address: ginsuast@wakehealth.edu

Clin Lab Med 44 (2024) 455–463
https://doi.org/10.1016/j.cll.2024.04.007
0272-2712/24/© 2024 Elsevier Inc. All rights reserved.

such as sample handling, pipetting, and data analysis can be seamlessly executed with precision and speed. This not only accelerates turnaround times but also allows laboratory professionals to focus on more complex tasks that require their expertise.

Accuracy and reproducibility are paramount in clinical diagnostics, and automation serves as a key catalyst in achieving these goals. By minimizing human intervention, automated systems reduce the likelihood of variability introduced during manual processing. Standardized protocols and controlled conditions ensure that each analysis is performed consistently, leading to reliable and reproducible results. This level of precision is particularly critical in areas such as molecular diagnostics and immunoassays, where small deviations can have significant clinical implications.

The advent of robotic technologies has further elevated the capabilities of automated clinical laboratories.[4] Robotics not only streamlines sample handling but also enables integration of high-throughput workflows. The ability to process a large number of samples simultaneously enhances the laboratory's capacity, allowing for scalability and improved resource utilization. This scalability is particularly beneficial in the context of surges in testing demand, such as during pandemics or large-scale screening programs.

Thoughtful and appropriate implementation of laboratory automation often results in multiple advantages, such as the standardization of processes, hands-on time-saving for laboratory personnel, improved pipetting precision (and oftentimes accuracy), in addition to the biosafety gains from requiring less manual handling of potentially hazardous reagents/samples. The use of automation in clinical flow cytometry laboratories is still limited compared to other clinical laboratory sections, such as chemistry, hematology, and microbiology where total laboratory automation (TLA; or near-TLA) is commonplace.

Flow cytometry workflow automation can be divided in several areas: preanalytic (sample preparation/wash, cocktail making), analytical (data acquisition and analysis), and postanalytic (data transfer and comprehensive reporting with ancillary studies).

This article delves into the multifaceted impact of automation on clinical flow cytometry, exploring the benefits, challenges, and future implications of these transformative technologies.

SAMPLE PREPARATION
Dissociation of Tissue

Flow cytometry is performed on single-cell suspensions. Tissues, including core biopsies, need to be disaggregated before they are stained and acquired. The quality of results in the flow cytometric analysis of any tissue depends upon the quality of the prepared suspension. Most clinical flow cytometry laboratories perform manual disaggregation using a variety of tools to release cells from the binding stroma. A few automated mechanical disaggregation systems are designed to standardize this process and increase efficiency in sample preparation.

The Medimachine system (BD Biosciences, San Jose, CA) is one such compact system. It consists of 3 components: the Medimachine itself and the "Medicons" and "Filcons" which are the disposable components used for cutting and filtering, respectively. The size of tissue recommended is ≤10 mm³ free of fat and necrosis. Disaggregation takes between 10 seconds to 4 minutes depending on the tissue type used and the cell suspension needed. Filtering is done by the operator manually using a syringe and the Filcon.

The gentleMACS Dissociators (Miltenyi Biotec, Auburn, CA) can process 2 or 8 (gentleMACS Octo) samples in parallel. They use preset optimized programs for tissue dissociation or homogenization for a variety of specific applications/tissue types. These systems utilize proprietary tubes (C Tubes or M Tubes) in a closed and sterile system, providing extra user safety and minimizing cross-contamination. Miltenyi also markets MACS Tissue Dissociation Kits with optimized enzyme mixes for preserving cell integrity and surface epitopes. The heaters (available on the Octo) enable enzyme incubation directly on the instrument. It is worth noting that these systems are used mostly in research laboratories and can be used to homogenize tissues for protein and nucleic acid extraction. Similar dissociation systems are available from other vendors, such as RWD.

The Cell Washer

Washing the cells is a common and important step in many flow cytometric assays, such as leukemia/lymphoma immunophenotyping and PNH testing. It is typically performed using a benchtop centrifuge prior to staining to wash off the lysis buffer, remove excess Ig from the cells suspension to allow for clear(er) staining for Ig LC (kappa/lambda) on B cells, and after staining to remove excess/unbound antibodies. Manual washing is labor-intensive and time-consuming. Using a cell washer (eg, Helmer's CW series) is commonly used in blood banks/transfusion services. It can be programmed to perform a series of customizable steps including fill, spin, decant, and agitate. The cell washer saves time and effort by automating the manual wash steps.

Laboratories should optimize the performance of their washing by adjusting the various settings and should also evaluate the cell recovery. Users have noticed significant cell loss when prewashing whole-blood specimens. In addition, laboratory tests should evaluate cross-tube contamination/spill.

Novel automated wash systems (eg, the laminar wash flow system from Curiox) promise significant improvement in debris removal and increasing the retention and viability of rare cell populations. Evaluating these systems in a clinical laboratory setting is in its early stages.

Lymphocyte Subset Assay Automation Devices

One of the main advantages of using automation in lymphocyte subset assay (LSA) is the minimization of interaction with potentially infectious samples. Both machines described later can handle samples with closed-tube sampling, thereby reducing exposure to biohazards. These devices proved very popular especially as the majority of LSA testing is for CD4 (and CD4/CD8 ratio) in HIV-positive patients.

The BD FACS SPA III is a sample and antibody aliquoting system that can be programmed from a connected stand-alone Windows-operated computer to transfer blood and reagents into daughter tubes, adds lysing solution, and mixes the sample according to a preprogrammed or custom protocol to automate workflow for lyse-no-wash flow cytometric assays.

The precision of pipetting should be evaluated periodically (recommended monthly) to ensure the accuracy of results.

The BD FACS lyse wash assistant is designed for assays that require wash step(s). It enables automated batch processing of up to 40 sample tubes per run.

Beckman Coulter's PrepPlus 2 is a similar workstation that can be programmed to pipette reagents, samples, controls, and counting beads into daughter tubes. The standard instrument has a single sample probe which moves in the X, Y, and Z axes and one modular digital pump for transferring fluids. It is controlled from an LCD monochromatic touchscreen on an interlinked TQ-Prep machine, which also holds the Immunoprep lysing reagents and performs the RBC lysis step.

While both the SPA-III and the PrepPlus 2/TQ-Prep sample preparation systems can be used for leukemia/lymphoma immunophenotyping, they are approved as in vitro diagnostic (IVD) devices only with specific lyse-no-wash applications created and marked by the devices' respective manufacturers.

Current Generation of Sample Preparation Systems

In the 2020s, the increased demand for automation in flow cytometry coupled with the significant staff shortages experienced across most health care sectors as a result of the COVID-19 pandemic, major cytometry manufacturers built modern sample preparation systems that were marketed as "walkaway" solutions.[1] The 3 main systems currently in the market are briefly reviewed later. Naturally, none of the systems are classed as IVD, and the laboratory is responsible for validating the performance of the system based on the application it is used for, in a fit-for-purpose manner. The systems do, however, support laboratory compliance with 21 CFR Part 11. Although the manufacturers have published typically very low (around = 0.2% specimen to specimen and = 0.01% reagent to reagent) carryover rates for their respective systems, the actual carryover for any specific assay invariably depends on the protocol used, the number of washes programmed into the assay, and the gating strategy.[1]

All systems have robust audit trails, and the ability to track the antibodies and/or reagents used via barcodes; however, these are manufacturer-specific. Laboratories using reagents from different manufacturers need to add a "custom" barcode and program in the reagent manually to allow the system to identify the "foreign" product. In addition, these systems can be connected to a local area network and interfaced to the LIS to receive patient information and test orders.[1]

The PS-10 sample preparation system (Sysmex, Lincolnshire, IL) was designed to automate staining, RBC lysis, and cocktailing of antibody reagents. Although the main unit itself does not have cell washing capabilities, the system is paired with a Helmer cell washer for lyse/wash procedures. Both units (and also Sysmex's XF-1600 cytometer) utilize the same centrifuge rotor to streamline the workflow and not require the moving around of secondary tubes, hence reducing the potential of a mix-up error.

The system has an onboard refrigerated storage for antibody and cocktail vials during daily use, but the vials must be uncapped manually, and recapped when the system is not in use. The pipetting probes have liquid-level sensors for level monitoring to alert the user when a reagent is running low (<25 tests) and when depleted.

BD's FACSDuet sample preparation system originally lacked a wash module and was used for processing specimens requiring lyse-no-wash assays only. A FACSDuet "Premium" model was released in 2023 which included onboard washing and centrifugation to accommodate lyse-wash assays. The integration of the FACSDuet with the FACSLyric cytometer allows the uninterrupted preparation and acquisition of specimens. It has a reagent rack "recall" option that improves reagent tracking and management. The Duet allows the user to load multiple vials of the same reagent (as primary and backup) to avoid errors related to insufficient reagents. The FACSDuet system can be run in a stand-alone manner, not physically connected to the cytometer; however, the user must manually transfer the prepared secondary tube carrier after it has been prepared on the FACSDuet and load it onto the cytometer for acquisition.

Both the PS-10 and FACSDuet can be used in the automation of creating antibody panel premixes (cocktails). This procedure, which has been traditionally performed by the laboratory (stressful, time-consuming, and costly when errors are made) or by the manufacturer (very expensive and needs to be requested with plenty of time in advance), is automated and barcode controlled using these SPS. The information for the single-color reagents and the on-board made cocktails is stored on the systems for re-use and easy traceability of data.

The CellMek SPS sample preparation system (Beckman Coulter, Miami, FL) was the first of the instruments to have an integrated cell wash module hence allowing the option to run lyse-wash and lyse-no-wash assays. It has an onboard computer and a touchscreen interface, with controls available only to operate the system. A stand-alone Windows-operated computer is required for designing or editing panels using CellMek's design panel software. In addition to liquid reagents, the CellMek has holders for Beckman's 12 well dry premixed custom antibody panel cartridges (DURACartridge).

Antibodies are stored in a refrigerated module on the CellMek and it supports the use of pierceable caps. This negates the need to open reagent vials, leave them capless during operation, or to remove and store the reagents racks at the end of each day of use. The CellMek keeps track of the volume for each reagent by calculating the remaining volume based on the original volume and the summation of volumes used because its pipetting probes do not have liquid-level sensors. Therefore, Beckman Coulter warns users to never use reagents in the CellMek SPS system that have been used to prepare samples manually. Upon completion of a processing run, the CellMek automatically generates an acquisition "worklist" that can be transferred to compatible Beckman cytometers (Navios, Navios EX, and DXFlex).

FLOW CYTOMETERS

Automation of the cytometers has largely been limited to the implementation of loader devices that allow users to program the software to acquire tubes in a predefined order in which specific assays/protocols are run for each sample (tube or well). Most modern cytometers are equipped with either a carousel or a rack, which is loaded by the user. Specific stoppage criteria are set so that acquisition of all specimens can continue without supervision or having to switch tubes manually. The use of multi-well plates instead of individual tubes has become more common in clinical laboratories. Newer cytometer models support the acquisition from a variety of plates. Some BD cytometer models can be retrospectively equipped with a plate acquisition device known as high-throughput sampler.

Automated data analysis depends on the complexity of the assay and the data. IVD lymphocyte subset enumeration assays are typically built with an autogate algorithm that identifies lymphocytes and their subset with the option to adjust the gates manually by the user before the results are finalized. Leukemia/lymphoma and other high complexity immunophenotyping assays are typically gated manually.

Automation of instrument setup, assay performance, and fluorescence compensation are available on most modern software. Tightly characterized fluorescent beads can be used to standardize light scatter intensity, fluorescence intensity, and hydrodynamic focusing by determining the values of forward scatter, side scatter, fluorescence intensity, and coefficient of variance when the fluorospheres are tested using laboratory and application-specific instrument settings. The cytometer's acquisition software monitors and automatically adjusts the instrument settings needed to obtain the values for each of the desired parameters of the fluorospheres.

Modern laboratories with very high workload (such as Münchner Leukämielabor, Munich, Germany) have collaborated with robotics companies to create custommade robots that automate the processes of specimen preparation in 96 well plates and loading the plates onto the cytometer (CytoFLEX, Beckman Coulter).

The AQUIOS CL (Beckman Coulter) is a "Load & Go" single-laser flow cytometer that performs a range of applications that use a no-wash sample preparation process, such as lymphocyte subset immunophenotyping and CD34+ stem cell enumeration. It uses a 5 position cassette to load blood specimen tubes onto its autoloader and combines sample preparation and analysis in one platform, which helps reduce the footprint of instruments. Although the AQUIOS is capable of performing cell counts volumetrically, it still requires counting beads for its CD34+ stem cell enumeration application.

Image-based fluorescence cell counters, which use high-sensitivity monochrome CCD cameras, such as the ADAM-II (NanoEntek, Seoul, South Korea), have been marketed as simple, automated devices to measure the percentage and absolute number of cells in normal and mobilized peripheral blood.

DATA ANALYSIS

The creation of analysis templates that incorporate a set of scattergrams, gates, and statistics allows for a semiautomated analysis of data acquired using the same panel. Organizing the analysis template logically and using standardized colors for specific subpopulations allows for quicker (and typically easier) interpretation of the results by the pathologists. The technologists can transfer the raw data files (as .FCS or .LMD) and load these to the analysis template and then review the plots and adjust the gates as necessary.

Introduction to Artificial Intelligence-assisted Data Analysis

The traditional way of analyzing/interpreting multicolor flow cytometric data by visually inspecting all (or a selection of) histograms and/or bivariate dot plots has served the clinical flow laboratories well. The use of hierarchical and Boolean gating, pattern recognition, back gating, and other techniques are valuable tools for laboratory scientists and pathologists. However, manual gating requires subjective decisions, limiting reproducibility; with the increase of the number of markers and fluorochromes used in clinical diagnostics–currently reaching over 40 parameters–the number of possible plot permutations exponentially increases. This is especially true with the application of full-spectrum cytometry. Manually analyzing high-dimensional datasets and capturing the expression of several markers simultaneously for each cell become extremely difficult if not impossible.

Some standard clinical analysis software already offers users tools to help analyze multiparametric data using built-in algorithms. Infinicyt (Cytognos/BD) has an "Automatic Population Separator" (APS), which is based on principal component analysis. It uses the information from all the parameters included in the FCS file to provide the best cell cluster separation and automatically identifies the markers that are most significant for this separation. The APS plots are configurable and allow the user to see the contribution of each parameter to the cluster separation. Gating can be made on the APS diagram.

Dimensionality Reduction and Clustering Algorithms

The introduction of dimensionality reduction algorithms that transform data from a high-dimensional space into a low-dimensional space allows for low-dimensional representation while retaining many meaningful properties of the original data and reduces data size. Clustering algorithms group cells based on similarity of expression patterns to recapitulate manual gating with the advantages of being able to "see" all the cells' features at once; not limited by 2 dimensional (2D) hierarchical gating.

Such algorithms create 2D maps on which cells are close to each other based on their overall immunophenotype. The interpretation of these maps relies on the identification of clusters of cells with a defined phenotype. Multiple dimensionality reduction algorithms are currently used in flow cytometry, albeit mostly in research settings, but will clearly offer significant advantages to clinical laboratories in the near future. Dimensionality reduction and clustering algorithms fall under the "unsupervised" category of machine learning (ML). Supervised ML requires reducing flow data to population-level representations, such as FlowSOM data, that can be passed to a classifier, such as random forests, neural networks, support vector machines, and deep learning.

The most commonly used artificial intelligence (AI)/ML tools in flow cytometry are listed in **Table 1**.

The first step of single-cell data analysis is data exploration, which is usually achieved through dimension reduction and followed by visualization, clustering, cell-type assignment, differential expression analyses, and so forth (https://www.nature.com/articles/s41467-023-37478-w).

Data preprocessing is almost invariably needed prior to applying any data reduction or clustering algorithm. It is a crucial part of the entire high-dimensional data analysis workflow and includes data cleaning, scaling, gating, downsampling, normalization, and merging. Some of these steps are highly recommended, and others are optional depending on the question, on the dataset and on the algorithms that will be run downstream. FCS Express (De Novo Software/Dotmatics, Pasadena, CA) offers multiple cleaning algorithms and downsampling methods, in addition to common high-dimensionality analysis tools

The application of automated data analysis, aided by DR, clustering, AI and ML in the setting of minimal/measurable residual disease (MRD) detection has shown promise. Multiple groups have shown that high correlations between results from manual gating and automated analysis can be achieved for MRD detection of B-ALL, AML, and CLL.[5–8]

LABORATORY INFORMATION (MANAGEMENT) SYSTEMS

The introduction and near-universal utilization of laboratory/hospital data management systems has had the largest impact on improving laboratory efficiencies. Creating 1- or 2 way interface links between the cytometry analysis software and the patients' medical records streamlined the process of data entry and simultaneously reduced the frequency of errors commonly associated with manual transcription. Most modern systems operate software that supports common workflows for

Table 1
Summary of common dimensionality reduction and clustering algorithms currently applied in flow cytometric applications

Dimensionality Reduction Algorithms	Clustering Algorithms
t-distributed stochastic neighbor embedding (t-SNE)	Spanning-tree progression analysis of density-normalized events
Hierarchical stochastic neighbor embedding (h-SNE)	Flow cytometry self-organizing map (FlowSOM)
Uniform manifold approximation and projection	Scalable weighted iterative flow-clustering technique
Opt-SNE	flowMeans
tSNE-CUDA	and many more

clinical pathology as well as anatomic pathology environments. Flow cytometry often spans both environments, but it can be successfully built in either. One of the key decisions to make when acquiring and building a new LIS is the need for integrated reporting which allows for the simultaneous viewing and editing of morphology, cytogenetics, molecular diagnostics, and flow cytometry together. Barcode-enabled workflows should allow laboratory techs to track specimens within and across sites beginning at the point of collection. Barcoding also ensures accurate specimen handling, processing, and resulting.

DISCUSSION

Automation in laboratory medicine has been present at different levels for many years, transforming traditionally time-consuming and labor-intensive processes into more cost-efficient, precise, and accurate ways of testing. Laboratory automation is necessary in order to address issues such as shortage of technologists, standardization and improve documentation and increased throughput.

Flow cytometry is not immune to the problems faced by other areas in the laboratory, and therefore, solutions involving automation are becoming increasingly important and available in this field. One of the key advantages of automation in flow cytometry is the ability to handle large sample sizes with minimal human intervention. Automated sample preparation, staining, and analysis streamline the workflow, reducing the potential for errors and increasing reproducibility of results.

Automated systems in flow cytometry not only enhance the speed of analysis but also contribute to the standardization of procedures. Consistency in sample handling and data acquisition is critical to producing reliable and comparable results across different patient samples and laboratories. Automation helps in achieving this consistency by precisely controlling numerous variables subject to change, minimizing manual variations. Furthermore, automation in FCM improves the overall accuracy of cell identification and analysis by using automated gating strategies, leading to a more reliable identification of cell populations. This is particularly beneficial in evaluation of low-level populations and MRD, where manual gating may introduce subjectivity and variability. In addition to improving efficiency and accuracy, automation contributes to the reduction of operator fatigue and optimization of resource utilization. By automating routine and repetitive tasks, operators can focus on more intellectually demanding aspects such as panel design, data interpretation, and validation of results, enhancing the overall productivity.

Despite the many advantages of automation, it is important to recognize some of the challenges associated with it. Few important considerations include implementation costs, the need to specialized training, and the potential introduction of new technical issues in to the already established workflows and information technology infrastructure. Additionally, the integration of automation should not compromise the flexibility required in the clinical setting for adapting to diverse sample types, setups, and protocols.

Looking ahead, the future of automation in clinical laboratories holds promising prospects. Continuous advancements in AI and ML are poised to enhance the analytical capabilities of automated systems. Smart algorithms can assist in data interpretation, pattern recognition, and even predictive analytics, further augmenting the role of clinical laboratories in personalized medicine and precision diagnostics.

SUMMARY

In summary, automation in flow cytometry represents a transformative advancement in the field. With diverse options available allowing for different degrees of automation from sample preparation to analysis, the benefits of increased throughput, improved accuracy, and reduced manual labor contribute to increased efficiency and reproducibility of results. As technology continues to evolve, the integration of the different platforms available for flow cytometry automation is likely to become more prevalent, shaping the future of cellular analysis and transforming the field in a positive way.

CLINICS CARE POINTS

- Flow cytometry has seen significant advances in automation with numerous options available ranging from sample preparation to analysis.
- Major preparation systems available in the market are the Beckman Coulter CellMek, the Sysmex PS10, and the BD FACSDuet.
- These systems can improve efficiency and reproducibility of results, allowing operators to focus on other more challenging tasks such as panel design and validation and data analysis.
- Additionally, multiple AI protocols for data analysis are being developed and validation in the clinical setting will improve the power of clinical flow cytometry.

DISCLOSURE

The authors have nothing to disclose.

REFERENCES

1. Al-Attar A, Kumar KR, Untersee D, et al. Automation in flow cytometry: guidelines and review of systems. Cytometry B Clin Cytom 2023. https://doi.org/10.1002/cyto.b.22125.
2. Hawker CD. Laboratory automation: total and subtotal. Clin Lab Med 2007;27(4): 749–70.
3. Kricka LJ, Savory J. International year of Chemistry 2011. A guide to the history of clinical chemistry. Clin Chem 2011;57(8):1118–26.
4. Thurow K, Gu X, Gode B, et al. Integrating mobile robots into automated laboratory processes: a suitable workflow management system. SLAS Technol 2021;26(2): 232–5.
5. R Reiter M, Diem M, Schumich A, et al, International Berlin-Frankfurt-Münster (iBFM)-FLOW-network and the AutoFLOW consortium. Automated flow cytometric MRD assessment in childhood acute B- lymphoblastic leukemia using supervised machine learning. Cytometry A 2019 Sep;95(9):966–75.
6. Salama ME, Otteson GE, Camp JJ, et al. Artificial intelligence enhances diagnostic flow cytometry workflow in the detection of minimal residual disease of chronic lymphocytic leukemia. Cancers 2022 May 21;14(10):2537.
7. Weijler L, Kowarsch F, Wodlinger M, et al. UMAP based anomaly detection for minimal residual disease quantification within acute myeloid leukemia. Cancers 2022; 14(4). https://doi.org/10.3390/cancers14040898.
8. Lewis JE, Cooper LAD, Jaye DL, et al. Automated deep learning-based diagnosis and molecular characterization of acute myeloid leukemia using flow cytometry. Mod Pathol 2024 Jan;37(1):100373.

Flow Cytometric Assessment of Malignant Hematologic Disorders

Connor M. Hartzell, MD, Aaron C. Shaver, MD, PhD,
Emily F. Mason, MD, PhD*

KEYWORDS

- Flow cytometry • Hematologic malignancy • Clonality • TRBC1
- Minimal residual disease

KEY POINTS

- Flow cytometry is an integral component to the diagnostic workup of hematologic malignancies.
- The fifth edition of the World Health Organization classification has proposed revised criteria for assigning lineage in acute leukemia.
- Flow cytometric analysis of myeloid maturation and monocyte subsets can aid in the diagnosis of myelodysplastic syndrome (MDS) and myelodysplastic/myeloproliferative neoplasms (MDS/MPN).
- Minimal residual disease assessment by flow cytometry is the standard of care for B-lymphoblastic leukemia and is becoming an important factor in post-therapy monitoring in acute myeloid leukemia.

INTRODUCTION

Multiparameter flow cytometry (MPF), which uses light scatter and fluorescent signals to quantitate expression levels of multiple antigens on individual cells within mixed single cell suspensions, is an integral element of the diagnostic evaluation of hematologic disease. By detecting patterns of antigen expression, MPF allows for the detection of cell lineage, clonality, and aberrancy, among other properties. MPF rapidly provides information about abnormal cell populations, within hours of tissue sampling, potentially days to weeks before additional morphologic and genetic data are available, which can direct the need for additional testing and

Department of Pathology, Microbiology & Immunology, Vanderbilt University Medical Center, 445 Great Circle Road, Nashville, TN 37228, USA
* Corresponding author.
E-mail address: emily.f.mason@vumc.org

Clin Lab Med 44 (2024) 465–477
https://doi.org/10.1016/j.cll.2024.04.008
0272-2712/24/© 2024 Elsevier Inc. All rights reserved.
labmed.theclinics.com

facilitate the initiation of therapy. This article will explore the utility of MPF in the clinical evaluation of hematologic malignancies and discuss emerging applications that hold the potential to enhance the power of this technology in diagnosing and monitoring disease.

PRINCIPLES OF FLOW CYTOMETRY

The use of MPF in the evaluation of hematologic malignancies requires fresh samples in a single-cell suspension. Thus, common sample types include peripheral blood, bone marrow (BM) aspirate, or lymph node and other tissue samples that have been dissociated. In the absence of fresh BM aspirate, single cells can, in some cases, be dissociated from an additional BM core biopsy placed in RPMI (Roswell Park Memorial Institute) medium. Samples are stained with antibodies targeting cell surface or, with proper preparation of target cells, intracellular antigens of interest, which are conjugated to fluorescent molecules or dyes. As the single-cell suspension passes through the flow cytometer, lasers of different wavelengths excite the fluorescent molecules, which then emit light at varying wavelengths.[1] The emitted light passes through filters, reaching detectors within the flow cytometer (photomultiplier tubes), which detect the emitted fluorescent light as well as visible light scatter, including forward scatter (FSC), an indication of cell size, and side scatter (SSC), an indication of internal complexity or granularity within a cell. These light signals are then converted into digital data signals, which can be analyzed using various computer software programs. Over time, with the development of new reagents for antibody conjugation and flow cytometers with increasing numbers of lasers, the number of "colors," or parallel signal types that can be analyzed, has increased from 2 or 4 in early instruments to a standard of 8 to 12 in modern analyzers, with more available in more sophisticated instruments.

MPF provides valuable data in the diagnosis of numerous hematopoietic processes, and peripheral blood MPF may be indicated in a number of settings, particularly in the context of cytoses, including lymphocytosis, monocytosis, or circulating blasts. MPF can also detect abnormal T-cell clones or other hematopoietic processes contributing to peripheral eosinophilia.[2,3] However, neutrophilia as well as polycythemia, thrombocytosis, and basophilia are generally not indications for peripheral blood MPF, as hematopoietic neoplasms that might be associated with these cytoses typically do not show diagnostic or aberrant features detectable by MPF.[4] Peripheral blood MPF can also aid in the evaluation of peripheral cytopenias by detecting B-cell or T-cell lymphoproliferative disorders as a cause for abnormal cell counts.

Allocation of tissue samples for flow cytometry is generally indicated whenever lymphoma or other hematologic malignancy is in the differential diagnosis. Importantly, multiple factors may lead to false-negative results when analyzing tissue samples by MPF. In particular, abnormal populations may only focally involve tissue specimens, may include relatively few lesional cells within non-neoplastic background populations, or may be associated with areas of necrosis or fibrosis. Sample processing and disaggregation lead to loss or decrease of some cell types, leading to challenges in using MPF to evaluate plasma cell neoplasms, which require analysis of a large number of cells. Additionally, MPF evaluation of lymphomas with rare malignant cells, such as classic Hodgkin lymphoma, requires careful analysis, including analysis of the associated non-neoplastic cell populations.[5] Given the utility of properly performed MPF, it is indicated as a component of most BM evaluations performed for the assessment of hematolymphoid neoplasms.

UTILITY OF FLOW CYTOMETRY IN THE ASSESSMENT OF HEMATOLOGIC MALIGNANCIES
Determination of Maturation Stage and Lineage

MPF represents one of the best tools to determine lineage and maturation stage of cell populations because it allows for the evaluation of multiple antigens on a single cell. For example, co-expression of markers of immaturity along with lineage-defining markers on a blast population aids in the classification of acute leukemia. Although phenotypes may vary, markers of immaturity include dim CD45 expression, positivity for CD34, and low SSC. Normal myeloid blasts also express CD117 and HLA-DR (**Fig. 1**A; red population). Lymphoblasts often express terminal deoxynucleotidyl transferase (TdT), although this is not lineage specific and can also be positive in abnormal myeloblasts. Features of immaturity in B cells include lack of surface light chain (LC) expression, bright expression of CD10 and CD38, and heterogeneous to negative CD20 expression (**Fig. 1**B; green population). Immature T cells may be negative for CD34 but may show positivity for CD1a in addition to cytoplasmic but not surface CD3 expression (**Fig. 1**C; green population).

Determination of blast lineage in the context of acute leukemia is critical in determining additional necessary testing and appropriate therapy. Certain well-known

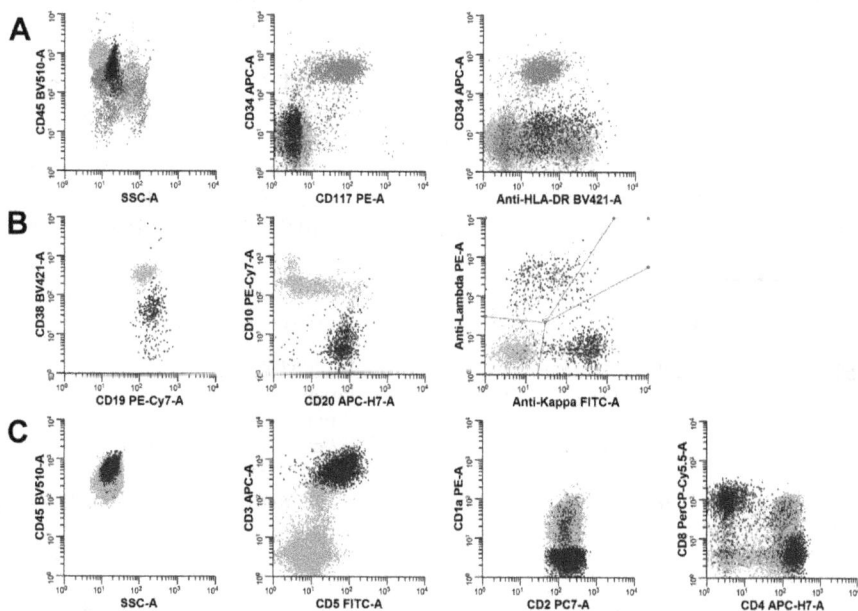

Fig. 1. Immunophenotypic findings for normal immature cell populations. (*A*) Normal myeloblasts (red) show dim expression of CD45, positivity for CD34, CD117, and HLA-DR, and low side scatter (SSC). Myeloblasts: red; lymphocytes: green; monocytes: blue; granulocytes: orange. (*B*) Normal hematogones (benign B-cell precursors; green) are positive for CD19, show bright expression of CD10 and CD38 with heterogeneous CD20 expression, and lack surface light chain expression. Mature B cells (blue) show polytypic expression of kappa and lambda light chains. (*C*) Normal immature T cells (thymocytes; green) show dim CD45 expression with positivity for CD2 and CD1a. Surface CD3 is negative, and these cells are generally double negative or double positive for CD4 and CD8. As T cells mature (purple), they gain surface CD3 expression, lose expression of CD1a, and show single positivity for either CD4 or CD8.

markers are strongly associated with particular lineages in both normal and neoplastic populations: myeloperoxidase (MPO), CD13, CD15, and CD33 with myeloid cells; CD19, CD20, and CD22 with B lymphocytes; and CD2, CD3, CD4, CD5, CD7, and CD8 with T lymphocytes. However, early in the study of acute leukemias, it became apparent that some markers that show strong lineage fidelity in normal cell types — for example, CD13 and CD33 for myeloid cells or CD2 and CD7 for T/natural killer (NK) lymphocytes — are often aberrantly expressed on acute leukemia cells belonging to other lineages.

In order to address this problem of lineage infidelity, classification systems, which rely heavily of MPF, have been developed to determine blast lineage in these cases of acute leukemia of ambiguous lineage (**Table 1**). Similar to prior systems, the International Consensus Classification[6] and the fifth edition of the World Health Organization (WHO) classification (WHO5)[7] define myeloid lineage by expression of cytoplasmic MPO or evidence of monocytic differentiation, including expression of at least 2 of the following: CD11c, CD14, CD64, lysozyme, and nonspecific esterase. T lineage is defined by cytoplasmic or surface CD3 expression. B-lineage assignment requires either: (1) 'strong' expression of CD19 in combination with strong expression of at least 1 of the following: CD10, CD22, or CD79a; or (2) 'weak' expression of CD19 with strong expression of at least 2 of these 3 markers. However, in considering the possibility of a B-lineage component in a case of T-lineage acute lymphoblastic leukemia (T-ALL), CD79a expression is not considered evidence of B lineage, as it can be expressed in T-ALL.

The WHO5 elaborates on these lineage assignment criteria to address the required level of antigen expression intensity. Overall, antigen expression on blasts should be considered in relation to expression levels on background normal cell populations. More specifically, blasts should be considered positive for a lineage-defining marker when the expression level of that marker on blasts exceeds 50% of the level of expression (on a linear scale) that is seen on background normal cells of that lineage (**Fig. 2**;

Table 1
Immunophenotypic criteria for assigning blast lineage for mixed phenotype acute leukemia

Lineage	Criterion	Comments
Myeloid	Myeloperoxidase or	Intensity in part exceeds 50% of mature neutrophil level[a]
	Monocytic differentiation	≥2 of nonspecific esterase, CD11c, CD14, CD64, lysozyme
B-lymphoid	Strong CD19 or	CD19 intensity in part exceeds 50% of normal B-cell progenitors[a]
		Plus ≥1 also strongly expressed: CD10, CD22, CD79a[b]
	weak CD19	CD19 intensity does not exceed 50% of normal B-cell progenitors[a]
		Plus ≥2 also strongly expressed: CD10, CD22, CD79a[b]
T-lymphoid	CD3 (cytoplasmic or surface)	CD3 intensity in part exceeds 50% of mature T-cells progenitors by flow cytometry[a]
		Immunohistochemistry positive with non-zeta chain reagent

[a] Intensity level as specified per the 5th edition WHO classification.
[b] CD79a should not be considered evidence of B lineage differentiation when considering B/T mixed phenotype acute leukemia.

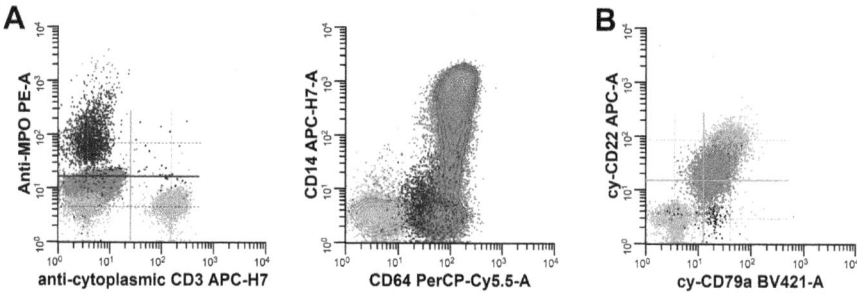

Fig. 2. New criteria for lineage assignment in mixed phenotype acute leukemia. Per the fifth edition of the World Health Organization classification, blasts should be considered positive for a lineage-defining marker when the expression level of that marker on blasts exceeds 50% of the level of expression (on a linear scale) that is seen on background normal cells of that lineage. (A) Blasts show a slight shift in cytoplasmic CD3 expression over background B cells and granulocytes, but do not reach 50% of the expression level (*solid green line*) seen in normal T cells. Blasts just meet the threshold of myeloperoxidase (MPO) expression at a level of 50% of normal granulocytes (*solid blue line*). Blasts also show bright expression of CD14 and CD64, consistent with acute myeloid leukemia with monocytic differentiation. (B) A case of B-lymphoblastic leukemia, where blasts are positive for cytoplasmic CD22 and cytoplasmic CD79a at levels greater than 50% (*solid green lines*) of that seen in normal B cells. Blasts: red; granulocytes: blue; lymphocytes: green.

red populations). 'Weak' expression of CD19 on B lymphoblasts would be considered positivity for CD19 that does not meet this threshold. Importantly, as genetic data become increasingly incorporated into the diagnosis of hematologic malignancies,[8] immunophenotypic data collected by MPF will likely be integrated with genetic results for the most accurate determination of blast lineage in acute leukemia of ambiguous lineage in the future.

Detection of Clonality and Aberrancy

MPF can be particularly valuable in the diagnosis of hematologic malignancies as a method for identifying clonality and/or aberrancy. Traditionally, clinical MPF assays have been used to detect clonality predominantly in B cell and plasma cell populations, via evaluation of immunoglobulin kappa LC (KLC) and lambda LC (LLC) expression.[9] During normal B-cell development, the process of VDJ recombination leads to exclusive expression of a single LC in any given B cell.[10] As such, reactive populations of B cells should contain a mixture of KLC-expressing and LLC-expressing cells, while clonal B-cell populations will show singular expression of either KLC or LLC, or may lack LC expression altogether.

Conversely, until recently, demonstration of T-cell clonality by MPF had relied predominantly on a cumbersome assay analyzing the usage of various variable regions of the T-cell receptor (TCR) beta chain,[11] which was not routinely performed in clinical practice. However, the availability of an antibody directed to the TCR beta chain constant region 1 (TRBC1) now allows for a much simpler method for T-cell clonality assessment. Similar to the exclusive expression of KLC or LLC in B cells, the constant region of the TCR beta chain in alpha/beta T cells is expressed exclusively from either the TRBC1 or the TRBC2 locus.[12] As such, mixed populations of alpha/beta T cells include TRBC1-positive and TRBC2-positive populations, whereas a clonal T-cell population will show exclusive expression of either TRBC1 or TRBC2.[13] The recent development of an antibody against TRBC1 has enabled assessment of clonality in

T cells in a similar fashion to LC assessment in B cells, by evaluating for T cell populations showing monophasic TRBC1 expression, that is, populations with restricted positivity or negativity for TRBC1[14] (**Fig. 3**; red populations). A threshold of 85% restricted expression (>85% of a population either positive or negative for TRBC1) has been suggested to indicate a clonal population.[15] Importantly, the utility of TRBC1 expression as a marker of clonality relies heavily on the ability to isolate the T-cell population of interest from background-reactive T cells, in order to then assess TRBC1 expression specifically on that population. Therefore, MPF panels should be designed using multiple T-cell antigens, in addition to TRBC1, to best allow for identification of the neoplastic T-cell population, based on abnormal expression patterns of T-cell antigens. Additionally, TRBC1 is not useful in detecting clonality in gamma/delta T cells or NK cells, which do not express the TCR beta chain.

The significance of clonal T-cell (and B cell) populations must be interpreted within clinical context. Clonal T-cell populations may be seen in the setting of a reactive immune response, autoimmunity, as a paraneoplastic phenomenon, or in the post-transplant setting, among others. These populations often show an immunophenotype resembling T-large granular lymphocyte leukemia and may be best classified as T-cell clones of uncertain significance when identified in patients without definitive evidence of T-cell neoplasia (for example, in the absence of cytopenias).[15] Additionally, studies have shown that small T-cell clones can be identified within otherwise healthy patients.[15] Indeed, clones representing less than 5% of total lymphocytes may not need to be routinely reported. Reactive clonal populations are typically smaller than their malignant counterparts and may diminish overtime in conjunction with the fading stimulus.[16,17]

In addition to clonality, immunophenotypic aberrancy, or deviation from the predicted immunophenotypic expression pattern, is useful in the diagnosis of malignant hematologic disorders. Aberrancy may be associated with antigen gain/overexpression, antigen loss/underexpression, cross-lineage expression, and/or maturation

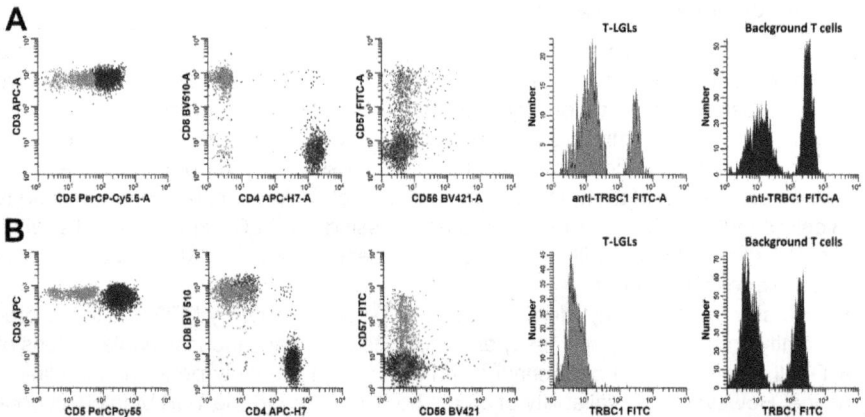

Fig. 3. Utility of T-cell receptor beta chain constant region 1 (TRBC1) expression in identifying clonal T-cell populations by flow cytometry. (*A*) A mixed population of reactive T cells, with a subpopulation of T-large granular lymphocytes (T-LGLs) (*red*) showing decreased CD5 expression and heterogeneous CD57 expression. This T-LGL population shows mixed TRBC1-positive and TRBC1-negative subsets, consistent with a polyclonal population. (*B*) A clonal T-LGL population (*red*), also with decreased CD5 expression and heterogeneous CD57 expression, shows uniform negativity for TRBC1.

discrepancies.[18–21] For example, acute myeloid leukemia (AML) with t(8;21); RUN-X1::RUNX1T1 frequently shows aberrant expression of B-lymphoid markers, including CD19, as well as particularly bright CD34 expression.[18] Early T-cell precursor (ETP) ALL is a subtype of T-ALL and therefore typically demonstrates expression of cytoplasmic CD3, without expression of MPO. However, other myeloid and early stem cell antigens, such as CD34, HLA-DR, CD117, CD13, and CD33, are frequently aberrantly expressed in this disease.[22] Myeloblasts in AML with mutated NPM1 are often negative for CD34 and HLA-DR; this particular immunophenotype is commonly associated with TET2 or IDH1/2 co-mutations and may indicate a more favorable prognosis in this disease.[23]

Multiple systems have been developed that incorporate immunophenotypic aberrancy identified by MPF into the diagnosis of myelodysplastic syndrome (MDS).[24] Abnormalities in expression patterns of CD11b, CD13, and CD16 in maturing myeloid elements are common in patients with MDS[25,26] (**Fig. 4**). The Ogata scoring system[27] evaluates 4 MPF parameters, assigning one point for each (**Table 2**). A score of ≥ 2 has been strongly associated with a diagnosis of MDS. Finally, MPF on peripheral blood has been shown to distinguish chronic myelomonocytic leukemia (CMML) from reactive monocytoses.[28] Monocyte subsets can be defined by the expression of CD14 and CD16, including CD14$^+$/CD16$^-$ classical, CD14$^+$/CD16$^+$ intermediate, and CD14^{low}/CD16$^+$ nonclassical monocytes. CMML characteristically shows an increased classical monocyte fraction, with a value of 94% classical monocytes being a highly sensitive and specific marker for CMML.

Detection of Measurable Residual Disease

The use of MPF to detect small abnormal cell populations within a heterogeneous sample has become a critical component of post-therapy disease monitoring for certain hematologic malignancies. The presence or absence of minimal or measurable residual disease (MRD) at various time points after the initiation of treatment can impact therapeutic decision-making for multiple diseases, including ALL, AML, chronic lymphocytic leukemia, and multiple myeloma.[29] For B-lineage ALL (B-ALL), in particular, MRD detection is well established as the most important predictor of prognosis and is now routinely incorporated into risk-adapted treatment protocols.[30,31] MPF MRD analysis in the context of AML is more complex, in part due to the absence of a single centralized study group, like the Children's Oncology Group, to drive the development of a single standardized assay, as was the case for B-ALL. As such, a standard panel for MPF AML MRD analysis has not emerged, with different centers pursuing overlapping but distinct strategies. The utility of MRD assessment in AML is an area of ongoing research, with the goal of incorporating these data into routine clinical care in the relatively near future.[32]

MPF for detection of MRD involves collecting large numbers of events (500,000–1 million or more) to detect very rare populations to a level of 10^{-4} to 10^{-5} (1 in 10,000–100,000 cells).[31] Doing so relies on identification of an immunophenotypically aberrant population, based on levels of antigen expression or an abnormal pattern of antigen expression for a given lineage and stage of maturation. This 'leukemia-associated immunophenotype' (LAIP) is typically identified at diagnosis and used to track disease over the course of treatment. However, acute leukemias are well known to show phenotypic shifts over time in response to therapy. The use of steroids in induction therapy for ALL has been associated with leukemic cell maturation and a shift to a more mature immunophenotype,[29] and AML blast populations can show not only phenotypic but also clonal evolution over time.[33] Thus, in addition to LAIP-focused analyses, a 'different-from-normal' approach, which relies on standardized antibody

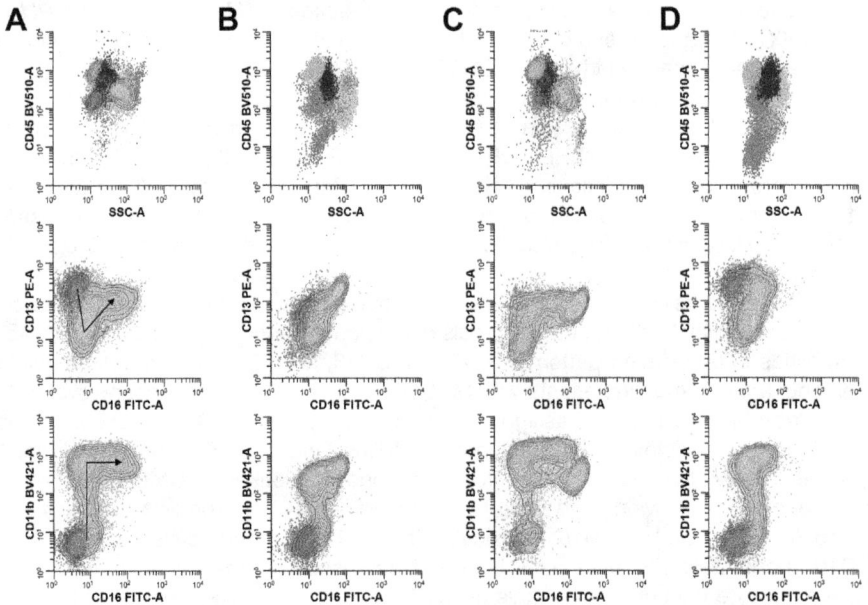

Fig. 4. Flow cytometric evidence of abnormal myeloid maturation. (*A*) Myeloid precursors show a stereotypical pattern of CD11b, CD13, and CD16 acquisition as they mature from the blast stage to the neutrophil stage. (*B–D*) In myelodysplastic syndrome (MDS), myeloid precursors may show asynchronous or abnormal expression patterns of these markers as a feature of dysplasia. Panel B shows decreased expression of CD16. Panel C shows bright expression of CD11b and CD16 on subsets of granulocytes and abnormal, asynchronous acquisition of CD13 and CD16. Panel D shows left-shifted myeloid maturation, with minimal acquisition of CD16, as well as decreased side scatter (SSC) in myeloid elements, which correlates with cytoplasmic hypogranularity. Blasts: red; granulocytes: yellow; monocytes: blue; lymphocytes: green.

panels and a strong understanding of normal expression patterns in maturing hematopoietic cells to identify abnormal leukemic cells, is also helpful. A detailed review of the technical aspects of MRD flow cytometry is beyond the scope of this article, but several recent articles have addressed this topic.[34–36]

Importantly, sample quality can greatly impact the sensitivity of MPF MRD analysis, particularly with respect to paucicellularity and hemodilution of BM samples. Paucicellularity may preclude collection of adequate events to reach a sensitivity of 0.01%, as

Table 2
Ogata scoring system for evaluating myelodysplastic syndrome by flow cytometry

Immunophenotypic parameter[a]	Cutoff Value
CD34+ myeloblasts, % of nucleated cells	>2%
% B cells among all CD34+ cells	<5%
CD45 MFI^{lymphocytes}/CD45 MFI$^{CD34 + myeloblasts}$	$\leq$4 or $\geq$7.5
Granulocyte SSC/lymphocyte SSC	<6

[a] Each parameter meeting the cutoff value is given a score of 1.

is standard for MPF MRD assays. Because hematopoietic malignancies often involve the BM to a greater extent than the peripheral blood, hemodilution will lead to an underestimation of the level of MRD.[29] Standardized methods to quantify the degree of hemodilution are lacking.[29] However, for samples that show features of significant paucicellularity or hemodilution, a comment addressing these limitations should be included in the flow cytometry report to aid clinical decision-making.

Another important consideration with respect to MPF MRD testing is the use of novel therapies targeting surface molecules utilized in MRD analysis. In particular, anti-CD19 therapies for B-ALL can lead to loss of CD19 expression,[37] significantly impacting MPF MRD analysis, which has typically relied heavily on CD19 expression to identify abnormal B-lymphoblast populations.[38] In this context, additional B-cell markers, such as CD22, CD24, and CD79a, can be incorporated into MRD analysis, although therapies targeting CD22 are now also incorporated into B-ALL therapy. Given the potential complexity of MPF MRD analysis, incorporation of molecular MRD testing, such as quantitative polymerase chain reaction and next-generation sequencing techniques, may be beneficial. Studies looking at both AML and B-ALL suggest that MPF and molecular MRD testing are complementary techniques that provide independent prognostic value and improve risk stratification.[39,40]

FUTURE DIRECTIONS

With the increasing diversity of MPF reagents, higher "color" capacity of new instruments, and complexity of analysis comes the need for more sophisticated technologies and tools. Collection and interpretation of traditional (or 'polychromatic') MPF data requires compensating for overlap between the light signals emitted by various dyes or fluorochromes[41] (**Fig. 5**A). This typically involves manually adjusting the

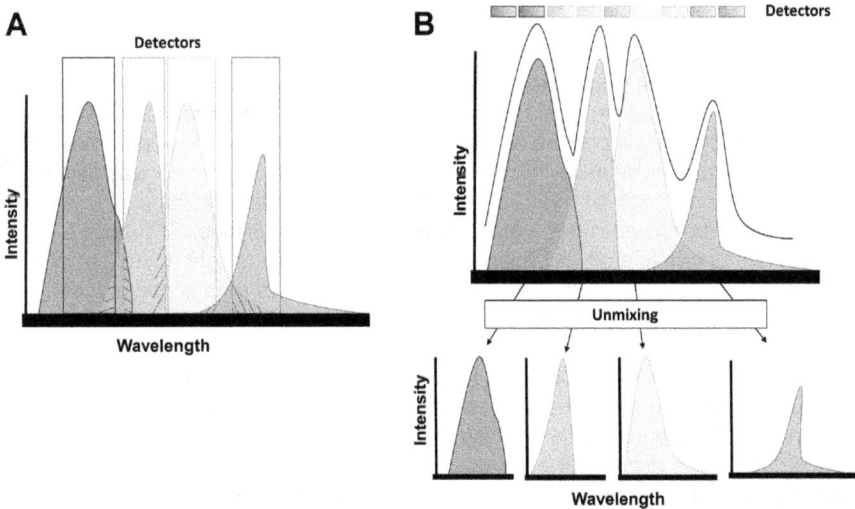

Fig. 5. Conventional versus spectral flow cytometry. (*A*) With conventional flow cytometry, detectors (*rectangles*) register light signals at specific wavelengths. Spectral overlap between various fluorochromes (*hatched areas*) is corrected manually through compensation adjustments. (*B*) Spectral flow cytometry uses a larger number of detectors to analyze the full spectrum of fluorescent light emitted by all fluorochromes in a sample. The complete spectrum data is subsequently unmixed, generating data on each individual component within the sample.

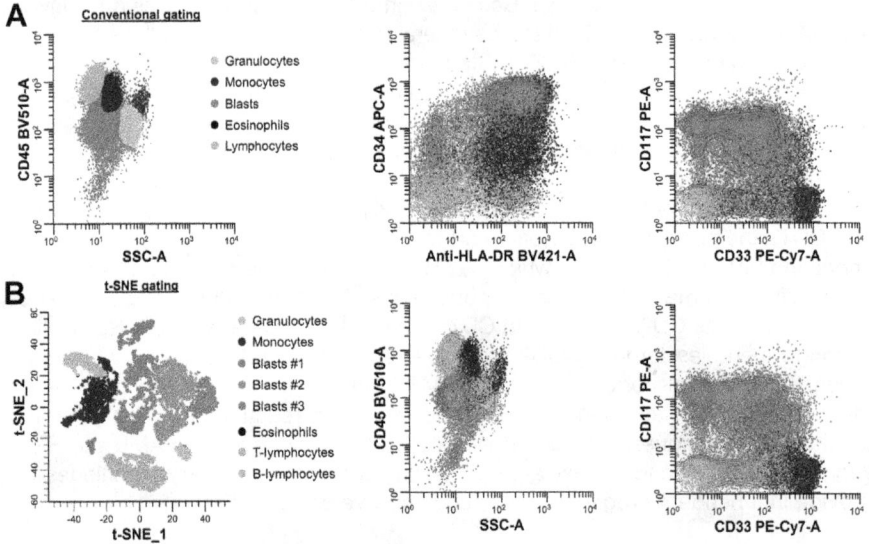

Fig. 6. Conventional and t-stochastic neighborhood embedding (t-SNE) gating in AML with monocytic differentiation. (*A*) A conventional gating strategy relying on CD45/SSC and CD34 expression may not always cleanly separate abnormal populations, particularly in cases of AML with monocytic differentiation, where blasts and immature monocytes can show a spectrum of expression for multiple markers. (*B*) Using tSNE analysis to consider all parameters in a single analysis, it is possible to more cleanly separate out multiple subpopulations all within the CD45 dim 'blast' gate. This type of analysis can potentially facilitate minimal or measurable residual disease (MRD) analysis at later time points, when some but not all blast subpopulations might persist.

data to correct for the component of a given signal that is generated from spectral overlap, which requires expertise and can impact accuracy and reproducibility of results. This challenge will only be amplified as increasing numbers of parameters are incorporated into a given assay. Spectral flow cytometry (SFC), which was developed 2 decades ago but is not yet widely used in clinical flow cytometry practice, represents an alternative technique that is not constrained by these issues. SFC uses a larger number of detectors to analyze the full spectrum of fluorescent light emitted by all fluorochromes in a sample[42] (**Fig. 5**B). The complete spectrum data is subsequently unmixed, using software and a database of the spectrum for individual dyes, generating data on each individual component within the sample.

In addition to novel data collection techniques, the use of more complex MPF assays will require enhanced data analysis tools. Conventional manual gating and visualization via 2-dimensional (2-D) histograms becomes labor intensive and less reproducible as the number of parameters included in an assay increases. This technique also potentially misses important information that can be ascertained using newer, multidimensional computational methods for analyzing MPF data. These computational approaches can incorporate dimensionality reduction, which allows for visualization of multidimensional data in a 2-D space, and clustering, which can highlight and group cell populations based on overall multiparameter expression patterns.[43] Principle component analysis (PCA) and t-stochastic neighborhood embedding (t-SNE) are 2 common methods that reduce dimensionality of data and group similar cells based on expression levels of all analyzed markers (**Fig. 6**). These and other emerging techniques hold the potential to enable more complex clinical assays and sophisticated data analysis to enhance MRD assays as well as other MPF panels (see also article "Automation in Flow Cytometry").

SUMMARY

Flow cytometry is an essential component of the diagnosis of hematologic malignancies. In addition to characterizing abnormal cell populations, MPF results can also indicate the need for additional testing, predict response to targeted therapy, and provide prognostic information. As the complexity of MPF assays increases, emerging computational methods for data collection and analysis will allow users to fully capitalize on all that MPF has to offer.

CLINICS CARE POINTS

- By evaluating multiple antigens on individual cells within mixed samples, MPF allows for the determination of cell lineage, stage of maturation, and aberrancy or clonality
- TRBC1 expression can be used to identify clonal T cell populations, which must be interpreted in the context of clinical findings and other laboratory results
- MRD detection represents the most important prognostic indicator in B-ALL; MPF MRD assays require complex analysis, as well as knowledge of prior therapy, and are complementary to molecular techniques
- Emerging computational techniques will aid analysis of complex MPF assays

DISCLOSURE

The authors have nothing to disclose.

REFERENCES

1. McKinnon KM. Flow cytometry: an overview. Curr Protoc Immunol 2018;120:5 1 1–5 1 11.
2. Carpentier C, Verbanck S, Schandene L, et al. Eosinophilia associated with CD3(-)CD4(+) T cells: characterization and outcome of a single-center cohort of 26 patients. Front Immunol 2020;11:1765.
3. Cogan E, Schandene L, Crusiaux A, et al. Brief report: clonal proliferation of type 2 helper T cells in a man with the hypereosinophilic syndrome. N Engl J Med 1994;330(8):535–8.
4. Davis BH, Holden JT, Bene MC, et al. 2006 Bethesda International Consensus recommendations on the flow cytometric immunophenotypic analysis of hematolymphoid neoplasia: medical indications. Cytometry B Clin Cytom 2007;72(Suppl 1):S5–13.
5. Fromm JR, Thomas A, Wood BL. Flow cytometry can diagnose classical hodgkin lymphoma in lymph nodes with high sensitivity and specificity. Am J Clin Pathol 2009;131(3):322–32.
6. Weinberg OK, Arber DA, Dohner H, et al. The International Consensus Classification of acute leukemias of ambiguous lineage. Blood 2023;141(18):2275–7.
7. Khoury JD, Solary E, Abla O, et al. The 5th edition of the world health organization classification of haematolymphoid tumours: myeloid and histiocytic/dendritic neoplasms. Leukemia 2022. https://doi.org/10.1038/s41375-022-01613-1.

8. Alexander TB, Gu Z, Iacobucci I, et al. The genetic basis and cell of origin of mixed phenotype acute leukaemia. Nature 2018;562(7727):373–9.

9. Weinberg DS, Pinkus GS, Ault KA. Cytofluorometric detection of B cell clonal excess: a new approach to the diagnosis of B cell lymphoma. Blood 1984; 63(5):1080–7.

10. Tonegawa S. Somatic generation of antibody diversity. Nature 1983;302(5909): 575–81.

11. Beck RC, Stahl S, O'Keefe CL, et al. Detection of mature T-cell leukemias by flow cytometry using anti-T-cell receptor V beta antibodies. Am J Clin Pathol 2003; 120(5):785–94.

12. Bjorkman PJ. MHC restriction in three dimensions: a view of T cell receptor/ligand interactions. Cell 1997;89(2):167–70.

13. Maciocia PM, Wawrzyniecka PA, Philip B, et al. Targeting the T cell receptor beta-chain constant region for immunotherapy of T cell malignancies. Nat Med 2017; 23(12):1416–23.

14. Shi M, Jevremovic D, Otteson GE, et al. Single Antibody detection of T-cell receptor alphabeta clonality by flow cytometry rapidly identifies mature T-cell neoplasms and monotypic small CD8-positive subsets of uncertain significance. Cytometry B Clin Cytom 2020;98(1):99–107.

15. Shi M, Olteanu H, Jevremovic D, et al. T-cell clones of uncertain significance are highly prevalent and show close resemblance to T-cell large granular lymphocytic leukemia. Implications for laboratory diagnostics. Mod Pathol 2020;33(10):2046–57.

16. Kussick SJ, Kalnoski M, Braziel RM, et al. Prominent clonal B-cell populations identified by flow cytometry in histologically reactive lymphoid proliferations. Am J Clin Pathol 2004;121(4):464–72.

17. Kroft SH, Harrington AM. How i diagnose mature T-cell proliferations by flow cytometry. Am J Clin Pathol 2022;158(4):456–71.

18. Porwit-MacDonald A, Janossy G, Ivory K, et al. Leukemia-associated changes identified by quantitative flow cytometry. IV. CD34 overexpression in acute myelogenous leukemia M2 with t(8;21). Blood 1996;87(3):1162–9.

19. Wells DA, Benesch M, Loken MR, et al. Myeloid and monocytic dyspoiesis as determined by flow cytometric scoring in myelodysplastic syndrome correlates with the IPSS and with outcome after hematopoietic stem cell transplantation. Blood 2003;102(1):394–403.

20. Khalidi HS, Medeiros LJ, Chang KL, et al. The immunophenotype of adult acute myeloid leukemia: high frequency of lymphoid antigen expression and comparison of immunophenotype, French-American-British classification, and karyotypic abnormalities. Am J Clin Pathol 1998;109(2):211–20.

21. Wood BL. Myeloid malignancies: myelodysplastic syndromes, myeloproliferative disorders, and acute myeloid leukemia. Clin Lab Med 2007;27(3):551–75, vii.

22. Coustan-Smith E, Mullighan CG, Onciu M, et al. Early T-cell precursor leukaemia: a subtype of very high-risk acute lymphoblastic leukaemia. Lancet Oncol 2009; 10(2):147–56.

23. Mason EF, Hasserjian RP, Aggarwal N, et al. Blast phenotype and comutations in acute myeloid leukemia with mutated NPM1 influence disease biology and outcome. Blood Adv 2019;3(21):3322–32.

24. Porwit A, Bene MC, Duetz C, et al. Multiparameter flow cytometry in the evaluation of myelodysplasia: analytical issues: recommendations from the european leukemianet/international myelodysplastic syndrome flow cytometry working group. Cytometry B Clin Cytom 2023;104(1):27–50.

25. Stetler-Stevenson M, Arthur DC, Jabbour N, et al. Diagnostic utility of flow cytometric immunophenotyping in myelodysplastic syndrome. Blood 2001;98(4):979–87.
26. Kussick SJ, Fromm JR, Rossini A, et al. Four-color flow cytometry shows strong concordance with bone marrow morphology and cytogenetics in the evaluation for myelodysplasia. Am J Clin Pathol 2005;124(2):170–81.
27. Della Porta MG, Picone C, Pascutto C, et al. Multicenter validation of a reproducible flow cytometric score for the diagnosis of low-grade myelodysplastic syndromes: results of a European LeukemiaNET study. Haematologica 2012;97(8):1209–17.
28. Selimoglu-Buet D, Wagner-Ballon O, Saada V, et al. Characteristic repartition of monocyte subsets as a diagnostic signature of chronic myelomonocytic leukemia. Blood 2015;125(23):3618–26.
29. Wood BL. Principles of minimal residual disease detection for hematopoietic neoplasms by flow cytometry. Cytometry B Clin Cytom 2016;90(1):47–53.
30. Borowitz MJ, Devidas M, Hunger SP, et al. Clinical significance of minimal residual disease in childhood acute lymphoblastic leukemia and its relationship to other prognostic factors: a Children's Oncology Group study. Blood 2008; 111(12):5477–85.
31. Saygin C, Cannova J, Stock W, et al. Measurable residual disease in acute lymphoblastic leukemia: methods and clinical context in adult patients. Haematologica 2022;107(12):2783–93.
32. Walter RB. Perspective on measurable residual disease testing in acute myeloid leukemia. Leukemia 2023. https://doi.org/10.1038/s41375-023-02084-8.
33. Zeijlemaker W, Gratama JW, Schuurhuis GJ. Tumor heterogeneity makes AML a "moving target" for detection of residual disease. Cytometry B Clin Cytom 2014; 86(1):3–14.
34. Wood BL. Acute myeloid leukemia minimal residual disease detection: the difference from normal approach. Curr Protoc Cytom 2020;93(1):e73.
35. Borowitz MJ, Wood BL, Keeney M, et al. Measurable residual disease detection in B-acute lymphoblastic leukemia: the children's oncology group (COG) method. Curr Protoc 2022;2(3):e383.
36. Tettero JM, Freeman S, Buecklein V, et al. Technical aspects of flow cytometry-based measurable residual disease quantification in acute myeloid leukemia: experience of the european leukemiaNet MRD working party. Hemasphere 2022;6(1):e676.
37. Chen X, Gao Q, Roshal M, et al. Flow cytometric assessment for minimal/measurable residual disease in B lymphoblastic leukemia/lymphoma in the era of immunotherapy. Cytometry B Clin Cytom 2023;104(3):205–23.
38. Kovach AE, Wood BL. Updates on lymphoblastic leukemia/lymphoma classification and minimal/measurable residual disease analysis. Semin Diagn Pathol 2023;40(6):457–71.
39. Jongen-Lavrencic M, Grob T, Hanekamp D, et al. Molecular minimal residual disease in acute myeloid leukemia. N Engl J Med 2018;378(13):1189–99.
40. Wood B, Wu D, Crossley B, et al. Measurable residual disease detection by high-throughput sequencing improves risk stratification for pediatric B-ALL. Blood 2018;131(12):1350–9.
41. Robinson JP. Flow cytometry: past and future. Biotechniques 2022;72(4):159–69.
42. Robinson JP, Ostafe R, Iyengar SN, et al. Flow cytometry: the next revolution. Cells 2023;12(14). https://doi.org/10.3390/cells12141875.
43. Duetz C, Bachas C, Westers TM, et al. Computational analysis of flow cytometry data in hematological malignancies: future clinical practice? Curr Opin Oncol 2020;32(2):162–9.

Flow Cytometry-based Immune Phenotyping of T and B Lymphocytes in the Evaluation of Immunodeficiency and Immune Dysregulation

Alan A. Nguyen, MD[a], Craig D. Platt, MD, PhD[b],*

KEYWORDS

- Flow cytometry • Inborn errors of immunity • Primary immunodeficiency
- Immune dysregulation

KEY POINTS

- Flow cytometry is used to define the underlying cellular basis for infection susceptibility and/or autoimmunity/autoinflammation.
- In patients with immunodeficiency, flow cytometry can be used to establish risk of infection, while in patients with immune dysregulation, the technique can be used to monitor disease activity and response to therapies.
- Flow cytometry can be used in conjunction with genetic testing to resolve variants of uncertain significance and validate genetic testing results.
- Flow cytometry may aid in the identification of aberrant immune pathways in patients with a suspected inborn error of immunity who lack a genetic diagnosis.

INTRODUCTION

Inborn errors of immunity (IEIs) are a group of approximately 500 congenital disorders that impair immune cell development and/or function. These include primary immunodeficiencies, which present with increased susceptibility to infection, and primary immune regulatory disorders, which present with autoimmunity, autoinflammation, lymphoproliferation, and/or atopy as predominant symptoms.[1,2] A method used to evaluate patients with suspected immunodeficiency or immune dysregulation entails using flow cytometry on peripheral blood. This technique is used for the enumeration of immune cells, measurement of relative proportions of cellular populations,

[a] Division of Immunology, Boston Children's Hospital, Harvard Medical School, Fegan Building 6th Floor, Boston, MA 02115, USA; [b] Division of Immunology, Boston Children's Hospital, Harvard Medical School, 1 Blackfan Circle, Karp Building 10th Floor, Boston, MA 02115, USA
* Corresponding author.
E-mail address: craig.platt@childrens.harvard.edu

Clin Lab Med 44 (2024) 479–493
https://doi.org/10.1016/j.cll.2024.04.009   labmed.theclinics.com
0272-2712/24/© 2024 Elsevier Inc. All rights reserved, including those for text and data mining, AI training, and similar technologies.

assessment of expression of specific proteins, and evaluation of cellular function, allowing clinicians and researchers to define the underlying cellular basis for infection susceptibility and/or autoimmunity/autoinflammation.[3–5]

While flow cytometers vary in their capabilities, the general principles involved are similar across instruments. Cells are suspended in a fluid and labeled with fluorescent antibodies or dyes specific to the molecules present on the cells of interest. They are then drawn into the flow cytometer and are focused by a sheath fluid to create a single file of individual cells that flow past one or more lasers at a rate of hundreds to thousands of cells per second. The light emitted by the fluorescent molecules are detected, converted to electrical signals, processed, and displayed in histograms and scatter plots to reveal characteristics of the cells and proteins of interest.[3,5]

A fully comprehensive overview of flow cytometry is not practical in this format. Instead, this primer aims to equip practicing clinicians—primarily clinical immunologists, rheumatologists, and infectious disease specialists—with a foundational understanding of T and B cell immunophenotyping, thereby unlocking its diagnostic and management potential for patients with suspected immunodeficiency and/or immune dysregulation.

LYMPHOCYTE SUBSETS

Lymphocyte subset evaluation is the most ordered and widely available flow cytometry test and is essential to any evaluation of cellular immunity. This test includes enumeration of $CD3^+$ T cells (including separate enumeration of $CD4^+$ and $CD8^+$ T cells), $CD19^+$ B cells, and $CD16^+$ and/or $CD56^+$ natural killer (NK) cells. While most flow cytometry results are qualitative, lymphocyte subset data routinely includes absolute cell counts as well as percentages. The most common method for cell enumeration entails adding a standardized number of counting beads to a known volume of cell suspension prior to acquisition. The absolute cell count is then calculated based on the ratio of cells to counting beads.[3]

It is important to keep in mind that normal ranges for most lymphocyte populations vary substantially by age (eg, a T cell count of 900 cells/μL, while normal in an adult, should raise concern for an IEI in an otherwise well-appearing infant). It is, therefore, essential that age-specific reference ranges be used.[6] Equally important is that flow cytometry results represent a snapshot in time. Lymphocyte numbers can vary dramatically based on infection, other critical illness, or use of systemic corticosteroids, highlighting the need to interpret the data within the clinical context of the patient.[4]

T-CELL ENUMERATION

T cells are identified by the expression of the CD3 complex (comprised of CD3εγ, CD3εδ, and CD3ζζ), usually via an antibody that recognizes CD3ε, and are commonly enumerated as part of the lymphocyte subset analysis described earlier.[7] T-cell lymphopenia may be identified at any age, though special attention is paid to patients with T-cell lymphopenia identified during infancy—these patients may have severe combined immunodeficiency (SCID), a life-threatening disorder if not treated by bone marrow transplantation or gene therapy within the first year of life.[8]

As universal newborn screening for SCID has been in place in the United States since 2018 (using quantitative polymerase chain reaction to detect T-cell recombination excision circles in dried blood spots), the vast majority of infants born with SCID in the United States are identified shortly after birth.[8] After a positive newborn screen, confirmatory testing is performed using flow cytometry for T-cell enumeration (together with naïve/memory phenotyping) to quickly stratify risk.[9] Patients with classic SCID have absent or very low number of T cells, whereas mild-to-moderate T-cell lymphopenia can be seen in other primary and secondary disorders described in later sections.[2,10]

Concurrent B and NK cell enumeration can be used to narrow the differential diagnosis in patients with suspected SCID while genetic testing is still pending.[9] For instance, low or absent T cells with preserved B and NK cells (T⁻B⁺NK⁺ SCID) would indicate a differential diagnosis including interleukin (IL)-7 receptor deficiency, deficiency of any of the CD3 chains (γ, δ, ε, and ζ) or thymic defects including complete DiGeorge or CHARGE syndrome—this later distinction is critical as patients with athymia are treated with thymus transplant rather than stem cell transplant. Patients with T⁻B⁻NK⁺ SCID typically have a disorder of VDJ recombination including defects in RAG1/RAG2, or radiosensitive forms of SCID including Artemis deficiency and DNA ligase IV deficiency—identifying patients with radiosensitive SCID is essential given the complications from ionizing radiation and myeloablative conditioning regimens seen in these patients. T⁻B⁺NK⁻ SCID should raise concern for X-linked SCID or janus kinase 3 (JAK3) deficiency. Adenosine deaminase (ADA) deficiency is the most common cause of T⁻B⁻NK⁻ SCID.[2]

Consideration of CD4⁺ and CD8⁺ T-cell subset enumeration results is also essential. Low CD4⁺ T cells, with preserved CD8⁺ T cell number (often described as an inverted CD4⁺/CD8⁺ ratio because CD4 cells outnumber CD8 T cells in most healthy individuals) are seen in a variety of primary and secondary disorders including human immunodeficiency virus (HIV)/acquired immunodeficiency syndrome and major histocompatibility complex (MHC) class II deficiency—this is also a nonspecific finding in many combined immunodeficiencies or chronic infections.[11,12] Low CD8⁺ T cells with preserved CD4⁺ T cells is somewhat less common but may indicate either MHC class I deficiency or ZAP-70 deficiency.[13] CD4⁺ and CD8⁺ T-cell enumeration also aids in the determination of the risk of opportunistic infection. For instance, the degree of CD4 lymphopenia is used to determine whether prophylaxis for pneumocystis jirovecii pneumonia (PJP) pneumonia should be initiated,[14] and the degree of CD8 lymphopenia may be used to determine the eligibility for live vaccines in patients with partial DiGeorge syndrome.[15]

T-CELL MEMORY PHENOTYPING

Mature CD4⁺ and CD8⁺ T cells that have completed development and have exited the thymus but have not yet encountered antigen are referred to as naïve T cells, while T cells that have encountered antigens and become activated are referred to as memory T cells.[16] CD45RA and CD45RO serve as markers of naïve and memory T cells, respectively, though additional markers including CCR7 and CD62 ligand (CD62L) are useful in defining subsets of memory T cells.[16] In **Fig. 1**, we demonstrate how CD45RA⁻ memory cells are further distinguished into central memory T cells expressing CCR7 (which home toward secondary lymphoid tissue), and effector memory T cells (which home toward peripheral organs).[16] This strategy also identifies terminally differentiated T effector memory cells that re-express CD45RA, a population referred to as TEMRAs—these are effector cells with poor proliferative abilities, increased features of senescence, and higher susceptibility to apoptosis.[17] TEMRAs have been shown to expand in patients with persistent viral infections such as cytomegalovirus and Epstein–Barr virus, and in patients with autoimmune disorders such as rheumatoid arthritis.[18,19]

Determination of the relative proportion of naïve and memory T cells is of particularly high clinical utility in the evaluation of patients with suspected SCID. This allows for the

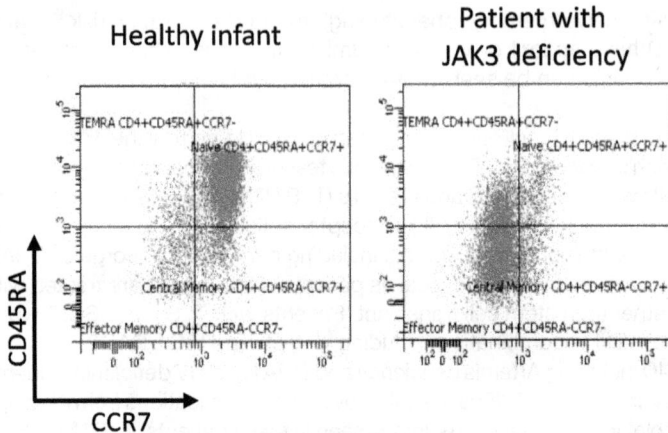

Fig. 1. Naïve/memory phenotyping of CD4$^+$ T cells using CD45RA and CCR7 in a healthy control (left) and a patient with leaky SCID due to JAK3 deficiency (right). Cells displayed are CD3$^+$CD4$^+$ T cells. Note the paucity of CD45RA$^+$CCR7$^+$ CD4 T cells in the right panel.

detection of oligoclonal expansion or maternal engraftment (both associated with low naïve T cell percentages), which may lead to falsely reassuring absolute T-cell counts.[10] Patients with CD45RA$^+$ CCR7$^+$ naïve CD4 T cells below 50% are at far greater risk of having SCID or another combined immunodeficiency compared with those infants with naïve CD4 T cells above 50%.[9] Patients with T-cell lymphopenia and naïve T cells above 50% are far more likely to have another underlying etiology such as prematurity, congenital heart disease, partial DiGeorge syndrome, or trisomy 21.[9] Normal or elevated numbers of naïve T cells are reassuring in most cases; however, they cannot entirely preclude a T-cell defect. In rare cases, high naive T cells in the context of opportunistic infection will indicate a defect in T-cell differentiation.[20]

Evaluation of recent thymic emigrants (RTEs) has overlapping utility with the naïve/memory phenotyping described earlier. RTEs are the youngest subset of naïve T cells, commonly defined as CD4$^+$CD31$^+$CD45RA$^+$, which distinguishes these cells from proliferated peripheral naïve T cells.[21] Like naïve T cells, RTEs are abundant in early childhood and decrease with age; they contain high T-cell receptor excision circle numbers, indicative of T cell receptor rearrangement.[22] RTEs are often used to evaluate thymic dysfunction in conditions such as partial DiGeorge syndrome,[23] CHARGE syndrome,[24] or in neonatal thymectomy.[25]

Assessment of naïve T-cell percentage is not limited to infants and is useful in patients of any age being assessed for immune dysregulation. Decreased naïve T-cell percentage has been described in immune dysregulation disorders, including Evan's syndrome (regardless of whether an underlying genetic defect is identified), common variable immunodeficiency (CVID) with noninfectious complications, CTLA4 deficiency, and activated PIK delta syndrome.[26–29] Naïve T-cell percentage may normalize with effective treatment, though in general, naïve T-cell percentage is not as reliable a biomarker of disease activity as follicular T-cell percentage (discussed in a subsequent section) or serum biomarkers of T-cell activation such as soluble IL2-receptor.[29–31]

DOUBLE-NEGATIVE T CELLS

While most T cells in peripheral blood express either CD4 or CD8, it is typical to see up to 10% of T cells negative for both markers. While most circulating T cells express the $\alpha\beta$ T-cell receptor (TCR), T cells expressing the $\gamma\delta$ TCR typically comprise the majority of these "double-negative" T cells (**Fig. 2**).[32] $\gamma\delta$ T cells have more limited TCR diversity than their $\alpha\beta$ counterparts but respond to infections more rapidly, particularly at mucosal surfaces where many antigens are first encountered.[32] Significant expansion of $\gamma\delta$ T cells can be in response to infection but may also be indicative of autoimmune disorders or hematologic malignancy.[32]

"Double-negative" $\alpha\beta$ T cells typically comprise less than 1.2% of total CD3[+] cells in healthy individuals. Expansion of double-negative $\alpha\beta$ T cells is less common and is best described in patients with autoimmune lymphoproliferative syndrome (ALPS; see **Fig. 2**).[33,34] Patients with ALPS present with nonmalignant lymphadenopathy, splenomegaly, hepatomegaly, immune-mediated cytopenias, and a significantly increased risk of secondary malignancy.[34] The most common cause of ALPS is a defect in the first apoptosis signal (FAS) receptor pathway, leading to impaired cell death and an expansion of autoreactive double-negative $\alpha\beta$ T cells. It should be noted that most patients

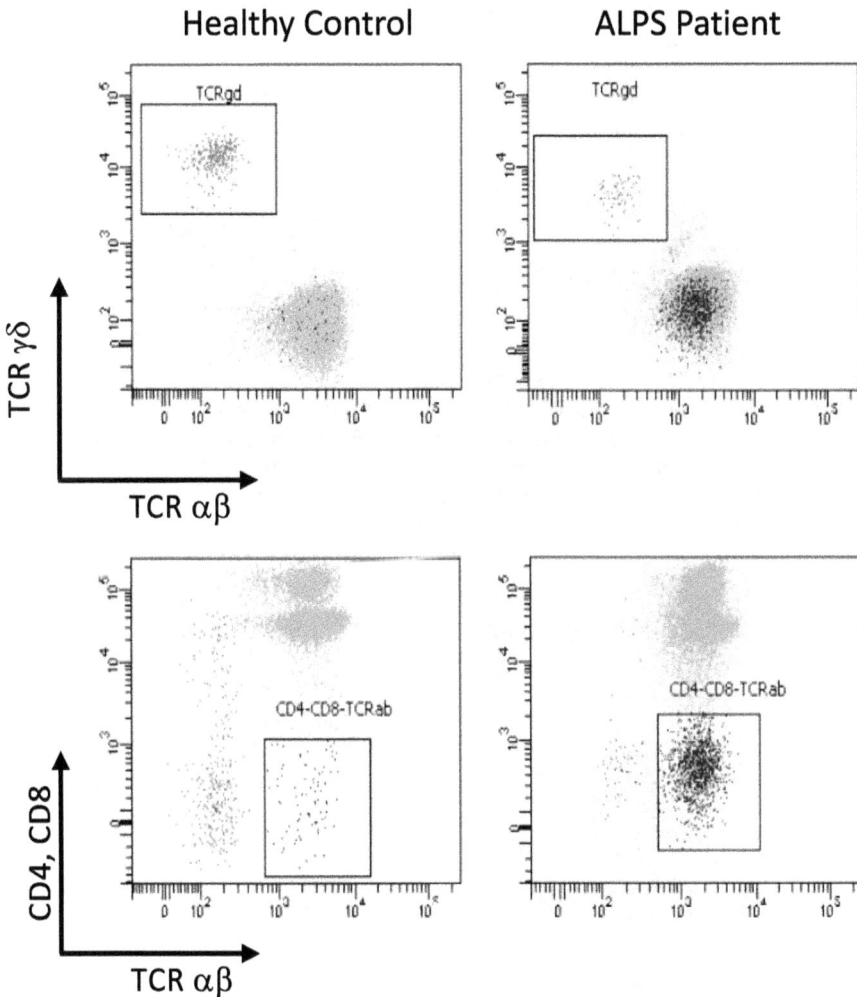

Fig. 2. Analysis of double-negative T cells in a healthy control (left panels) and in a patient with ALPS (right panels). Cells displayed are CD3[+] T cells. Note the expansion of $\alpha\beta$ T cells that are negative for CD4 and CD8 in the lower right panel.

with modest expansion of $\alpha\beta$ double-negative T cells do not have ALPS—patients with more common disorders including systemic lupus erythematosus (SLE) and Sjogren's syndrome may also have elevated numbers of DN T cells.[33] When used as a diagnostic test for ALPS, double-negative T-cell evaluation should, therefore, be performed in conjunction with other ALPS biomarkers including vitamin B12, soluble FAS ligand, IL-10, and IL-18.[35]

REGULATORY T CELLS

Regulatory T cells (Tregs) are a subset of CD4[+] T cells that maintain peripheral tolerance, down modulating the immune response though the production of cytokines including IL-10 and transforming growth factor beta and expression of inhibitory receptors including CTLA4.[36,37] The gold standard for Treg identification is FOXP3 expression, a transcription factor that is necessary for Treg differentiation (**Fig. 3**). Some clinical laboratories avoid the complexity of intracellular staining for this marker, instead identifying CD25[+]CD127[low] CD4 T cells as Tregs. Treg deficiencies, sometimes referred to as "tregopathies," are a subset of disorders caused by genetic defects that impair Treg development, survival, and/or function leading to multiorgan autoimmunity.[38] The prototypical tregopathy is FOXP3 deficiency, which leads to immune dysregulation, polyendocrinopathy, and enteropathy X-linked (IPEX) syndrome.[39] Other disorders impacting Treg number include CTLA4 haploinsufficiency, lipopolysaccharide-responsive beige-like anchor protein (LRBA) deficiency, and BTB and CNC homology 2 (BACH2) haploinsufficiency.[40,41] However, the impact on Treg number may be subtle in disorders other than IPEX syndrome, limiting the clinical utility of the test.

FOLLICULAR HELPER T CELLS

Follicular helper T (Tfh) cells are a subtype of CD4[+] T cells in secondary lymphoid organs that promote the formation of germinal centers and differentiation of B cells into antibody secreting cells. Upon upregulation of CXCR5 and downregulation of CCR7, Tfh cells migrate to B follicles where they regulate antigen-specific B-cell responses via costimulatory molecules including CD40 L, CD28, OX40, inducible T-cell costimulator (ICOS), and PD1.[42,43] Expansion of circulating Tfh (cTFh) cells (which correlate with germinal center formation) has been described in a variety autoimmune disorders

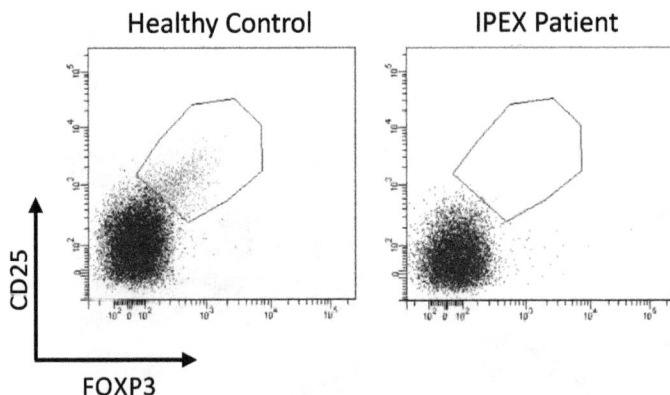

Fig. 3. Analysis of Tregs from a healthy control (left panel) and Tregs from a patient with IPEX syndrome (right panel). Cells displayed are CD3[+]CD4[+] T cells. Note the lack of CD25[+]FOXP3[+] Tregs in the right panel.

(eg, SLE, rheumatoid arthritis, type I diabetes, and Evan's syndrome), as well as monogenic immune dysregulation syndromes (eg, cytotoxic T-lymphocyte-associated protein [CTLA] haploinsufficiency, LRBA deficiency, and STAT1 gain of function; **Fig. 4**).[26,30,44,45] Importantly, effective immunosuppressive therapy leads to normalization of cTFh percentage in many cases, making this an excellent biomarker of disease activity for patients with immune dysregulation.[30,44,46]

B-CELL ENUMERATION

While B-cell function can be evaluated at the most basic level using immunoglobulin levels and vaccine responses, B-cell flow cytometry allows for more detailed evaluation of immunodeficiency seen in hypogammaglobulinemia or agammaglobulinemia, and may identify biomarkers of immune dysregulation.[3,5,47] B-cell phenotyping begins with B-cell enumeration, typically as part of lymphocyte subset analysis. The most common marker used to identify B cells is CD19, present on all B cell subsets except long-lived plasma cells that reside in the bone marrow. While B cells express CD20 slightly later in development, 98% of B cells are double positive for both CD19 and CD20.[48] These markers may generally be used interchangeably for the purposes of flow cytometry on peripheral blood; however, specific use may be considered to assess the possibility of genetic deficiency of CD19 or CD20, or loss of CD19 or CD20 expression as a mechanism of resistance in patients treated with anti-CD20 monoclonal antibody (eg, rituximab) or CD19-specific chimeric antigen receptor T cells.[2,49] Severe B-cell lymphopenia may be seen in patients who have been treated with these B cell-depleting therapies, as well as genetic disorders including X-linked agammaglobulinemia, autosomal recessive agammaglobulinemias, and PU.1 deficiency.[50,51] However, most immunodeficiencies and immune dysregulation syndromes present with normal numbers of B cells—the additional phenotyping described below helps with characterization of these disorders.

B-CELL NAÏVE/MEMORY PHENOTYPING

After development in the bone marrow, naive B cells circulate in the blood and lymphatic system. Naïve B cells are commonly defined as cells that (1) do not express

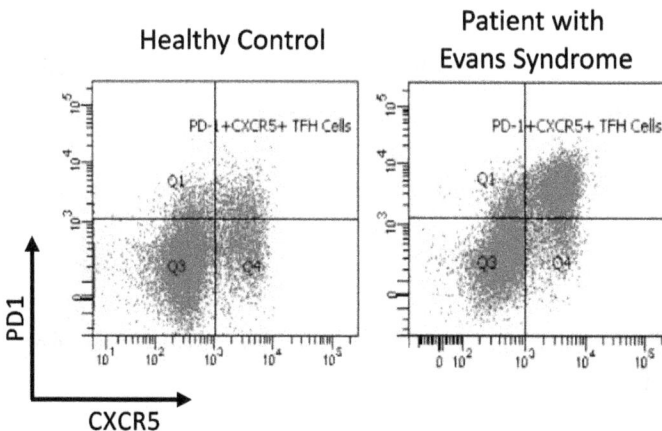

Fig. 4. Analysis of PD1$^+$CXCR5$^+$ cTFh cells from a healthy control (left) and from a patient with Evans syndrome (right). Cells displayed are CD4$^+$ T cells. Note expansion of PD1$^+$CXCR5$^+$ cells in the right panel.

the memory marker CD27 and (2) have not undergone class switching and express the membrane-bound immunoglobulins IgM and immunoglobulin (Ig) D. Memory B cells are commonly defined by the presence of the marker CD27, with "switched memory" B cells additionally demonstrating loss of IgD and IgM expression, as they have undergone isotype switching (**Fig. 5**).[48]

Patients with hyper-IgM syndromes have low or undetectable IgD⁻CD27⁺ switched memory B cells due to poor or absent isotype switching. Switched memory B cells are also decreased in other disorders that impact B-cell activation and differentiation including CVID.[52] After B-cell-depleting therapy such as rituximab, recovery of switched memory B cells has been shown to serve as a more useful marker of endogenous IgG production than B-cell number.[53–55] In patients receiving immunoglobulin replacement after B cell-depleting therapy, trending switched memory B cell percentage may aid in decisions regarding the need for ongoing immunoglobulin replacement. While recovery of switched memory B cells is associated with a reduced risk of hypogammaglobulinemia in these patients, this finding is also associated with the risk of relapse in autoimmune disorders, including multiple sclerosis and nephrotic syndrome.[53–55]

The use of CD27 as a memory marker is complicated by significant numbers of circulating IgM⁺IgD⁺CD27⁺ B cells with an Ig repertoire that has been generated without prior antigen exposure.[56,57] This population is often referred to as "non-switched" or "unswitched" memory cells, or as "IgM memory cells." However, as gene expression profiling and surface marker expression have demonstrated that circulating IgM⁺IgD⁺CD27⁺ B cells correspond with splenic marginal zone B cells, these circulating cells are also defined as circulating marginal zone B cells.[58,59] These cells produce "natural" antibodies with broad specificity but low affinity to both bacterial and self-antigens. They are particularly important to the response against T-cell independent antigens and encapsulated bacteria.[60–62]

As the spleen plays an essential role in maintenance of unswitched memory B cells, enumeration of this population been proposed as a proxy for splenic B-cell function.[60,63,64] While not all patient populations with asplenia and low unswitched memory B cells appear to be at increased risk of invasive infections, low memory B cells, and unswitched memory B cells in particular, have been described as a risk factor for community-acquired severe bacterial infections in patients with heterotaxy.[63,65]

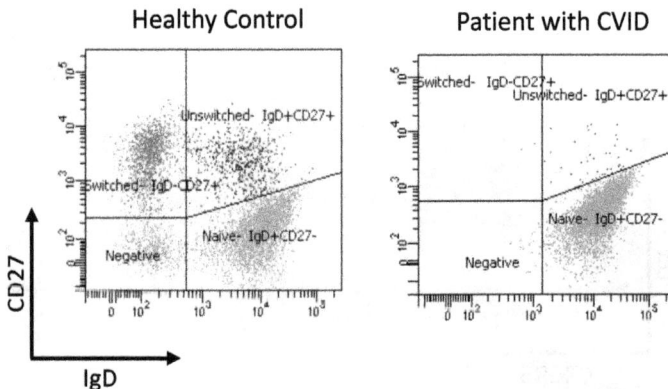

Fig. 5. Naïve/memory phenotyping of B cells using CD27 and IgD from healthy control (left) and from a patient with CVID (right). Gating applied to CD19⁺ B cells. Note the paucity of memory B cells in the right panel.

Patients without any apparent anatomic spleen defect may also have decreased numbers of both switched and unswitched memory B cells, including patients with hypogammaglobulinemia and chronic infections such as HIV.[66–70]

TRANSITIONAL B CELLS

Transitional B cells are the most immature subset of naive B cells in peripheral blood, completing the final stages of maturation after exiting the bone marrow. In healthy individuals, transitional B cells include self-reactive B cells that have yet to undergo negative selection.[48] Expansion of transitional B cells has been demonstrated in a wide array of disorders including SLE, Sjögren's syndrome, juvenile dermatomyositis, CTLA4 haploinsufficiency, LRBA deficiency, activated phosphatidylinositol 3-kinase (PI3K) delta syndrome, and STAT3 gain of function.[71,72] In **Fig. 6**A, we identify transitional B cells based on high levels of CD24 and CD38, though these cells may also be identified by high expression of CD10, and IgM. Transitional B cells have been

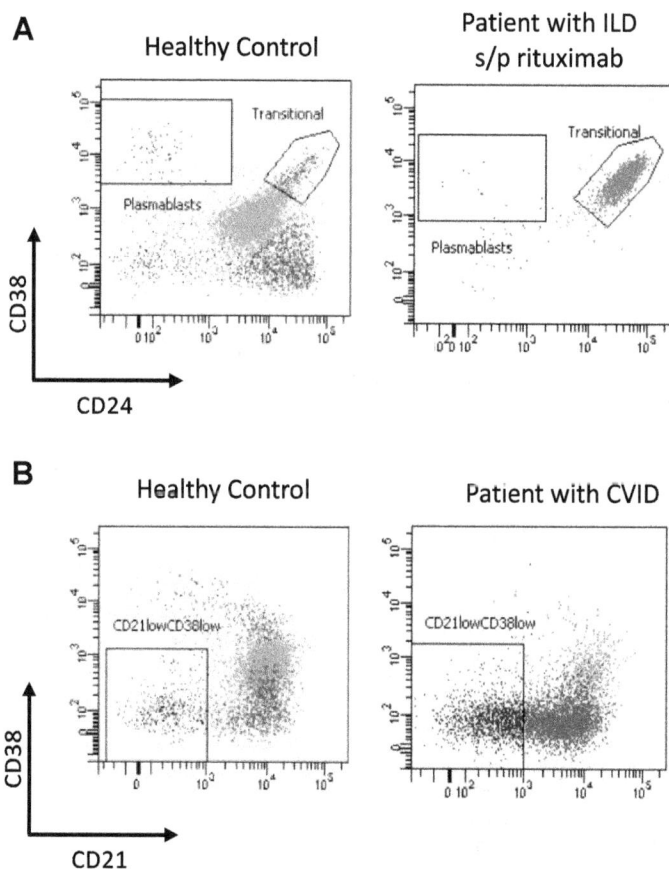

Fig. 6. Assessment of transitional B cells and plasmablasts from a healthy control (left) and from a patient with interstitial lung disease 8 months after use of rituximab. Gating applied to CD19[+] B cells. Note that nearly all B cells have a transitional B cell phenotype in the right panel (A). Assessment of CD21[low] B cells from a healthy control (left) and from a patient with CVID and splenomegaly (right). Cells displayed are CD19[+] B cells. Note the expansion of CD21[low]CD38[low] B cells in the right panel (B).

described as having 3 subsets (T1, T2, and T3), representing progressive stages of maturation. CD21 expression may be used to distinguish between stages of transitional T1 and T2 B cells, the latter expressing higher levels of CD21. T3 cells are not easily distinguished from mature naïve B cells.[71]

PLASMABLASTS

The terminal differentiation of B cells generates antibody secreting cells including both short-lived plasmablasts and long-lived plasma cells.[73] Plasma cells are generally inaccessible to flow cytometry performed on peripheral blood (exceptions being in some patients with active infection, autoimmunity, or malignancy).[48] Plasmablasts, often defined as $CD19^+CD38^+CD24^-$ can be detected in peripheral blood (see **Fig. 6**A). The cells can alternatively be identified as either $CD19^+CD20^-CD38^+$ or $CD19^+CD38^+CD27^+$.[48] Low circulating plasmablasts have been described in patients with CVID or other disorders that impair terminal B cell differentiation.[74] Expanded plasmablast populations have been described in patients with type I diabetes, IgG4-related disease, and anti-neutrophil cytoplasmic antibodies (ANCA)-associated vasculitis.[75-77]

CD21[low] B CELLS

$CD21^{low}$ B cells are a heterogenous B-cell subset that is present in healthy individuals but expanded in a wide array of autoimmune disorders including SLE, rheumatoid arthritis, systemic sclerosis, Sjögren's syndrome, multiple sclerosis, and Crohn's disease.[78,79] In patients with CVID, an association between $CD21^{low}CD38^{low}CD11c^+$ B cell expansion and an increased risk of splenomegaly and multisystem autoimmunity has been described (use of CD38 distinguishes these cells from T1 transitional B cells, described earlier; see **Fig. 6**A).[78] Expansion of $CD21^{low}$ B cells has also been described in patients with chronic infection including hepatitis C virus and HIV, malaria, and severe acute respiratory syndrome coronavirus 2.[78,79] It is important to note that the expanded $CD21^{low}$ cells seen in patients with one condition are not necessarily equivalent to those seen in other conditions. CD11c, FcRL4, and Tbet have been used to define subsets of $CD21^{low}$ B cells on a research basis.[78]

CONCLUSIONS AND FUTURE DIRECTIONS

Flow cytometry is indispensable for evaluating patients suspected to have immunodeficiency and/or immune dysregulation. However, the flexibility in assay design, while a significant strength, is also a limitation. There are multiple valid definitions of any given cellular population and, with few exceptions, a lack of standardization between most clinical laboratories. This complicates interpretation by clinicians and makes it more difficult to use data from multiple centers in clinical research. Other limitations include the need for highly trained technicians and ordering clinicians who are trained in interpretation of the results. Reviews like this one are aimed at helping the later limitation, particularly given the increasing recognition that the flow cytometry assays are not only useful for patients presenting to immunology, rheumatology, and infectious disease clinics, but increasingly hematology, pulmonology, gastroenterology, and endocrinology clinics as well.

It is important to note that while the assays discussed in this review are clinically available, many more tests are only available on a research basis. In some cases, the lack of clinical availability may be due to technical complexity or the difficulty of working with shipped samples. However, for research-based assays that are reproducible and robust with clear clinical utility, efforts must be made to quickly adapt and validate these tests for use in clinical settings.

CLINICS CARE POINTS

- Age-specific reference ranges must be used when interpreting lymphocyte subset data, as normal values vary significantly with age.
- Naïve/memory T cell phenotyping is used to help distinguish between primary and secondary causes of T cell lymphopenia in patients identified to be at risk of severe combined immunodeficiency by newborn screening.
- In patients who have received B cell-depleting therapies, combining B cell enumeration with naïve/memory B cell phenotyping can provide a more comprehensive assessment of B cell reconstitution and potential for recovery of immunoglobulin production than relying on B cell enumeration alone.
- In patients with antibody deficiency, the presence of expanded populations of memory T cells, circulating T follicular helper cells, transitional B cells, and/or CD21low B cells may signal the presence of ongoing autoimmune complications or an increased risk of developing such complications.

DISCLOSURE

A. A. Nguyen is a staff physician at Boston Children's Hospital and Instructor of Pediatrics at Harvard Medical School. C. D. Platt is a staff physician and Medical Director of Flow Cytometry at Boston Children's Hospital, and Assistant Professor of Pediatrics at Harvard Medical School. The spouse of C. D. Platt is employed by Quest Diagnostics. A. A. Nguyen has nothing to disclose.

REFERENCES

1. Notarangelo LD, Bacchetta R, Casanova JL, et al. Human inborn errors of immunity: an expanding universe. Sci Immunol 2020;5(49). https://doi.org/10.1126/sciimmunol.abb1662.
2. Tangye SG, Al-Herz W, Bousfiha A, et al. Human inborn errors of immunity: 2022 update on the classification from the international union of immunological societies expert committee. J Clin Immunol 2022;42(7):1473–507.
3. Abraham RS, Aubert G. Flow cytometry, a versatile tool for diagnosis and monitoring of primary immunodeficiencies. Clin Vaccine Immunol 2016;23(4):254–71.
4. Farmer JR, DeLelys M. Flow cytometry as a diagnostic tool in primary and secondary immune deficiencies. Clin Lab Med 2019;39(4):591–607.
5. Kanegane H, Hoshino A, Okano T, et al. Flow cytometry-based diagnosis of primary immunodeficiency diseases. Allergol Int 2018;67(1):43–54.
6. Shearer WT, Rosenblatt HM, Gelman RS, et al. Lymphocyte subsets in healthy children from birth through 18 years of age : the Pediatric AIDS Clinical Trials Group P1009 study. J Allergy Clin Immunol 2003;112(5):973–80.
7. Mariuzza RA, Agnihotri P, Orban J. The structural basis of T-cell receptor (TCR) activation: an enduring enigma. J Biol Chem 2020;295(4):914.
8. Thakar MS, Logan BR, Puck JM, et al. Measuring the effect of newborn screening on survival after haematopoietic cell transplantation for severe combined immunodeficiency: a 36-year longitudinal study from the Primary Immune Deficiency Treatment Consortium. Lancet 2023;402(10396):129–40.

9. Hale JE, Platt CD, Bonilla FA, et al. Ten years of newborn screening for severe combined immunodeficiency (SCID) in Massachusetts. J Allergy Clin Immunol Pract 2021;9(5):2060–7.e2.

10. Dvorak CC, Haddad E, Heimall J, et al. The diagnosis of severe combined immunodeficiency (SCID): the primary immune deficiency treatment consortium (PIDTC) 2022 definitions. J Allergy Clin Immunol 2023;151(2):539–46.

11. Hanna S, Etzioni A. MHC class I and II deficiencies. J Allergy Clin Immunol 2014; 134(2):269–75.

12. Fischer A, Notarangelo LD, Neven B, et al. Severe combined immunodeficiencies and related disorders. Nat Rev Dis Prim 2015;1(1):1–18.

13. Roifman CM, Dadi H, Somech R, et al. Characterization of ζ-associated protein, 70 kd (ZAP70)-deficient human lymphocytes. J Allergy Clin Immunol 2010; 126(6). https://doi.org/10.1016/j.jaci.2010.07.029.

14. Stern A, Green H, Paul M, et al. Prophylaxis for Pneumocystis pneumonia (PCP) in non-HIV immunocompromised patients. Cochrane Database Syst Rev 2014; 2014(10). https://doi.org/10.1002/14651858.CD005590.PUB3.

15. Kimberlin DW, Barnet ED, Lynfield R, et al, editors. Red book: 2021–2024 report of the committee on infectious diseases. 32nd ed.; 2021.

16. Mahnke YD, Brodie TM, Sallusto F, et al. The who's who of T-cell differentiation: human memory T-cell subsets. Eur J Immunol 2013;43(11):2797–809.

17. Brummelman J, Pilipow K, Lugli E. The single-cell phenotypic identity of human CD8+ and CD4+ T cells. Int Rev Cell Mol Biol 2018;341:63–124.

18. Hofstee MI, Cevirgel A, de Zeeuw-Brouwer ML, et al. Cytomegalovirus and Epstein-Barr virus co-infected young and middle-aged adults can have an aging-related T-cell phenotype. Sci Rep 2023;13(1). https://doi.org/10.1038/S41598-023-37502-5.

19. Di Mitri D, Azevedo RI, Henson SM, et al. Reversible senescence in human CD4+CD45RA+CD27- memory T cells. J Immunol 2011;187(5):2093–100.

20. Schmidt-Supprian M, Courtois G, Tian J, et al. Mature T cells depend on signaling through the IKK complex. Immunity 2003;19(3):377–89.

21. Kohler S, Thiel A. Life after the thymus: CD31+ and CD31- human naive CD4+ T-cell subsets. Blood 2009;113(4):769–74.

22. Junge S, Kloeckener-Gruissem B, Zufferey R, et al. Correlation between recent thymic emigrants and CD31+ (PECAM-1) CD4+ T cells in normal individuals during aging and in lymphopenic children. Eur J Immunol 2007;37(11):3270–80.

23. Ricci S, Masini M, Valleriani C, et al. Reduced frequency of peripheral CD4+CD45RA+CD31+ cells and autoimmunity phenomena in patients affected by Del22q11 syndrome. Clin Immunol 2018;188:81–4.

24. Assing K, Nielsen C, Kirchhoff M, et al. CD4+ CD31+ recent thymic emigrants in CHD7 haploinsufficiency (CHARGE syndrome): a case. Hum Immunol 2013; 74(9):1047–50.

25. Van Den Broek T, Delemarre EM, Janssen WJM, et al. Neonatal thymectomy reveals differentiation and plasticity within human naive T cells. J Clin Invest 2016;126(3):1126–36.

26. Kumar D, Prince C, Bennett CM, et al. T-follicular helper cell expansion and chronic T-cell activation are characteristic immune anomalies in Evans syndrome 2022;139(3):369–83.

27. Schwab C, Gabrysch A, Olbrich P, et al. Phenotype, penetrance, and treatment of 133 cytotoxic T-lymphocyte antigen 4–insufficient subjects. J Allergy Clin Immunol 2018;142(6):1932–46.

28. Bateman EAL, Ayers L, Sadler R, et al. T cell phenotypes in patients with common variable immunodeficiency disorders: associations with clinical phenotypes in comparison with other groups with recurrent infections. Clin Exp Immunol 2012; 170(2):202.

29. Lucas CL, Kuehn HS, Zhao F, et al. Dominant-activating, germline mutations in phosphoinositide 3-kinase p110δ cause T cell senescence and human immuno-deficiency. Nat Immunol 2014;15(1):88.

30. Alroqi FJ, Charbonnier LM, Baris S, et al. Exaggerated follicular helper T-cell re-sponses in patients with LRBA deficiency caused by failure of CTLA4-mediated regulation. J Allergy Clin Immunol 2017. https://doi.org/10.1016/j.jaci.2017.05.022.

31. Kumar D, Nguyen TH, Bennett CM, et al. mTOR inhibition attenuates cTfh cell dysregulation and chronic T-cell activation in multilineage immune cytopenias. Blood 2023;141(3):238–43.

32. Fonseca S, Pereira V, Lau C, et al. Human peripheral blood gamma delta T cells: report on a series of healthy caucasian Portuguese adults and comprehensive re-view of the literature. Cells 2020;9(3). https://doi.org/10.3390/CELLS9030729.

33. Li H, Tsokos GC. Double-negative T cells in autoimmune diseases. Curr Opin Rheumatol 2021;33(2):163–72.

34. Matson DR, Yang DT. Autoimmune lymphoproliferative syndrome: an overview. Arch Pathol Lab Med 2020;144(2):245–51.

35. Caminha I, Fleisher TA, Hornung RL, et al. Using biomarkers to predict the pres-ence of FAS mutations in patients with features of the autoimmune lymphoprolifer-ative syndrome. J Allergy Clin Immunol 2010;125(4):946.

36. Sakaguchi S, Miyara M, Costantino CM, et al. FOXP3+ regulatory T cells in the human immune system. Nat Rev Immunol 2010;10(7):490–500.

37. Alroqi FJ, Chatila TA. T Regulatory cell biology in health and disease. Curr Allergy Asthma Rep 2016;16(4):1–8.

38. Cepika AM, Sato Y, Liu JMH, et al. Tregopathies: monogenic diseases resulting in regulatory T-cell deficiency. J Allergy Clin Immunol 2018;142(6):1679–95.

39. Borna S, Meffre E, Bacchetta R. FOXP3 deficiency, from the mechanisms of the dis-ease to curative strategies. Immunol Rev 2023. https://doi.org/10.1111/imr.13289.

40. Afzali B, Grönholm J, Vandrovcova J, et al. BACH2 immunodeficiency illustrates an association between super-enhancers and haploinsufficiency. Nat Immunol 2017;18(7):813–23.

41. Gámez-Díaz L, Grimbacher B. Immune checkpoint deficiencies and autoimmune lymphoproliferative syndromes. Biomed J 2021;44(4):400–11.

42. Kurata I, Matsumoto I, Sumida T. T follicular helper cell subsets : a potential key player in autoimmunity. Immunol Med 2021;44(1):1–9.

43. Laurent C, Fazilleau N, Brousset P. A novel subset of T-helper cells: follicular T-helper cells and their markers. Haematologica 2010;95(3):356–8.

44. LaBere B, Nguyen AA, Habiballah SB, et al. Clinical utility of measuring CD4+ T follicular cells in patients with immune dysregulation. J Autoimmun 2023; 140(August):103088.

45. Caldirola MS, Martínez MP, Bezrodnik L, et al. Immune monitoring of patients with primary immune regulation disorders unravels higher frequencies of follicular T cells with different profiles that associate with alterations in B cell subsets. Front Immunol 2020;11:576724.

46. Lo B, Zhang K, Lu W, et al. Patients with LRBA deficiency show CTLA4 loss and immune dysregulation responsive to abatacept therapy. Science (1979) 2015; 349(6246):436–40.

47. Bonilla FA, Khan DA, Ballas ZK, et al. Practice parameter for the diagnosis and management of primary immunodeficiency. J Allergy Clin Immunol 2015;136(5): 1178–86.

48. Kumánovics A, Sadighi Akha AA. Flow cytometry for B-cell subset analysis in immunodeficiencies. J Immunol Methods 2022;509(August). https://doi.org/10.1016/j.jim.2022.113327.

49. Pavlasova G, Mraz M. The regulation and function of CD20: an "enigma" of B-cell biology and targeted therapy. Haematologica 2020;105(6):1494–506.

50. Smith T, Cunningham-Rundles C. Primary B-cell immunodeficiencies. Hum Immunol 2019;80(6):351–62.

51. Le Coz C, Nguyen DN, Su C, et al. Constrained chromatin accessibility in PU.1-mutated agammaglobulinemia patients. J Exp Med 2021;218(7). https://doi.org/10.1084/jem.20201750.

52. Ahn S, Cunningham-Rundles C. Role of B cells in common variable immune deficiency. Expet Rev Clin Immunol 2009;5(5):557–64.

53. Novi G, Bovis F, Fabbri S, et al. Tailoring B cell depletion therapy in MS according to memory B cell monitoring. Neurology(R) neuroimmunology & neuroinflammation 2020;7(5). https://doi.org/10.1212/NXI.0000000000000845.

54. Colucci M, Carsetti R, Cascioli S, et al. B cell reconstitution after rituximab treatment in idiopathic nephrotic syndrome. J Am Soc Nephrol 2016;27(6):1811–22.

55. Fribourg M, Cioni M, Ghiggeri G, et al. CyTOF-enabled analysis identifies class-switched B cells as the main lymphocyte subset associated with disease relapse in children with idiopathic nephrotic syndrome. Front Immunol 2021;12:726428.

56. Klein U, Rajewsky K, Küppers R. Human immunoglobulin (Ig)M+IgD+ peripheral blood B cells expressing the CD27 cell surface antigen carry somatically mutated variable region genes: CD27 as a general marker for somatically mutated (memory) B cells. J Exp Med 1998;188(9):1679–89.

57. Bautista D, Vásquez C, Ayala-ramírez P, et al. Differential expression of IgM and IgD discriminates two subpopulations of human circulating IgM + IgD + CD27 + B Cells that differ phenotypically , functionally , and genetically. Front Immunol 2020;11(May):1–19.

58. Weller S, Braun MC, Tan BK, et al. Human blood IgM "memory" B cells are circulating splenic marginal zone B cells harboring a prediversified immunoglobulin repertoire. Blood 2004;104(12):3647–54.

59. Hendricks J, Bos NA, Kroese FGM. Heterogeneity of memory marginal zone B cells. Crit Rev Immunol 2018;38(2):145–58.

60. Capolunghi F, Rosado MM, Sinibaldi M, et al. Why do we need IgM memory B cells? Immunol Lett 2013;152(2):114–20.

61. Tangye SG, Good KL. Human IgM+CD27+ B cells: memory B cells or "memory" B cells? J Immunol 2007;179(1):13–9.

62. Weill JC, Weller S, Reynaud CA. Human marginal zone B cells. Annu Rev Immunol 2009;27:267–85.

63. Cameron PU, Jones P, Gorniak M, et al. Splenectomy associated changes in IgM memory B cells in an adult spleen registry cohort 2011;6(8). https://doi.org/10.1371/journal.pone.0023164.

64. Kruetzmann S, Rosado MM, Weber H, et al. Human immunoglobulin M memory B cells controlling streptococcus pneumoniae infections are generated in the spleen 2003;197(7). https://doi.org/10.1084/jem.20022020.

65. Chiu SN, Shao PL, Wang JK, et al. Low immunoglobulin M memory B-cell percentage in patients with heterotaxy syndrome correlates with the risk of severe bacterial infection. Pediatr Res 2016;79(2):271–7.

66. Carsetti R, Rosado MM, Donnanno S, et al. The loss of IgM memory B cells correlates with clinical disease in common variable immunodeficiency. J Allergy Clin Immunol 2005;115(2):412–7.
67. Agematsu K, Futatani T, Hokibara S, et al. Absence of memory B cells in patients with common variable immunodeficiency. Clin Immunol 2002;103(1):34–42.
68. Sánchez-Ramón S, Radigan L, Yu JE, et al. Memory B cells in common variable immunodeficiency: clinical associations and sex differences. Clin Immunol 2008; 128(3):314–21.
69. D'Orsogna LJ, Krueger RG, McKinnon EJ, et al. Circulating memory B-cell subpopulations are affected differently by HIV infection and antiretroviral therapy. AIDS 2007;21(13):1747–52.
70. Morrow M, Valentin A, Little R, et al. A splenic marginal zone-like peripheral blood CD27+B220- B cell population is preferentially depleted in HIV type 1-infected individuals. AIDS Res Hum Retroviruses 2008;24(4):621–33.
71. Zhou Y, Zhang Y, Han J, et al. Transitional B cells involved in autoimmunity and their impact on neuroimmunological diseases. J Transl Med 2020;18(131):1–12.
72. Abraham RS. How to evaluate for immunodeficiency in patients with autoimmune cytopenias: laboratory evaluation for the diagnosis of inborn errors of immunity associated with immune dysregulation. Hematology: the American Society of Hematology Education Program 2020;2020(1):661.
73. Nutt SL, Hodgkin PD, Tarlinton DM, et al. The generation of antibody-secreting plasma cells. Nat Rev Immunol 2015;15(3):160–71.
74. Chovancova Z, Vlkova M, Litzman J, et al. Antibody forming cells and plasmablasts in peripheral blood in CVID patients after vaccination. Vaccine 2011; 29(24):4142–50.
75. Wallace ZS, Mattoo H, Carruthers M, et al. Plasmablasts as a biomarker for IgG4-related disease, independent of serum IgG4 concentrations. Ann Rheum Dis 2015;74(1):190–5.
76. Ling Q, Shen L, Zhang W, et al. Increased plasmablasts enhance T cell-mediated beta cell destruction and promote the development of type 1 diabetes. Mol Med 2022;28(1):1–16.
77. Elmér E, Smargianaki S, Pettersson Å, et al. Increased frequencies of switched memory B cells and plasmablasts in peripheral blood from patients with ANCA-associated vasculitis. J Immunol Res 2020;2020.
78. Gjertsson I, Mcgrath S, Grimstad K, et al. A close-up on the expanding landscape of CD21-/low B cells in humans. Clin Exp Immunol 2022;210:217–29.
79. Isnardi I, Ng YS, Menard L, et al. Complement receptor 2/CD21− human naive B cells contain mostly autoreactive unresponsive clones. Blood 2010;115(24):5026.

Applications of Flow Cytometry in Diagnosis and Evaluation of Red Blood Cell Disorders

Alexis Dadelahi, PhD[a,b], Taylor Jackson, DO[a,b],
Archana M. Agarwal, MD[a,c,d], Leo Lin, MD, PhD[a,e,f,g,h],
Anton V. Rets, MD, PhD[a,d,i], David P. Ng, MD[a,d,j,k,*]

KEYWORDS

- Flow cytometry • Red blood cell disorder • Band 3 • Fetal–maternal hemorrhage
- Paroxysmal nocturnal hemoglobinuria

KEY POINTS

- Flow cytometric analysis is a technique with high sensitivity, specificity, and throughput, making it a valuable tool for analyzing peripheral blood cells.
- Clinical flow cytometry plays a central role in the diagnosis and monitoring of multiple red blood cells abnormalities such as paroxysmal nocturnal hemoglobinuria, fetal–maternal hemorrhage, and hereditary spherocytosis.
- Using widely available consensus guidelines, flow cytometric analysis is becoming more standardized across different laboratories leading to improved test result portability and continuity of care for patients.

INTRODUCTION

Flow cytometric analysis (FCA) is a vital component of clinical laboratory diagnostics, and its role in clinical medicine continues to expand as the technology evolves. Unlike

[a] Department of Pathology, University of Utah, 15 N. Medical Drive East, Suite 1100, Salt Lake City, UT 84112, USA; [b] ARUP Laboratories, Salt Lake City, UT, USA; [c] Special Hematology, ARUP Laboratories, Salt Lake City, UT, USA; [d] Hematopathology, ARUP Laboratories, Salt Lake City, UT, USA; [e] Research and Innovation, ARUP Laboratories, Salt Lake City, UT, USA; [f] Immunologic Flow Cytometry, ARUP Laboratories, Salt Lake City, UT, USA; [g] Immunology, ARUP Laboratories, Salt Lake City, UT, USA; [h] PharmaDx, Research & Innovation ARUP Laboratories, 500 Chipeta Way, MS 115, Salt Lake City, UT 84108, USA; [i] Immunohistochemistry and Histology, ARUP Laboratories, Salt Lake City, UT, USA; [j] Applied Artificial Intelligence and Bioinformatics, ARUP Laboratories, Salt Lake City, UT, USA; [k] Hematologic Flow Cytometry, ARUP Laboratories, Salt Lake City, UT, USA
* Corresponding author. 500 Chipeta Way, MC G04-115, Salt Lake City, UT 84108.
E-mail address: david.ng@aruplab.com

Clin Lab Med 44 (2024) 495–509
https://doi.org/10.1016/j.cll.2024.04.010
0272-2712/24/© 2024 Elsevier Inc. All rights reserved.

many other methods currently used in the clinical laboratory setting, FCA is unique in that it permits the direct assessment of individual cell in large numbers on a high throughput platform, allowing for access to a broad range of information pertinent to patient care, such as immunophenotyping, cell number and distribution, and even insight into cell function. While modern-day flow cytometers are highly sophisticated instruments capable of interrogating thousands of cells per second with simultaneous multiparameter measurement and analysis, many of the basic fundamentals of modern day FCA have been clinically relevant for over 70 years. For instance, in 1947, the first air flux cytometers, capable of detecting 0.5 μm events by scattered light, were developed in response to the US Army's desire for a system capable of rapid detection of bacterial biowarfare agents in aerosols. By 1950, the first fluorescein isothiocyanate (FITC) antibody conjugation was described,[1] a concept that remains a cornerstone of FCA today. Almost 30 years later, new fluorochromes that could be employed in multicolor flow cytometry were developed, and, combined with the production of monoclonal antibodies targeting blood lymphoid antigens, modern FCA was born.[1]

While the basic analytical capacity of flow cytometric analyzers has greatly expanded over time, the fundamental principles involved in FCA remain largely unchanged. Simply, a cell suspension is forced into a stream of fluid with a set flow rate with thousands of cells passing through the beam of a laser one by one at the interrogation point. Populations of cells of interest are recognized by the measurement of different parameters based on the behavior of the light beam as it passes through the cell (forward scatter [FSC] and side scatter [SSC]), as well as the signal emission of any fluorescent marker detected with an optical collection system on the flow cytometer. Low-angle light diffusion is known as FSC, and the magnitude of FSC is roughly correlated to the relative size of the cell passing through the beam. SSC refers to the light diffusion, which occurs at larger angles (collected at 90° of the laser beam) and results from diffusion, reflection, and refraction due to the structural complexity of a cell. SSC correlates with the granularity of a cell population.[1] Thus, granulocytes are typically identified based on having higher SSC compared to lymphocyte populations.

Red blood cells (RBCs) are significantly smaller than white blood cells (WBCs); however, it is not possible to easily discriminate between RBCs and leukocytes using FSC and SSC alone.[2] Many cytometers are equipped with both blue (488 nm) and violet (405 nm) lasers, which allows for easy differentiation of RBCs and WBCs based on a unique scatter pattern in human whole blood when events are assessed in the context of blue versus violet SSC. Since RBCs contain hemoglobin, which readily absorbs violet light, they can be easily separated from WBCs that display a higher violet SSC[2] (**Fig. 1**). Finally, the application of antibodies conjugated with fluorochromes confers the ability to assess expression of several cellular markers simultaneously. By evaluating the presence or absence of a marker, coexpression with other markers of interest, and determining the level of intensity of the expression (ie, a dim signal correlates with a lower expression level of the protein of interest on/in a given cell), we can extract information regarding the types of cells present, the functional status of those cells, and the relative abundance with which they are occurring in a given sample of interest.

Based on this information, FCA can be utilized to investigate various aspects of a suspected disease state in the clinic. FCA has been most readily adapted to the detection of hematologic neoplasm due to the nature of the specimen (liquid-phase) with most hematologic neoplasms expressing identifiable proteins on their cell surface available for immunophenotyping. Flow cytometry has since become a mainstay in the diagnosis of hematologic neoplasms (see article Hartzell et al, "Flow Cytometric Assessment of Malignant Hematologic Disorders," in this issue).

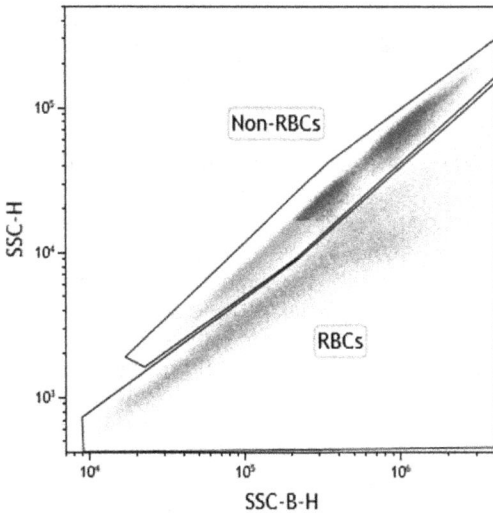

Fig. 1. Separation of RBCs from leukocytes using differential absorption of violet (405 nm) versus blue (488 nm) light.

FCA has also been extended to hematology analyzers. The current hematology analyzer in most hospital and reference laboratory settings utilizes the principle of flow cytometry to distinguish cells rapidly and in high volume in generation of complete blood counts (CBCs) and has largely replaced manual cell differentials. Many instruments are currently on the market, with most using flow cytometry as the method of choice for clinical CBCs (see article Shean et al, "Advances in Hematology Analyzers Technology," in this issue). While the potential applications for FCA are multiple and growing, the main thrust of this review is to elaborate and discuss the use of flow cytometry in the characterization and diagnosis of RBC disorders.

UTILITY OF FLOW CYTOMETRIC ANALYSIS IN PAROXYSMAL NOCTURNAL HEMOGLOBINURIA AND ASSOCIATED ANEMIA

Paroxysmal nocturnal hemoglobinuria (PNH) is an acquired clonal hematologic disorder caused by a deficiency or absence of glycosyl phosphatidylinositol-anchored membrane proteins (GPI-APs) on RBCs and WBCs, which can lead to recurrent episodic intravascular hemolysis and venous thrombosis. Disease is most often associated with somatic variants in the phosphatidylinositol glycan class A (*PIGA*) gene located on the X chromosome. The protein encoded by *PIGA* is essential for biosynthesis of the GPI-anchors required for tethering GPI proteins to the cell surface.[3] The absence or deficiency of GPI-APs increases cell sensitivity to complement-mediated cell lysis, resulting in varying degrees of RBC hemolysis and disease severity.[4,5] FCA of GPI-AP expression on RBCs and WBCs remains the gold standard for both diagnosis and monitoring of PNH, though it is important to bear in mind that the presence of a PNH clone alone is not sufficient for a diagnosis of PNH.[6-10]

In PNH, defective GPI anchoring is responsible for decreased expression of several (more than 15) proteins on the cell surface. Among them are decay-accelerating factor (CD55) and homologous restriction factor (CD59). Early methodology assessed expression levels of CD55 and CD59 on RBCs and WBCs.[7,8,11] Cells with reduced expression of CD55 and CD59 were classified as type II cells, while cells completely lacking GPI-AP expression were classified as type III cells. Type II and type III cells were used as an indicator of PNH clone size in support of a diagnosis of PNH when combined with other clinical signs and symptoms (ie, appropriate clinical setting, laboratory markers of hemolysis, unexplained thrombosis, and so forth[4]). While this strategy provided a reliable way for quantifying major PNH clones, it lacked adequate accuracy and sensitivity in patients with minor clones (<1%–4%). Additionally, assay resolution was hindered by the absence of RBC-specific and WBC-specific lineage markers.[6,11,12]

Minor PNH clones are often observed in patients with other causes of anemia such as aplastic anemia and some subsets of myelodysplastic syndrome.[4,5,11,13–15] Although these patients do not always exhibit clinical symptoms of PNH, detection and monitoring of these clones is critical[11,16] for diagnostic, prognostic, and therapeutic purposes. Moreover, smaller PNH clones in the RBC component may elude detection due to their susceptibility to hemolysis and/or their dilution in the setting of a recent RBC transfusion.[4,11] For these reasons, highly sensitive assays have been developed and are now recommended by the International Clinical Cytometry Society and European Society for Clinical Cell Analysis guidelines for detecting GPI-deficient cells in PNH and related disorders.[4,17,18]

FCA for quantifying PNH clones demands special considerations for analysis and interpretation for 2 reasons: the limited number (in some cases extremely) of events detected and the fact that the assay measures a population *lacking* a fluorescent signal. It is essential to exclude artifacts related to the assay from inclusion in the PNH-positive population. Multiparameter gating strategies (outlined in later discussion) are employed to reduce this risk, but each laboratory must ensure the established cutoff for PNH-positive populations is substantially higher than the background rate in normal samples for the reportable population. Small populations of suspected PNH cells can be confirmed by collecting more events and observing an increase in PNH cells commensurate with the rise in measured events. However, if a change in the distribution of PNH-positive events from the initial collection is observed, results should be interpreted with caution.[6] It is also important to be mindful of setting a cutoff value for PNH-positive clone percentages well above the percentage of PNH phenotypic cells expected in normal individuals (2–6/million for RBCs and 2–10/million in WBCs). To address this issue, the suggested detection threshold for assay sensitivity is 0.01%, which is 5 to 10× higher than the detectable incidence of GPI-deficient cells in normal samples, enhancing the clinical utility of these results.[6,19] Finally, to increase confidence in the measurement of small PNH clones as determined by the Poisson distribution, it is suggested to collect at least 100,000 events with greater than 20 definitive GPI-negative events identified to achieve high sensitivity while mitigating the possible contribution of artifacts.[6,19] Up to 1 million events can be collected in cases where PNH type III events are detected within the first 100,000 cells.[11] The exact level of precision requisite for determining the actual percentage of PNH cells at the low end of sensitivity has yet to be determined, but collection of 50 events resulting in a standard deviation of ± 7 and a coeffecient of variation (CV) of 14% (governed by Poisson statistics) is the current recommendation. The lower limit of quantitation can then be calculated as 50 PNH cells/number of gated events acquired × 100% and the population of PNH cells reported.[6,19]

Modern assays employ both CD59 and the RBC-specific marker CD235a (glycophorin A) to delineate abnormal (types II and III) clones from normal (type I)[11] (**Fig. 2**). Similarly, WBCs are assessed using the leukocyte-specific marker CD45 in combination with at least 2 GPI-linked structures.[11,17] This latter point of using at least 2 markers cannot be overstated as different cell lineages and different stages of maturation will display different levels of GPI-linked proteins. Indeed, in the setting of left

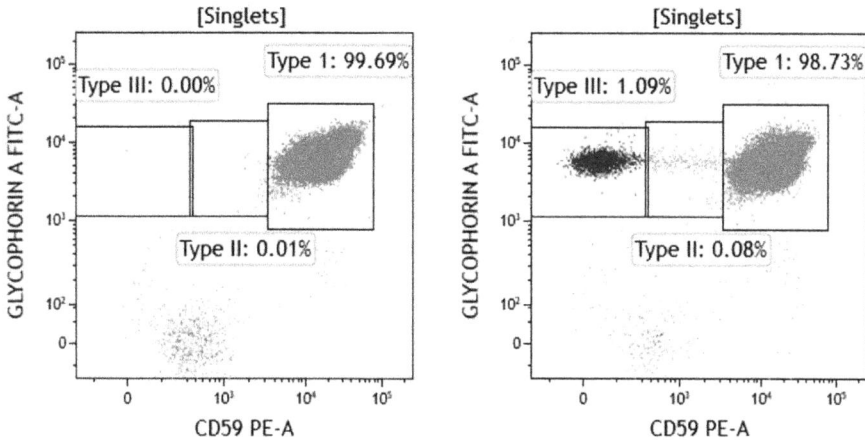

Fig. 2. Normal RBCs (Left), abnormal RBCs (*Right*) with moderate loss of CD59 consistent with a type III clone (*green population*), and near-complete loss of CD59 consistent with a type III clone (*blue population*).

shift, these analyses can be falsely positive, that is, showing decrease or loss of GPI-linked proteins not as the result of PNH but a significant population of immature cells (eg, CD24 or CD14 on immature granulocytes and monocytes, respectively).[17,20] This also implies that PNH assays cannot be performed in bone marrow specimens given the normal presence of immature forms. In modern assays, a fluorescent-labeled form (typically FITC or similar small molecule fluorophores) of the bacterially derived toxin proaerolysin, a virulence factor of *Aeromonas hydrophila*, which binds specifically to GPI anchor of proteins, is used in combination with either CD24 or CD157 (for neutrophils), or either CD14 or CD157 (for monocytes)[11,15,21,22] (**Table 1** and **Fig. 3**). Only type III clones are reported, as no clinical utility has been established for reporting type II clones among WBC populations.[6] Notably, the relative size of PNH clones

Table 1 Common antigens useful for detection of paroxysmal nocturnal hemoglobinuria clones among white blood cell populations		
Antigen	Target	Purpose
CD45	Leukocytes	Delineate monocytes/ neutrophils from platelets, cellular debris, and/or unlysed RBCs
CD64 (FcγI receptor)	Monocytes (mostly)	Monocyte gating
CD15	Neutrophil	Neutrophil gating
CD33	Monocytes and neutrophils	Gating, deprecated in modern literature
FLAER	GPI (monocytes and neutrophils)	GPI-linked
CD157	Monocytes/neutrophils	GPI-linked
CD16 (FcγIIIa receptor)	Monocytes (+, nonclassic subsets) and neutrophils (++)	GPI-linked, deprecated in modern literature
CD14	Monocyte	GPI-linked
CD24	Neutrophil	GPI-linked

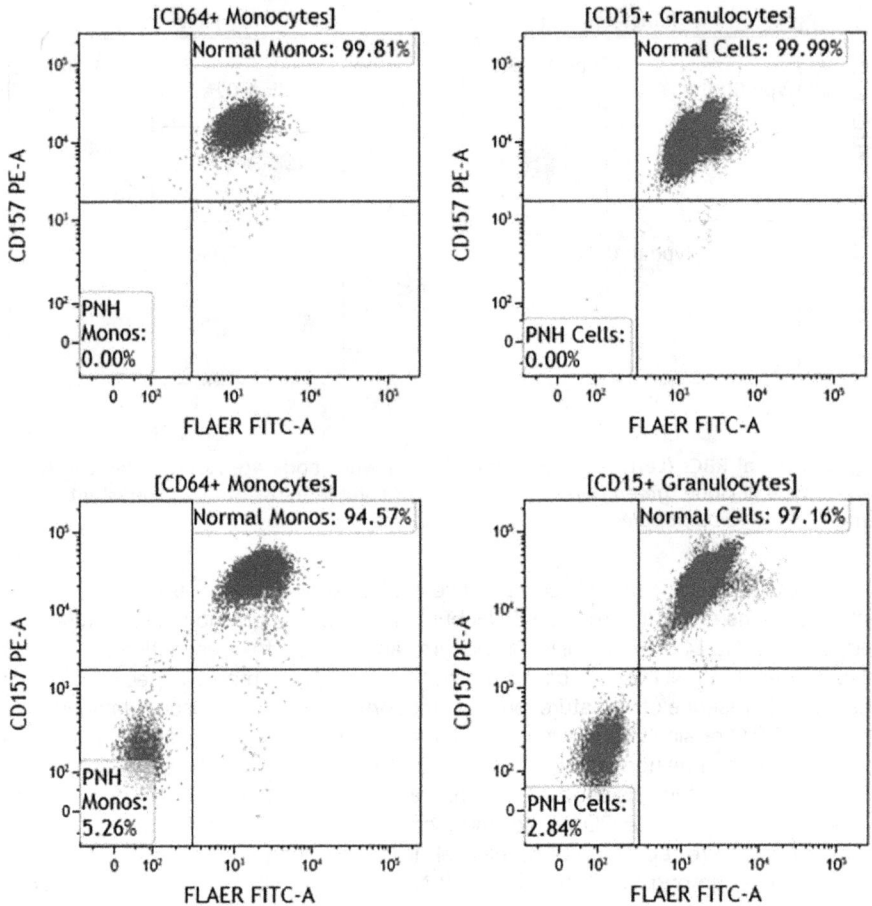

Fig. 3. Normal pattern of CD157 and FLAER on monocytes and granulocytes (*top*) and abnormal loss of FLAER and CD157 on monocytes and granulocytes (*bottom*).

may differ between the neutrophil and monocyte populations with monocytes often exhibiting larger clone sizes compared to neutrophils.[6,11,23] For this reason, monocytes may more accurately reflect the "true" PNH clone size as opposed to the neutrophil population and should always be reported when enough events are available for collection.[6,19] Currently, guidelines recommend reporting the quantitative data for PNH clones detected in WBCs (neutrophils and monocytes) and type II, type III, and total PNH clone proportions in RBCs to avoid falsely negative reports.[6]

FLOW CYTOMETRIC ANALYSIS OF FETAL HEMOGLOBIN

Similar to PNH, the ability of flow cytometric methods to rapidly and accurately identify and measure a target cell population has proven its utility in detecting the presence of RBCs with fetal hemoglobin (HbF) in the peripheral blood. HbF is the main Hb fraction in a fetus or newborn, though low-level HbF (1%–2%) synthesis remains throughout adult life and is restricted to a small subset of RBCs, referred to as "F-cells." HbF levels can be elevated in certain inherited hemoglobin disorders (eg, β-thalassemia, sickle cell anemia, and hereditary persistence of HbF[24–26]) or acquired conditions (a subset of myeloid neoplasms, treatment with medications such as hydroxyurea, and so forth). During pregnancy, however, the detection of increased levels of HbF in maternal circulation is indicative of a cross-placental transfer of fetal blood into the maternal circulation, or fetal–maternal hemorrhage (FMH).[27]

Low levels of FMH can occur during normal pregnancy, especially during labor and delivery, or after a traumatic event during pregnancy when the placenta is damaged.[25,27,28] In cases where rhesus factor (Rh)-negative mothers are exposed to Rh-positive fetal blood, the hemorrhage event can lead to alloimmunization of the mother (production of antibodies against Rh), which can have devastating consequences for future pregnancies such as hemolytic disease of the fetus and newborn, hydrops fetalis, and death.[25,27,28] Alloimmunization can be prevented by administration of anti-D immunoglobulin (Rho(D)) to the mother shortly after FMH occurs; however, the calculation of the correct dosage directly depends on the magnitude of the FMH detected. Since there are multiple potential causes of FMH and the volume of FMH can vary widely,[25,27] it is crucial to quickly and accurately quantify the amount of fetal blood in maternal circulation.

The traditional method for quantification of HbF is the Kleihauer–Betke test (KBT), which leverages the fact that fetal RBCs, predominantly containing HbF, are less resistant to acid elution than adult RBCs.[25] While the KBT requires minimal supplies and supporting instrumentation, it is labor intensive, requires enumeration of at least 2000 cells, and lacks standardization (eg, blood smear thickness, pH variations, interobserver/interhospital variance in result interpretation), all of which contribute to diminished accuracy and precision. Moreover, the presence of maternal F-cells can further confound result interpretation, at times leading to falsely elevated levels of FMH.[25,29–31] Overall, this method has been associated with both underestimation and overestimation of FMH.[25]

FCA in the context of FMH typically employs 1 of 2 strategies for identifying fetal cells in maternal circulation: (1) direct targeting and quantification of Rh factor or (2) staining and measurement of intracellular HbF. While the former offers some advantages, including shorter turnaround time and alleviation of maternal HbF confounding result interpretation,[27] it relies on an Rh status mismatch between mother and child to identify FMH. There is also the potential of overlooking the presence of Rh-positive cells due to reagent limitations in detecting weak D phenotypes, restricting the clinical utility of this approach.[25,27] Quantification of intracellular HbF ameliorates these issues. However, the need for fixation and permeabilization makes this strategy more technically challenging and time consuming compared to methods that rely on analysis of Rh on the RBC surface. As previously mentioned, F-cells retain HbF, representing an endogenous source of HbF in maternal circulation that requires careful use of controls to distinguish between maternal F-cells and HbF present in circulation because of FMH. Adult F-cells display heterogeneity in their hemoglobin production, typically containing a combination of adult hemoglobin (HbA) and HbF[32] **(Fig. 4)**. Excluding scenarios in which HbF is elevated in maternal circulation (ie, as a result of an inherited hemoglobin disorder such as sickle cell disease [SCD], β-thalassemia, and so forth), this allows for distinguishing between fetal-derived cells producing high levels of HbF and the lower HbF-expressing maternal F-cells that will show a distinctively dimmer peak upon analysis. To discriminate between these populations with high confidence, it is essential that controls are run concurrently to define the level of fluorescence attributed to fetal RBCs with high HbF content versus mid-to-low HbF expressing adult F-cells.[25] Using this practice, in most cases FCA can adequately distinguish between adult F-cells and fetal RBCs. Additionally, more RBCs can be analyzed faster by FCA compared to KBT leading to shorter turnaround times for test results and increased accuracy and reproducibility.[25]

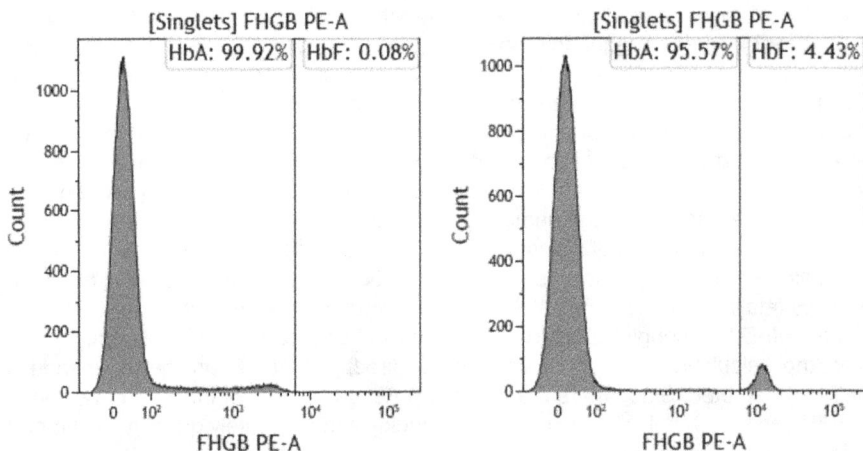

Fig. 4. (*Left*) Normal distribution of HbF F in peripheral blood RBCs. (*Right*) Abnormal population (~4.43%) of HbF F high RBCs consistent with FMH (peak just to the right of 10^4).

Compared to KBT or FCA methods targeting Rh for FMH quantification, FCA of HbF can also be of benefit in a broader range of clinical scenarios. Evaluation of HbF can aid in conditions characterized by elevated HbF in adults, such as tracking F-cell numbers in sickle cell anemia, which can be helpful for prognostic and therapeutic reasons. Despite these advantages, 94% of quantitative assays for FMH still utilize the KBT, likely due to the higher costs of FCA testing, the need for qualified technical staffing, and the difficulty associated with ensuring the availability of an FCA laboratory that provides rapid FMH testing around the clock.[29]

HEREDITARY SPHEROCYTOSIS/BAND 3 TESTING

Hereditary spherocytosis (HS) is a relatively common condition (prevalence of 1:2000 in some populations) and the most common cause of inherited hemolytic anemia.[33–38] It classically presents as hemolytic anemia, jaundice, and splenomegaly. The workup for hemolytic anemia includes complete blood count (CBC), documentation of hemolysis (eg, measurement of lactate dehydrogenase, indirect bilirubin, and haptoglobin), reticulocyte count, Coombs' test, and blood smear review. The diagnosis of HS historically relied on the correlation of clinical presentation and laboratory studies to achieve the correct diagnosis. Despite its relatively high prevalence, HS can be challenging to diagnose especially in neonates and in patients with autosomal recessive inheritance due to a lack of family history. Moreover, mild forms of the disease can be missed by routinely used diagnostic modalities.

Osmotic fragility testing (OFT) in conjunction with mean corpuscular hemoglobin concentration and review of RBC morphology have been utilized for many years to help diagnose HS. Flow cytometric methods have also been developed to aid the diagnosis of HS including flow cytometry osmotic fragility (FC-OFT) and flow cytometry eosin-5′-maleimide (FC-EMA) binding test. In comparison to OFT, both FC-OFT and FC-EMA have been shown to have greater sensitivity and specificity. However, the advanced technical requirements to perform these FC-based assays is a limiting factor at many institutions.

Several RBC proteins in the membrane skeleton protein complex may be involved in HS including ankyrin, alpha-spectrin and beta-spectrin, Band 3 protein (an anion channel protein), and protein 4.2.[39] Deficiency in these proteins leads to dysfunctional vertical cytoskeleton-membrane interactions and causes membrane instability and membrane loss. An increased surface-to-volume ratio, morphologically manifested as microspherocytosis, is also responsible for increased RBC fragility and RBC lysis (both in vivo and in vitro), resulting in the clinical manifestations of HS. The OFT, which demonstrates an abnormally high propensity of RBCs to in vitro lysis induced by hypotonic solutions, has low diagnostic specificity and does not allow one to distinguish between HS and other spherocytic disorders, or other causes of hemolysis such as autoimmune hemolytic anemia. In contrast, FC-OFT demonstrates higher sensitivity and specificity (97% and 95.8%, respectively[10]) when compared to traditional OFT in the diagnosis of HS.[40] Higher sensitivity makes FC-OFT a good screening test for HS.[41] Similar to traditional OFT, patient's RBCs are added to increasingly hypotonic saline. After incubation, the sample is run on the flow cytometer to determine the percentage of intact cells.[42]

Of the membrane proteins responsible for HS, Band 3 is essential for the stabilization of the cytoskeleton/membrane complex.[43] Mutations in the gene coding for the Band 3 protein can result in decreased protein in the membrane, resulting in the HS phenotype. In addition, aberrancies in other proteins that weaken the vertical membrane protein interaction also cause a decrease in RBC membrane Band 3 expression, as Band 3 is also lost during membrane fragmentation. Therefore, Band 3 is in many ways an ideal target for a flow cytometric detection of HS. Moreover, Band 3 is abundantly present on the surface of RBCs and can be targeted by the fluorescent dye EMA.[44] The decreased binding of EMA to Band 3 detected by decreased RBC EMA fluorescence is indicative of Band 3 loss from the RBC membrane (**Fig. 5**).[42] FC-EMA has high specificity and sensitivity (reportedly >90%) for HS diagnosis.[44–46] FC-EMA is also able to distinguish the RBCs in HS from the RBCs in hereditary pyropoikilocytosis (HPP) based on the differences in mean fluorescence intensity (MFI; the MFI for RBC EMA fluorescence is lower in HPP compared to HS).[44] This assay requires smaller specimen volume compared to traditional OFT making it ideal for pediatric and neonatal patients.[47–49]

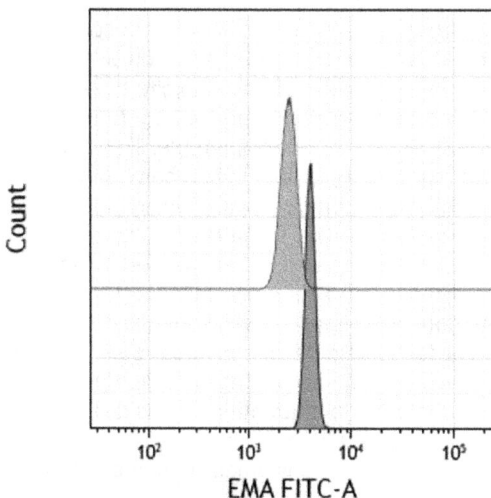

Fig. 5. Band 3 testing with EMA. Red: normal control, Green: abnormal patient sample with left-shifted MFI peak (decreased EMA binding).

Among the assays currently available for the evaluation of HS, FC-EMA has been shown to have increased sensitivity and a comparably high specificity.[50] A reduced MFI has predominantly been the single parameter used across the scientific community when FC-EMA is used for a diagnosis of HS.[51] An HS method comparison study evaluating FC-EMA showed that using a decrease in the MFI or increase in the coefficient of variation of the signal peak resulted in an assay sensitivity of 67% to 70% with specificities greater than 90%. When a decrease in the MFI and increase in the CV of the peak were evaluated in conjunction, HS assay sensitivity increased to 83% with a specificity still greater than 90%.[50]

The current recommendations for diagnosing HS include the initial evaluation of the CBC and RBC indices, review of the peripheral blood smear, hemolysis studies (indirect bilirubin, lactate dehydrogenase, haptoglobin, and reticulocytes), and Coombs' testing followed by confirmatory testing using one of the following methods: FC-EMA, OFT, glycerol lysis testing, or cryohemolysis. Flow cytometric methods have demonstrated superiority over traditional methods in diagnosing HS. Of note, in one of the articles reviewed,[41] for their HS test population, FC-OFT was performed concurrently with FC-EMA in children with clinically confirmed disease. While most affected patients' results were as expected by both methods, a small number did test positive on one method and negative on the other. Due to the low-specimen volumes needed for both FC-OFT and FC-EMA, it may be beneficial to perform both tests concurrently within the pediatric population. It would also be reasonable to perform these tests to identify patients eligible for definitive molecular confirmation of HS, as molecular testing is still significantly more expensive and has a longer turnaround time compared to the FC methods.[41]

IMAGING FLOW CYTOMETRY

In traditional hematologic flow cytometry, WBCs are identified and categorized by their FSC/SSC and fluorescence characteristics. Characterization of cells is based on detecting the scatter of light (FSC and SSC) as single cells are passed through a laser. The size and complexity differentiate the type of WBCs, and that data are displayed on a flow plot. Early flow cytometers used unstained cells characterization, but using the same principle, white cells treated with fluorescent dyes specific for surface proteins allowed for greater characterization with the addition of more lasers used at different wavelengths that would excite the fluorescent dyes attached to the cells. This allowed for greater number of targets per run while being able to still use a relatively small volume of patient sample. This method, however, was unable to incorporate the morphologic findings as has been evaluated by bright-field microscopy for decades. Morphologic evaluation by staining cells and inspection by bright-field microscopy continues to be the mainstay for RBC disorders but is limited by the relatively low numbers of cells assessed by an observer. This process is labor intensive, subjective, and requires advanced training to achieve competency.[52] The introduction of imaging flow cytometry combined these methods in which a digital camera takes photos of individual cells as they pass through the flow chamber, thereby enabling morphologic evaluation using bright-field, dark-field, and/or fluorescent images to characterize each cell.[53] Imaging flow cytometry offers the ability to morphologically evaluate orders of magnitude more cells that can help identify pathologic conditions where only a small percentage of the cells are of interest.

One of the settings where imaging flow cytometry has been used is SCD. In SCD, abnormal beta-chain results in Hb polymerization under hypoxic conditions causing the characteristic crescentic RBC shape. Imaging flow cytometry can characterize significantly more RBCs leading to increased sensitivity and accuracy in determining disease burden, especially in the posttreatment setting.[54]

Some infectious diseases affecting RBCs that are evaluated by light microscopy is another setting when imaging flow cytometry can be beneficial. Malaria, for example, has traditionally been identified by evaluation of thick and thin prep peripheral blood smears that is labor intensive and requires technical expertise in both the smear preparation and evaluation phases of testing. Flow cytometric methods of detection were developed in which DNA-specific fluorescent dyes added to the specimen would bind malarial DNA present in infected RBCs with uninfected RBCs not fluorescing; however, technical limitations still affected accurate detection of infected cells.[55] The advantage of imaging flow cytometry over conventional flow cytometry is the ability to morphologically identify erythrocytes containing *Plasmodium* organisms in a high throughput manner, while also generating multiple fluorescent images along with dark-field and bright-field images.[55]

The use of imaging flow cytometry is currently limited to large laboratories and research institutions. However, this technique offers the potential for increasing identification of challenging erythrocyte disorders that currently rely on lower throughput methods. Limitations of these methods include lower throughput compared with non-imaging flow cytometers (100s to 1000 of events per second [eps] compared with >10,000 eps) and the need for sophisticated analysis pipelines to segment and classify cell images requiring the development of machine learning tools designed with large, annotated images datasets, which are not currently available using traditional light microscopy methods.

SUMMARY

The use of flow cytometry shows a clear advantage in diagnosing multiple diseases of RBCs compared to other methods that have lower throughput with increased labor requirements and potentially lower specificity and sensitivity. In contrast, FCA offers exponentially higher throughput, both regarding the cell and sample numbers assessed, with superior sensitivity and specificity compared to previous methods of detection. Moreover, modern FCA assays can be readily standardized across laboratories and the potential for automation reduces the cost, labor, and time required by many older methods while improving the reproducibility and robustness of the results acquired. Together, these features have proven crucial in the application of FCA in the investigation and diagnosis of many abnormalities, particularly for rare RBC disorders such as subclinical PNH and sickle cell trait.

As with every method, potential advantages must be weighed against the disadvantages. Changes in medical technology often are slow moving and require education and adoption by clinicians. Importantly, a major factor in successful transition to newer methods is "buy in" by clinicians willing to adopt the use of these tests in lieu of the "traditional" assays. Integrating new technologies unavoidably comes with new/unfamiliar technical issues, which are often easy to address, but can diminish the ability to convince clinicians the assay is an improvement over the older methods it replaced. Furthermore, setting up a modern flow cytometry laboratory comes with significant personnel and hardware costs compared to older test methodologies. The advantage in the case of flow cytometry is that the technology itself is well established and the technical issues that arise are often predictable and addressable. Finally, investment in effective training and competency of the technical staff performing the tests is imperative and their expertise is not to be discounted.

CLINICS CARE POINTS

- FCA provides a rapid and accurate approach for measuring target cells of interest, and often offers enhanced sensitivity and specificity compared to traditional methodologies. These characteristics make FCA particularly useful in the context of RBC disorders which benefit from highly sensitive methods and/or those requiring prompt investigation, such as PNH and FMH.
- The rapidity and relative low cost of FCA can facilitate affordable screening prior to more expensive confirmatory molecular testing in some RBC disorders such as HS.
- Imaging flow cytometry enables the morphologic evaluation of cells in conjunction with traditional flow cytometry evaluation. This increases sensitivity and accuracy via higher throughput of cells relative to traditional methods. The addition of morphologic evaluation decreases the potential pitfalls of overcalling in the presence of non-specific binding within a specimen.
- Barriers to FCA include significant investment in instrumentation and well-trained personnel, as well as familiarity of these assays by ordering clinicians. Laboratories currently performing other flow cytometry assays can more easily adopt FCA testing for RBC disorders, leading to increased familiarity and more widespread adoption of the technology as the gold standard of care.

DISCLOSURE

Authors have nothing to disclose.

REFERENCES

1. Picot J, Guerin CL, Le Van Kim C, et al. Flow cytometry: retrospective, fundamentals and recent instrumentation. Cytotechnology 2012;64(2):109–30.
2. Rico LG, Salvia R, Ward MD, et al. Flow-cytometry-based protocols for human blood/marrow immunophenotyping with minimal sample perturbation. STAR Protoc 2021;2(4):100883.
3. Nafa K, Mason PJ, Hillmen P, et al. Bessler. Mutations in the PIG-A gene causing paroxysmal nocturnal hemoglobinuria are mainly of the frameshift type. Blood 1995;86(12).
4. Dezern AE, Borowitz MJ. ICCS/ESCCA consensus guidelines to detect GPI-deficient cells in paroxysmal nocturnal hemoglobinuria (PNH) and related disorders part 1 - clinical utility. Cytometry B Clin Cytometry 2018;94(1).
5. Charles P, Mitsuhiro O, Stephen R, et al. Diagnosis and management of paroxysmal nocturnal hemoglobinuria. Blood 2005;106(12).
6. Andrea I, Iuri M, Sutherland DR, et al. ICCS/ESCCA consensus guidelines to detect GPI-deficient cells in paroxysmal nocturnal hemoglobinuria (PNH) and related disorders part 3 - data analysis, reporting and case studies. Cytometry B Clin Cytometry 2018;94(1).
7. vdS CE, TW H, vtV-K ET, et al. Deficiency of glycosyl-phosphatidylinositol-linked membrane glycoproteins of leukocytes in paroxysmal nocturnal hemoglobinuria, description of a new diagnostic cytofluorometric assay. Blood 1990;76(9).
8. Hall SE, Rosse WF. The use of monoclonal antibodies and flow cytometry in the diagnosis of paroxysmal nocturnal hemoglobinuria. Blood 1996;87(12).
9. Richards SJ, Rawstron AC, Hillmen P. Application of flow cytometry to the diagnosis of paroxysmal nocturnal hemoglobinuria. Cytometry 2000;42(4).

10. Moyo VM, Mukhina GL, Garret ES, et al. Natural history of paroxysmal nocturnal haemoglobinuria using modern diagnostic assays. Br J Haematol 2004;126(1).
11. Sutherland DR, Andrea I, Iuri M, et al. ICCS/ESCCA consensus guidelines to detect GPI-deficient cells in paroxysmal nocturnal hemoglobinuria (PNH) and related disorders part 2 - reagent selection and assay optimization for high-sensitivity testing. Cytometry B Clin Cytometry 2018;94(1).
12. Sutherland DR, N Kuek, Juan AO, et al. Use of a FLAER-based WBC assay in the primary screening of PNH clones. Am J Clin Pathol 2009;132(4).
13. Azra R, Farhad R, Anjay R, et al. A prospective multicenter study of paroxysmal nocturnal hemoglobinuria cells in patients with bone marrow failure. Cytometry B Clin Cytometry 2014;86(3).
14. Marta M, FS Alex, Enrique C, et al. Diagnostic screening of paroxysmal nocturnal hemoglobinuria: prospective multicentric evaluation of the current medical indications. Cytometry B Clin Cytometry 2017;92(5).
15. Sutherland DR, Keeney M, Illingworth A. Practical guidelines for the high-sensitivity detection and monitoring of paroxysmal nocturnal hemoglobinuria clones by flow cytometry. Cytometry B Clin Cytometry 2012;82(4).
16. Pilar Maria H-C, Julia A, Maria Luz S, et al. Normal patterns of expression of glycosylphosphatidylinositol-anchored proteins on different subsets of peripheral blood cells: a frame of reference for the diagnosis of paroxysmal nocturnal hemo-globinuria. Cytometry B Clin Cytometry 2006;70(2).
17. Michael J B, Fiona E C, Joseph A D, et al. Guidelines for the diagnosis and moni-toring of paroxysmal nocturnal hemoglobinuria and related disorders by flow cy-tometry. Cytometry B Clin Cytometry 2010;78(4).
18. Pu JJ, Hu R, Mukhina GL, et al. The small population of PIG-A mutant cells in myelodysplastic syndromes do not arise from multipotent hematopoietic stem cells. Haematologica 2012;97(8).
19. Brando B, Gatti A, Preijers F. Flow cytometric diagnosis of paroxysmal nocturnal hemoglobinuria: pearls and pitfalls - a critical review article. EJIFCC 2019;30(4): 355–70.
20. Sutherland DR, Kuek N, Davidson J, et al. Diagnosing PNH with FLAER and multi-parameter flow cytometry. Cytometry B Clin Cytometry 2007;(3):72B.
21. Sutherland DR, Illingworth A, Keeney M, et al. High-sensitivity detection of PNH red blood cells, red cell precursors, and white blood cells. Current protocols in cytometry 2015. https://doi.org/10.1002/0471142956.cy0637s72.
22. Sutherland DR, Acton E, Keeney M, et al. Use of CD157 in FLAER-based assays for high-sensitivity PNH granulocyte and PNH monocyte detection. Cytometry B Clin Cytometry 2014;86(1).
23. Zhang Y, Ding J, Gu H, et al. Diagnosis of paroxysmal nocturnal hemoglobinuria with flowcytometry panels including CD157: data from the real world. Cytometry B Clin Cytometry 2020;98(2):193–202.
24. Kaufman DP, Khattar J, Lappin SL. Physiology, fetal hemoglobin. Text 2023. Avail-able at: https://www.ncbi.nlm.nih.gov/books/NBK500011/.
25. Kim YA, Makar RS. Detection of fetomaternal hemorrhage. Am J Hematol 2012;87(4).
26. Othman J, Orellana D, Chen LS, et al. The presence of F cells with a fetal pheno-type in adults with hemoglobinopathies limits the utility of flow cytometry for quan-titation of fetomaternal hemorrhage. Cytometry B Clin Cytometry 2018;94(4): 695–8.
27. Ward RY. ICCS eNewsletter. 2023. Available at: https://www.cytometry.org/newsletters/eICCS-2-2/article3.php. [Accessed 4 November 2023].

28. Welsh KJ, From the Department of Pathology and Laboratory Medicine UoTHS-CaH, obotECotAoCLPa Scientists, Bai Y. From the Department of Pathology and laboratory medicine UoTHSCaH, Scientists obotECotAoCLPa. Pathology Consultation on patients with a large Rh Immune Globulin Dose requirement. Am J Clin Pathol 2023;145(6):744–51.

29. Karafin MS, Glisch C, Souers RJ, et al. Use of fetal hemoglobin quantitation for Rh-positive pregnant females: a National Survey and review of the Literature. Arch Pathol Lab Med 2019;143(12):1539–44.

30. WG Wood, Stamatoyannopoulos G, Lim G, et al. F-cells in the adult: normal values and levels in individuals with hereditary and acquired elevations of Hb F. Blood 1975;46(5).

31. Franco RS, Ysain Z, Palascak MB, et al. The effect of fetal hemoglobin on the survival characteristics of sickle cells. Blood 2006;(3):108.

32. Khandros E, Blobel GA. Heterogeneity of fetal hemoglobin production in adult red blood cells. Curr Opin Hematol 2021;28(3):164–70.

33. Barcellini W, Bianchi P, Fermo E, et al. Hereditary red cell membrane defects: diagnostic and clinical aspects. Blood Transfus 2011;9(3):274–7.

34. Bolton-Maggs PH. Hereditary spherocytosis; new guidelines. Arch Dis Child 2004;89(9):809–12.

35. Bolton-Maggs PH, Langer JC, Iolascon A, et al. General haematology task force of the British Committee for standards in H. Guidelines for the diagnosis and management of hereditary spherocytosis–2011 update. Br J Haematol 2012; 156(1):37–49.

36. Iolascon A, Avvisati RA. Genotype/phenotype correlation in hereditary spherocytosis. Haematologica 2008;93(9):1283–8.

37. Park ES, Jung HL, Kim HJ, et al. Hereditary hemolytic anemia in Korea from 2007 to 2011: a study by the Korean hereditary hemolytic anemia working party of the Korean Society of hematology. Blood Res 2013;48(3):211–6.

38. Perrotta S, Gallagher PG, Mohandas N. Hereditary spherocytosis. Lancet 2008; 372(9647):1411–26.

39. Tse WT, Lux SE. Red blood cell membrane disorders. Br J Haematol 1999; 104(1):2–13.

40. Shim YJ, Won DI. Flow cytometric osmotic fragility testing does reflect the clinical severity of hereditary spherocytosis. Cytometry B Clin Cytom 2014;86(6): 436–43.

41. Ciepiela O, Adamowicz-Salach A, Zgodzinska A, et al. Flow cytometric osmotic fragility test: increased assay sensitivity for clinical application in pediatric hematology. Cytometry B Clin Cytom 2018;94(1):189–95.

42. Park SH, Park CJ, Lee BR, et al. Comparison study of the eosin-5'-maleimide binding test, flow cytometric osmotic fragility test, and cryohemolysis test in the diagnosis of hereditary spherocytosis. Am J Clin Pathol 2014;142(4): 474–84.

43. Peters LL, Shivdasani RA, Liu SC, et al. Anion exchanger 1 (band 3) is required to prevent erythrocyte membrane surface loss but not to form the membrane skeleton. Cell 1996;86(6):917–27.

44. King MJ, Telfer P, MacKinnon H, et al. Using the eosin-5-maleimide binding test in the differential diagnosis of hereditary spherocytosis and hereditary pyropoikilocytosis. Cytometry B Clin Cytom 2008;74(4):244–50.

45. Arora RD, Dass J, Maydeo S, et al. Flow cytometric osmotic fragility test and eosin-5'-maleimide dye-binding tests are better than conventional osmotic

fragility tests for the diagnosis of hereditary spherocytosis. Int J Lab Hematol 2018;40(3):335–42.

46. Stoya G, Gruhn B, Vogelsang H, et al. Flow cytometry as a diagnostic tool for hereditary spherocytosis. Acta Haematol 2006;116(3):186–91.

47. Christensen RD, Agarwal AM, Nussenzveig RH, et al. Evaluating eosin-5-maleimide binding as a diagnostic test for hereditary spherocytosis in newborn infants. J Perinatol 2015;35(5):357–61.

48. Crisp RL, Solari L, Gammella D, et al. Use of capillary blood to diagnose hereditary spherocytosis. Pediatr Blood Cancer 2012;59(7):1299–301.

49. King MJ, Behrens J, Rogers C, et al. Rapid flow cytometric test for the diagnosis of membrane cytoskeleton-associated haemolytic anaemia. Br J Haematol 2000; 111(3):924–33.

50. Crisp RL, Solari L, Vota D, et al. A prospective study to assess the predictive value for hereditary spherocytosis using five laboratory tests (cryohemolysis test, eosin-5'-maleimide flow cytometry, osmotic fragility test, autohemolysis test, and SDS-PAGE) on 50 hereditary spherocytosis families in Argentina. Ann Hematol 2011;90(6):625–34.

51. Agarwal AM, Liew MA, Nussenzveig RH, et al. Improved harmonization of eosin-5-maleimide binding test across different instruments and age groups. Cytometry B Clin Cytom 2016;90(6):512–6.

52. Rees P, Summers HD, Filby A, et al. Imaging flow cytometry: a primer. Nat Rev Methods Primers 2022. https://doi.org/10.1038/s43586-022-00167-x.

53. McGrath KE, Bushnell TP, Palis J. Multispectral imaging of hematopoietic cells: where flow meets morphology. J Immunol Methods 2008;336(2):91–7.

54. Ozpolat T, Chang TC, Wu X, et al. Phenotypic analysis of erythrocytes in sickle cell disease using imaging flow cytometry. Cytometry 2022;101(5): 448–57.

55. Dekel E, Rivkin A, Heidenreich M, et al. Identification and classification of the malaria parasite blood developmental stages, using imaging flow cytometry. Methods 2017;112:157–66.

Flow Cytometry and Platelets

Andrew L. Frelinger III, PhD

KEYWORDS

- Blood platelet disorders • Platelet • Function tests • Platelet activation
- Flow cytometry • Phenotyping • Thrombocytopenia

KEY POINTS

- Clinical flow cytometry for patients with suspected inherited platelet function disorders is useful as part of a larger diagnostic workup.
- Platelet activation markers detected by flow cytometry predict risk for thrombosis or bleeding in selected populations.

BACKGROUND/INTRODUCTION

Platelet activation is important for the major role that platelets play in hemostasis and thrombosis, but it also occurs in a variety of pathologic conditions including acute coronary syndromes,[1,2] cystic fibrosis,[3] diabetes,[4,5] hemodialysis,[6] heparin-induced thrombocytopenia,[5,7] vaccine-induced thrombotic thrombocytopenia,[8,9] ischemic stroke,[10] myeloproliferative disorders,[11,12] preeclampsia,[13,14] sickle cell disease,[15] lupus,[16] sepsis,[17] and systemic inflammation.[18–20]

Platelets are small (1–3 μm) anucleate cells which, in healthy individuals, circulate in a resting or unactivated state. However, when activated by soluble agonists, high shear, extracellular matrix, or foreign cells, platelets undergo alterations in surface glycoprotein function and/or expression level and may release dense and alpha granule contents. At sites of vascular injury, platelets adhere to exposed collagen and von Willebrand Factor (vWF) via multiple receptors including platelet surface glycoprotein (GP) VI-Fc receptor γ (FcR γ)-chain complex, GPIaIIa (integrin α2β1), GPIb-IX-V.[21] This adhesion, along with soluble factors released by damaged tissue, triggers changes in the conformation of platelet surface GPIIb-IIIa[22] (integrin αIIbβ or CD41/CD61) leading to fibrinogen binding and platelet-platelet aggregation contributing to the formation of a hemostatic plug. Platelet activation also causes release of platelet dense granules, which contain mainly small molecules such as ADP, serotonin, and histamine which amplify platelet activation and aggregation. Strong platelet activation results in release of alpha granule contents, a second type of platelet

Center for Platelet Research Studies, Dana-Farber/Boston Children's Cancer and Blood Disorders Center, Boston Children's Hospital, 300 Longwood Avenue, Boston, MA 02115-5737, USA
E-mail address: Andrew.Frelinger@childrens.harvard.edu

Clin Lab Med 44 (2024) 511–526
https://doi.org/10.1016/j.cll.2024.04.011   labmed.theclinics.com
0272-2712/24/© 2024 Elsevier Inc. All rights reserved.

granule which contains adhesion proteins, cytokines, and growth factors including fibrinogen, vWF, platelet factor 4 (PF-4), β thromboglobulin, VEGF, and PDGF.[23] Granule release is accompanied by exposure on the platelet surface of granule membrane proteins: CD63[24] from dense granule membranes and CD62P and TLT-1 [TREM-like transcript-1][25-27] from alpha granule membranes. Once exposed on the platelet surface, P-selectin mediates the adhesion of activated platelets to monocytes, neutrophils, and endothelial cells by binding to P-selectin glycoprotein ligand-1 (PSGL-1) which is constitutively expressed on these cells. Because P-selectin exposure occurs simultaneously with release of inflammatory mediators such as PF-4 from alpha granules[23] and platelet surface P-selectin mediates recruitment of leukocytes to sites of inflammation,[28] platelet surface expression of P-selectin is considered to be pro-inflammatory.

Strong platelet agonists such as thrombin or the combination of thrombin and collagen[29,30] cause increased exposure of phosphatidylserine, a negatively charged phospholipid which allows binding of calcium ions and coagulation factors thereby enabling conversion of prothrombin to thrombin.[31] Thus, in addition to providing a hemostatic platelet plug, platelets also contribute to coagulation.

Clinical flow cytometry for patients with suspected inherited platelet function disorders is useful as part of a larger diagnostic workup.[32] Patients should receive a full clinical evaluation including a personal and family history of bleeding manifestations typical of inherited or acquired platelet function defects. Obtaining a bleeding score using a standardized methodology such as the ISTH-BAT[33] is useful. After exclusion of patients with severe thrombocytopenia, abnormal coagulation tests, or vWF, platelet function studies including flow cytometric analysis of platelet surface adhesion receptors and activation markers is appropriate. Clinical platelet function testing practices across Northern European centers were recently reviewed.[34] Flow cytometry was common amongst the participating centers (10/14) but is not well standardized.[35] **Table 1** identifies clinical conditions which exhibit alterations in platelet biomarkers detectable by flow cytometry.

GENERAL PRINCIPLES FOR PLATELET FLOW CYTOMETRY

The measurement of activation markers on platelets by flow cytometry requires the incubation of fluorescently-labeled probes, usually antibodies, specific for platelet surface or intracellular targets with a platelet-containing sample followed by dilution or fixation and flow cytometric analysis.[36,37] Both pre-analytical[38,39] and analytical variables (**Table 2**) may affect assay results including choice of anticoagulant, time between sample collection and analysis, flow cytometer calibration, and fluorescence compensation settings. While many of these issues are commonly addressed in protocols for other flow cytometry assays, they may be particularly problematic for platelet activation studies. For instance, care must be taken during sample collection because variability in blood sampling techniques can impact platelet activation.[40] Typically, blood for platelet studies is collected using a 21 g needle directly into EDTA or sodium citrate anticoagulant[41] after discarding the first 1 to 2 mL collected which may contain factors that activate platelets. However, some studies suggest that a discard is not required.[42] Citrate-anticoagulated blood is usually used for platelet activation studies because it contains micromolar levels of free calcium which is required to support platelet surface activated GPIIb-IIIa binding to fibrinogen and platelet-platelet aggregation. EDTA-anticoagulated blood can be used to evaluate inherited deficiencies in surface glycoproteins (eg, GPIIb and GPIIIa in GT or GPIb-IX-V in Bernard Soulier syndrome). Platelet activation may be assessed in platelet-rich plasma or washed

Table 1
Platelet biomarkers utilized in flow cytometric assays for assessing platelet activation and function

Platelet Biomarkers	Applications
Activation	
CD62P	Acute coronary syndromes[1,2]
CD63	Antiplatelet therapies[122-124]
CD107a	Cystic fibrosis[3]
PAC-1	Diabetes[5,7]
PDMPs	Heart transplant vasculopathy[4]
	Hemodialysis[6]
	Heparin-induced thrombocytopenia[125,126]
	Vaccine-induced thrombotic thrombocytopenia[8,9]
	Ischemic stroke[10]
	Myeloproliferative disorders[11,12]
	Percutaneous coronary intervention[127]
	Preeclampsia[13,14]
	Systemic inflammation[18-20]
Aggregation	
GPIb-IX-V complex	Bernard-Soulier syndrome[128,129]
• CD42a	
• CD42b	
• CD42d	
GPIIb/IIIa complex	Glanzmann thrombasthenia[128,130]
• CD41	
• CD61	
• PAC-1	
von Willebrand factor	Platelet-type von Willebrand disease[131]
Dense granule deficiency	
CD63	Hermansky Pudlak syndrome[24,132]
Mepacrine	Chediak–Higashi syndrome.[106,107]
Serotonin	Griscelli syndrome
	Wiskott-Aldrich syndrome[133]
	Thrombocytopenia with absent radii (TAR) syndrome[134]

platelets but whole blood is preferred to minimize possible in vitro activation and loss of platelet subpopulations.

Assessment of platelet activation markers on minimally manipulated samples is intended to evaluate the activation state of circulating platelets, which can be elevated as a result of a local in vivo insult such as myocardial infarction (MI)[43] or stroke[2,44] or systemic pathology such as diabetes,[45] peripheral vascular disease,[46] Alzheimer's,[47] or rheumatoid arthritis.[19] Ex vivo addition of platelet agonists allows the additional determination of platelet reactivity, that is, the sensitivity and maximal response of the patient's platelets to specific platelet agonists. Hyper-reactivity to ex vivo platelet stimulation has been reported in patients with diabetes, nephropathy,[48] and metastatic cancer.[49] In contrast, platelet hypo-reactivity has been reported in neonates,[50,51] while elderly individuals appear to have both hyper-reactivity to ADP and hypo-reactivity to thrombin.[52]

PLATELET AGGREGATION

Platelet activation by ADP, thrombin, or other agonists results in conformational changes in GPIIb-IIIa which allow it to bind to fibrinogen, thereby mediating platelet-platelet aggregation.[53-55] PAC-1, an IgM monoclonal antibody, preferentially recognizes

Table 2
Variables affecting assessment of platelet activation by flow cytometry

Stage	Variable	Options
Pre-analytical	Sample collection	Location (vein/artery/catheter), tourniquet, needle size, discard of initial draw
	Anticoagulant	EDTA, sodium citrate, heparin, *etc.*
	Container	Polypropylene, siliconized glass, size (surface area in contact with sample and area at liquid/gas interface)
	Sample type	Whole blood, PRP, washed platelets, fixed platelets
	Storage between collection and assay	Time, temperature, agitation (shipping via vacuum tubes)
Assay	Platelet count	Fixed dilution Normalized platelet count
	Buffer	Plasma vs buffer Calcium concentration
	Antibody/probes	Polyclonal; Monoclonal; Clone Source, fluorochrome, batch Concentration (saturation vs. separation index)
	Agonists	ADP, arachidonic acid, collagen, collagen-related peptide[135] (CRP) and cross-linked CRP, convulxin, thrombin, thrombin receptor activating peptide (PAR1-activating peptide, variants of SFLLRN[136]), PAR4-activating peptide (variants of GYPGQV,[137] AYPGKF,[138] A-Phe(4-F)-PGWLVKNG[139]), rhodocytin,[140] U46619,
	Order of operation	1) Probes 2) Agonist 3) Sample 4) Incubate 5) Fix 1) Agonist 2) Sample 3) Incubate 4) Probes 5) Fix 1) Agonist 2) Sample 3) Incubate 4) Fix 5) Probes Secondary stains
	Time and temperature	Activation kinetics vs. antibody binding kinetics 4° vs RT vs 37°C
	Stop	Dilution vs fixation Choice of fixative
	Storage between assay and analysis	Time; temperature
Analysis	Instrument	Model, lasers, filters, sensitivity, calibration
	Settings	Threshold, gating
	Compensation, unmixing	Single stain controls, FMO, isotype controls, manual/automated

(continued on next page)

Table 2 (continued)		
Stage	**Variable**	**Options**
Reporting	Qualitative	Normal/Abnormal; (L), (H)
	Quantitative	Mean, geometric mean, median
		Percent positive
		Reference range
	Interpretation	Experience

the activated conformation of GPIIb-IIIa.[56–59] Consequently, PAC-1 binding reliably detects activated platelets[58–60] and closely correlates with platelet aggregation.[61] Moreover, Food and Drug Administration-approved small molecule and antibody based fibrinogen receptor antagonists (eg, eptifibatide, tirofiban, abciximab) also block binding of PAC-1. Activated GPIIb-IIIa on platelets can also be detected using fluorescently conjugated fibrinogen[62–66] and stable preparations of fibrinogen labeled with a variety of fluorophores are commercially available.[67–70] However, because activated GPIIb-IIIa on circulating platelets binds rapidly to plasma fibrinogen (present at ~200–400 mg/dL), binding of fluorescent PAC-1 or fibrinogen to fresh blood or platelet-rich plasma (PRP) in the absence of an ex vivo added agonist is usually low. Fibrinogen bound to platelet surface activated GPIIb-IIIa can be detected using an anti-fibrinogen antibody[60,71–73] as an indirect measure of activated GPIIb-IIIa on circulating platelets. High concentration of plasma fibrinogen, which can compete with labeled PAC-1 and fibrinogen, can be accounted for by using high concentrations of labeled PAC-1 and fibrinogen or by washing the platelets to remove competing unlabeled fibrinogen. Binding of labeled PAC-1 or fibrinogen to platelets activated by ex vivo addition of agonist can be inhibited by certain therapeutic antiplatelet agents: fibrinogen receptor antagonists (abciximab, eptifibatide, tirofiban) inhibit PAC-1 and fibrinogen in response to all agonists; aspirin inhibits binding in response to arachidonic acid, platelet P2Y12 ADP receptor antagonists reduce binding in response to ADP, and so forth. **Fig. 1** shows an example of healthy donor whole blood stained with a panel of antibodies directed toward platelet surface markers in the presence of increasing concentrations of ADP or TRAP (thrombin receptor activating peptide). Results for individual markers can be reported as mean or median fluorescence intensity (antibody capture beads can be used to convert fluorescence values to molecules per platelet[74]), the percent of platelets positive for the marker, the EC_{50} for agonist stimulation or maximal marker expression. Details on the use of flow cytometry to monitor GPIIb-IIIa activation have been previously described.[37,61,75,76]

Light transmission aggregation of platelets in platelet-rich plasma[77,78] was the first robust and widely used test of platelet function making it the gold-standard against which new tests were measured. De Cuyper and colleagues, in 2013[79] and Vinholt and colleagues, in 2017[80] reported direct measurement of platelet-platelet aggregation by flow cytometry. Each group divided patient samples into two aliquots, labeled them with different fluorochromes, combined the labeled platelets together with healthy donor plasma, then added an agonist (see **Table 2**) and agitated (~1000 rpm) at 37°C. Aliquots of the aggregating samples were then fixed and analyzed by fluorescence flow cytometry. While this approach provides the functional endpoint of platelet-platelet aggregation, the sample manipulation, complex procedure, and time required have the potential to introduce artifact, ultimately making it less attractive than the measurement of activated GPIIb-IIIa in whole blood samples as described above.

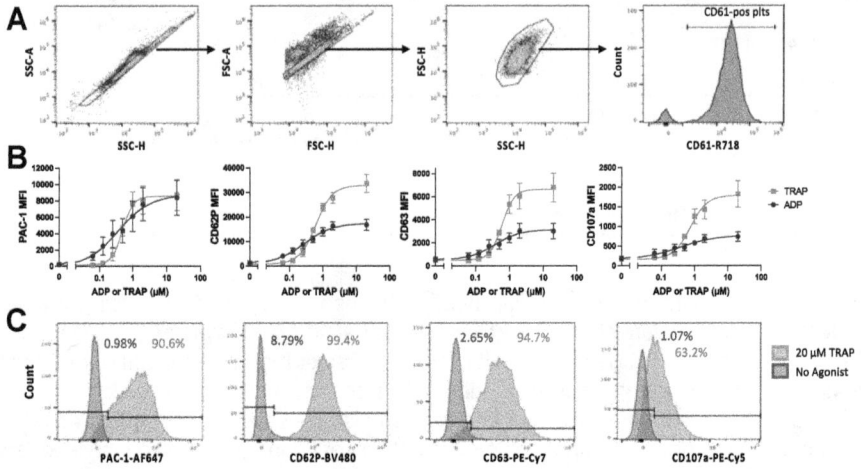

Fig. 1. Example of flow cytometric assessment of platelet activation markers by flow cytometry. Healthy donor blood activated *ex vivo* with ADP or TRAP in the presence of a panel of 16 fluorescent probes[120,121] against platelet surface markers and analyzed by flow cytometry on a Cytek Aurora Spectral Cytometer. (*A*) Gating: Following gating for singlets, platelets are identified based on characteristic forward- and side-light scatter profile and by CD61-positivity; (*B*) ADP- and TRAP-stimulated PAC-1, CD62P, CD63, and CD107a mean fluorescence of CD61-positive platelet events; (*C*) Gating for percent PAC1, CD62P, CD63 and CD107a -positive platelets in unstimulated (*blue*) and 20 μM TRAP (*red*) stimulated samples. Results are n = 3 means ±SEM. Panel markers not shown: annexin V, C3b, CD29, CD31, CD32, CD36, CD154, GPVI, TLR-9, TLT-1. Abbreviations: ADP, adenosine diphosphate; LAMP, lysosomal associated membrane protein; MFI, mean fluorescence intensity; TRAP, thrombin receptor agonist peptide; TLR, Toll-like receptor; TLT, TREM-like transcript.

PLATELET ACTIVATION (P-SELECTIN AND LEUKOCYTE-PLATELET AGGREGATES)

P-selectin (CD62P, PADGEM[81] GMP-140[82]) is a transmembrane glycoprotein which resides in Weibel-Palade bodies in endothelial cells and in alpha granules of platelets. Upon activation, these granules fuse with the plasma membrane, resulting in cell surface exposure of P-selectin[83] and release of alpha granule contents. In addition to acting as a marker for alpha granule release, once exposed, platelet surface P-selectin can bind to its counter-ligand, PSGL-1 which is constitutively expressed on the surface of certain leukocytes including monocytes, neutrophils, dendritic cells, and some lymphocytes thereby mediating the formation of heterotypic cell aggregates.[83] Platelet surface expression of P-selectin and P-selectin-dependent platelet-leukocyte aggregates (particularly platelet-monocyte and platelet-neutrophil aggregates) are clinically significant markers of platelet activation.[84] Following binding to PSGL-1, the extracellular domain of P-selectin can be released into the bloodstream as soluble P-selectin.[85] Thus, both platelet surface P-selectin and platelet-leukocyte aggregates are markers of recent in vivo platelet activation, although monocyte-platelet aggregates are a more sensitive marker of in vivo platelet activation than P-selectin.[84] Platelet surface P-selectin and leukocyte-platelet aggregates, unlike activated GPIIb-IIIa, can be measured in blood added to a fixative immediately after collection.[37,86] The ability of platelets to express platelet surface P-selectin and form platelet-leukocyte aggregates in response to *ex vivo* agonists can be measured using citrate anticoagulated blood. However, the level of platelet-leukocyte aggregates increases rapidly after blood collection[86] because even miniscule amounts of platelet surface P-selectin cause platelets to bind to monocytes and neutrophils. Platelet-monocyte and platelet-neutrophil aggregates are elevated in a number of clinical conditions including cardiovascular disease, diabetes, sickle cell disease, lupus, and multiple sclerosis.[87–90] Specific protocols for the measurement of leukocyte-platelet aggregates are available.[76,86,91–93]

PLATELET DENSE GRANULE RELEASE (CD63 AND MEPACRINE)

In contrast to alpha granules, which contain relatively more proteins than small molecules, platelet dense granules contain relatively more small molecules including adenine nucleotides (ADP, ATP, diadenosine polyphosphates), monoamines (serotonin, histamine), and calcium. The presence of high amounts of calcium in these granules gives them their characteristic dark/dense appearance in scanning electron microscopy.[94] Once released, ADP, serotonin, and histamine bind to their receptors on platelets, amplifying platelet activation and contributing to stable platelet aggregation.[95] Platelets from healthy donors have on average 6 to 7 dense granules per platelet,[94] but this number and/or the content of dense granules is reduced in patients with storage pool disease.[96] A deficit in platelet dense granule content can be detected by flow cytometric analysis of mepacrine, a fluorescent dye which binds to nucleotides present in dense granules.[96–100] The procedure is rapid, requiring only a short incubation of whole blood or isolated platelets with mepacrine followed by flow cytometric analysis.[97,100,101] Use of a compatible fluorescent platelet antibody (eg, CD41, CD61, CD42) to specifically identify platelets is recommended. Mepacrine loaded platelets can also be used to evaluate agonist-stimulated release of dense granule contents. In healthy individuals, thrombin and other strong platelet agonists cause release of ~80% of mepacrine.[97,100]

Decrease in the number of dense granules per platelet leads to reduced agonist-stimulated platelet surface expression of the dense granule membrane protein, CD63. Some individuals with storage pool disease show an isolated ADP deficit, an isolated serotonin deficit, or a deficit in both ADP and serotoinin.[96] While abnormalities in MRP4, a nucleotide transporter or VMAT, a monoamine transporter are suspected,[102] the underlying mechanism is unknown. In such individuals, agonist stimulated platelet surface CD63 may be normal. Platelet surface CD63 has been found to be higher on circulating platelets in adults[103] and adolescents[6] with Type II diabetes mellitus than on healthy individuals.

CD107a (LAMP-1) LYSOSOMAL GRANULE MEMBRANE MARKER

CD107a is a heavily glycosylated platelet lysosome membrane-associated protein that becomes expressed on the surface of platelets exposed to high concentrations of thrombin.[104] Lower thrombin concentrations which result in platelet alpha granule or dense granule release does not lead to platelet surface CD107a expression. CD107a is present in many cell types where it is important for lysosome biogenesis, lysosomal pH regulation, and autophagy.[105] In platelets, CD107a serves as a marker of platelet activation and lysosomal release.[104] Agonist-dependent platelet surface expression of CD107a is decreased in patients with Chediak-Higashi syndrome due to a defect in exocytosis pathways.[106–108] CD107a has also been proposed as a marker of decreased platelet function in stored platelets (platelet storage lesion).[109]

OTHER

Targeting of platelets by autoantibodies can lead to activation of the complement system and a reduction in platelet counts. Levels of C4d, a degradation product of the complement component C4, is present at elevated levels on platelets in patients with Lupus/antiphospholipid syndrome,[110,111] stroke,[112] and ITP.[113,114] While not a platelet activation marker per se, platelet surface C4d suggests complement activation and a plausible explanation for thrombocytopenia in certain clinical settings.

FcγRIIa is a low affinity platelet Fc receptor which binds IgG1 and IgG2[115] and amplifies platelet activation when ligands, such as immobilized fibrinogen, bind to GPIIb-IIIa.[116] The polymorphic variant, FcγRIIa$_{R131}$, binds IgG2 with lower affinity.[115] Levels of platelet surface FcγRIIa, measured using a quantitative flow cytometry assay,[117] were elevated in patients with acute MI, unstable angina, or ischemic stroke compared to healthy individuals.[118] Moreover, elevated platelet surface FcγRIIa levels of greater than 11,000 molecules/platelet independently predicted risk of MI, stroke, and death in patients with a prior MI.[117] While most other platelet tests report qualitative differences in antibody staining, platelet surface FcγRIIa is reported as molecules per platelet by comparison of fluorescence to antibody capture beads with precise number of binding sites per bead (Quantum Simply Cellular anti-mouse beads, Bangs Laboratories, Fishers, IN).[119]

SUMMARY

In summary, whole blood flow cytometry is a powerful laboratory technique for assessment of platelet activation and function. It is used to assess platelet activation, leukocyte-platelet aggregates, platelet aggregation, and measure dense granule release, among others. In addition to the rapid turn around time, this technique is not limited by low platelet counts. Clinical applications of whole blood flow cytometric assays of platelet function in various disease states may include identification of patients who would benefit from additional antiplatelet therapy and prediction of ischemic events. Flow cytometry can also be used for monitoring of glycoprotein IIb-IIIa antagonist therapy, diagnosis of inherited deficiencies of platelet surface glycoproteins, diagnosis of storage pool disease, diagnosis of heparin-induced thrombocytopenia, and measurement of the rate of thrombopoiesis.

CLINICS CARE POINTS

- A clean blood draw and gentle handling of specimens are required to avoid spontaneous platelet activation.
- Abnormal results should be confirmed by repeat testing to exclude possible interference by anti-platelet medications (most commonly, aspirin or non-steroidal anti-inflammatory drugs).

ACKNOWLEDGMENTS

We would like to acknowledge the contribution of Ms. Jacqueline R. Perry to this article.

DISCLOSURE

The author has nothing to disclose.

FUNDING

This work was supported in part by NIH K23 HL141651.

REFERENCES

1. Coulter SA, Cannon CP, Ault KA, et al. High levels of platelet inhibition with abciximab despite heightened platelet activation and aggregation during thrombolysis for acute myocardial infarction: results from TIMI (thrombolysis in myocardial infarction) 14. Circulation 2000;101(23):2690–5.

2. Stellos K, Bigalke B, Stakos D, et al. Platelet-bound P-selectin expression in patients with coronary artery disease: impact on clinical presentation and myocardial necrosis, and effect of diabetes mellitus and anti-platelet medication. J Thromb Haemost 2010;8(1):205–7.

3. O'Sullivan BP, Linden MD, Frelinger AL 3rd, et al. Platelet activation in cystic fibrosis. Blood 2005;105(12):4635–41.

4. Fateh-Moghadam S, Bocksch W, Ruf A, et al. Changes in surface expression of platelet membrane glycoproteins and progression of heart transplant vasculopathy. Circulation 2000;102(8):890–7.

5. Israels SJ, McNicol A, Dean HJ, et al. Markers of platelet activation are increased in adolescents with type 2 diabetes. Diabetes Care 2014;37(8): 2400–3.

6. Kawabata K, Nakai S, Miwa M, et al. Platelet GPIIb/IIIa is activated and platelet-leukocyte coaggregates formed in vivo during hemodialysis. Nephron 2002; 90(4):391–400.

7. Serebruany VL, Malinin A, Ong S, et al. Patients with metabolic syndrome exhibit higher platelet activity than those with conventional risk factors for vascular disease. J Thromb Thrombolysis 2008;25(2):207–13.

8. Handtke S, Wolff M, Zaninetti C, et al. A Flow cytometric assay to detect platelet activating antibodies in VITT after ChAdOx1 nCov-19 vaccination. Blood 2021. https://doi.org/10.1182/blood.2021012064.

9. Cesari F, Sorrentino S, Gori AM, et al. Detection of platelet-activating antibodies associated with vaccine-induced thrombotic thrombocytopenia by flow cytometry: an Italian experience. Viruses 2022;14(6). https://doi.org/10.3390/v14061133.

10. Grau AJ, Ruf A, Vogt A, et al. Increased fraction of circulating activated platelets in acute and previous cerebrovascular ischemia. Thromb Haemostasis 1998; 80(2):298–301.

11. Villmow T, Kemkes-Matthes B, Matzdorff AC. Markers of platelet activation and platelet-leukocyte interaction in patients with myeloproliferative syndromes. Thromb Res 2002;108(2–3):139–45.

12. Jensen MK, de Nully Brown P, Lund BV, et al. Increased circulating platelet-leukocyte aggregates in myeloproliferative disorders is correlated to previous thrombosis, platelet activation and platelet count. Eur J Haematol 2001;66(3): 143–51.

13. Janes SL, Goodall AH. Flow cytometric detection of circulating activated platelets and platelet hyper-responsiveness in pre-eclampsia and pregnancy. Clin Sci (Lond) 1994;86(6):731–9.

14. Konijnenberg A, van der Post JA, Mol BW, et al. Can flow cytometric detection of platelet activation early in pregnancy predict the occurrence of preeclampsia? A prospective study. Am J Obstet Gynecol 1997;177(2):434–42.

15. Frelinger AL 3rd, Jakubowski JA, Brooks JK, et al. Platelet Activation and Inhibition iN Sickle cell disease (PAINS) study. Platelets 2013;25(1):27–35.

16. Lood C, Tyden H, Gullstrand B, et al. Platelet activation and anti-phospholipid antibodies collaborate in the activation of the complement system on platelets in systemic lupus erythematosus. PLoS One 2014;9(6):e99386.

17. Woth G, Tokes-Fuzesi M, Magyarlaki T, et al. Activated platelet-derived micro-particle numbers are elevated in patients with severe fungal (Candida albicans) sepsis. Ann Clin Biochem 2012;49(Pt 6):554–60.

18. Gawaz M, Dickfeld T, Bogner C, et al. Platelet function in septic multiple organ dysfunction syndrome. Intensive Care Med 1997;23(4):379–85.

19. Joseph JE, Harrison P, Mackie IJ, et al. Increased circulating platelet-leucocyte complexes and platelet activation in patients with antiphospholipid syndrome, systemic lupus erythematosus and rheumatoid arthritis. Br J Haematol 2001; 115(2):451–9.

20. Russwurm S, Vickers J, Meier-Hellmann A, et al. Platelet and leukocyte activation correlate with the severity of septic organ dysfunction. Shock 2002;17(4): 263–8.

21. Lee RH, Stefanini L, Bergmeier W. Platelet signal transduction. In: Michelson AD, Cattaneo M, Frelinger III AL, et al, editors. Platelets. 4th edition. San Deigo: Elsevier; 2019. p. 329–47, chap 18.

22. Shattil SJ, Brass LF. Induction of the fibrinogen receptor on human platelets by intracellular mediators. J Biol Chem 1987;262(3):992–1000.

23. Flaumenhaft R, Sharda A. Platelet secretion. In: Michelson AD, Cattaneo M, Frelinger III AL, et al, editors. Platelets. 4th edition. San Diego: Elsevier; 2019. p. 349–70, chap 19.

24. Nishibori M, Cham B, McNicol A, et al. The protein CD63 is in platelet dense granules, is deficient in a patient with Hermansky-Pudlak syndrome, and appears identical to granulophysin. J Clin Invest 1993;91(4):1775–82.

25. Merten M, Thiagarajan P. P-selectin expression on platelets determines size and stability of platelet aggregates. Circulation 2000;102(16):1931–6.

26. Washington AV, Schubert RL, Quigley L, et al. A TREM family member, TLT-1, is found exclusively in the alpha-granules of megakaryocytes and platelets. Blood 2004;104(4):1042–7.

27. Morales-Ortiz J, Deal V, Reyes F, et al. Platelet-derived TLT-1 is a prognostic indicator in ALI/ARDS and prevents tissue damage in the lungs in a mouse model. Blood 2018;132(23):2495–505.

28. Pitchford SC, Momi S, Giannini S, et al. Platelet P-selectin is required for pulmonary eosinophil and lymphocyte recruitment in a murine model of allergic inflammation. Blood 2005;105(5):2074–81.

29. Alberio LJ, Clemetson KJ. All platelets are not equal: COAT platelets. Curr Hematol Rep 2004;3(5):338–43.

30. Dale GL. Coated-platelets: an emerging component of the procoagulant response. J Thromb Haemost 2005;3(10):2185–92.

31. Gasecka A, Nieuwland R, Siljander PR. Platelet-derived extracellular vesicles. In: Michelson AD, Cattaneo M, Frelinger III AL, et al, editors. Platelets. 4th edition. San Diego: Elsevier; 2019. p. 401–16, chap 22.

32. Gresele P, Subcommittee on Platelet Physiology of the International Society on Thrombosis and Hemostasis. Subcommittee on platelet physiology of the international society on thrombosis and hemostasis. Diagnosis of inherited platelet disorders: guidance from the SSC of the ISTH. J Thromb Haemost 2015;13(2):314–22.

33. Gresele P, Orsini S, Noris P, et al. Validation of the ISTH/SSC bleeding assessment tool for inherited platelet disorders: a communication from the Platelet Physiology SSC. J Thromb Haemost 2020;18(3):732–9.

34. Szanto T, Zetterberg E, Ramstrom S, et al. Platelet function testing: current practice among clinical centres in Northern Europe. Haemophilia 2022;28(4):642–8.

35. Frelinger AL, Rivera J, Connor DE, et al. Consensus recommendations on flow cytometry for the assessment of inherited and acquired disorders of platelet number and function: communication from the ISTH SSC Subcommittee on Platelet Physiology. J Thromb Haemost 2021;19(12):3193–202.

36. Blair TA, Frelinger IIIAL, Michelson AD. Flow cytometry. In: Michelson AD, Cattaneo M, Frelinger III AL, et al, editors. Platelets. 4th edition. San Diego: Elsevier; 2019. p. 627–52, chap 35.

37. Spurgeon BEJ, Linden MD, Michelson AD, et al. 3rd. Immunophenotypic analysis of platelets by flow cytometry. Curr Protoc 2021;1(6):e178.

38. Hindle MS, Cheah LT, Yates DM, et al. Preanalytical conditions for multiparameter platelet flow cytometry. Research and Practice in Thrombosis and Haemostasis 2023;7(7). https://doi.org/10.1016/j.rpth.2023.102205.

39. Mody M, Lazarus AH, Semple JW, et al. Preanalytical requirements for flow cytometric evaluation of platelet activation: choice of anticoagulant. Transfus Med 1999;9(2):147–54.

40. Rondina MT, Grissom CK, Men S, et al. Whole blood flow cytometry measurements of in vivo platelet activation in critically-Ill patients are influenced by variability in blood sampling techniques. Thromb Res 2012;129(6):729–35.

41. Pedersen OH, Nissen PH, Hvas AM. Platelet function investigation by flow cytometry: sample volume, needle size, and reference intervals. Platelets 2018; 29(2):199–202.

42. Welch EL, Crooks MG, Hart SP. Agreement between blood draw techniques for assessing platelet activation by flow cytometry. Platelets 2019;30(4):530–4.

43. Linden MD, Furman MI, Frelinger AL 3rd, et al. Indices of platelet activation and the stability of coronary artery disease. J Thromb Haemost 2007;5(4):761–5.

44. McCabe DJ, Harrison P, Mackie IJ, et al. Platelet degranulation and monocyte-platelet complex formation are increased in the acute and convalescent phases after ischaemic stroke or transient ischaemic attack. Br J Haematol 2004;125(6): 777–87.

45. Davi G, Patrono C. Platelet activation and atherothrombosis. N Engl J Med 2007; 357(24):2482–94.

46. Dopheide JF, Rubrech J, Trumpp A, et al. Leukocyte-platelet aggregates-a phenotypic characterization of different stages of peripheral arterial disease. Platelets 2016;1–10. https://doi.org/10.3109/09537104.2016.1153619.

47. Khezri MR, Esmaeili A, Ghasemnejad-Berenji M. Platelet activation and alzheimer's disease: the probable role of PI3K/AKT pathway. J Alzheim Dis 2022; 90(2):529–34.

48. Tarnow I, Michelson AD, Barnard MR, et al. Nephropathy in type 1 diabetes is associated with increased circulating activated platelets and platelet hyperreactivity. Platelets 2009;20(7):513–9.

49. Cooke NM, Egan K, McFadden S, et al. Increased platelet reactivity in patients with late-stage metastatic cancer. Cancer Med 2013;2(4):564–70.

50. Rajasekhar D, Barnard MR, Bednarek FJ, et al. Platelet hyporeactivity in very low birth weight neonates. Thromb Haemostasis 1997;77(5):1002–7.

51. Weiss LJ, Drayss M, Mott K, et al. Ontogenesis of functional platelet subpopulations from preterm and term neonates to adulthood: the PLINIUS study. Blood Adv 2023;7(16):4334–48.

52. Gnanenthiran SR, Pennings GJ, Reddel CJ, et al. Identification of a distinct platelet phenotype in the elderly: ADP hypersensitivity coexists with platelet PAR (Protease-Activated receptor)-1 and PAR-4-mediated thrombin resistance. Arterioscler Thromb Vasc Biol 2022;42(8):960–72.

53. Coller BS, Peerschke EI, Scudder LE, et al. Studies with a murine monoclonal antibody that abolishes ristocetin- induced binding of von Willebrand factor to platelets: additional evidence in support of GPIb as a platelet receptor for von Willebrand factor. Blood 1983;61(1):99–110.
54. Parise LV, Phillips DR. Reconstitution of the purified platelet fibrinogen receptor. Fibrinogen binding properties of the glycoprotein IIb-IIIa complex. J Biol Chem 1985;260(19):10698–707.
55. Bennett JS, Vilaire G. Exposure of platelet fibrinogen receptors by ADP and epinephrine. J Clin Invest 1979;64(5):1393–401.
56. Shattil SJ, Hoxie JA, Cunningham M, et al. Changes in the platelet membrane glycoprotein IIb.IIIa complex during platelet activation. J Biol Chem 1985; 260(20):11107–14.
57. Shattil SJ, Motulsky HJ, Insel PA, et al. Expression of fibrinogen receptors during activation and subsequent desensitization of human platelets by epinephrine. Blood 1986;68(6):1224–31.
58. Shattil SJ, Cunningham M, Hoxie JA. Detection of activated platelets in whole blood using activation-dependent monoclonal antibodies and flow cytometry. Blood 1987;70(1):307–15.
59. Abrams C, Shattil SJ. Immunological detection of activated platelets in clinical disorders. Thromb Haemostasis 1991;65(5):467–73.
60. Abrams CS, Ellison N, Budzynski AZ, et al. Direct detection of activated platelets and platelet-derived microparticles in humans. Blood 1990;75(1):128–38.
61. Frelinger AL 3rd. Using flow cytometry to monitor glycoprotein IIb-IIIa activation. Platelets 2018;1–7. https://doi.org/10.1080/09537104.2018.1478073.
62. Kasahara K, Takagi J, Sekiya F, et al. Analysis of distribution of receptors among platelets by flow cytometry. Thromb Res 1987;45(6):763–70.
63. Jackson CW, Jennings LK. Heterogeneity of fibrinogen receptor expression on platelets activated in normal plasma with ADP: analysis by flow cytometry. Br J Haematol 1989;72(3):407–14.
64. Hantgan RR. An investigation of fibrin-platelet adhesive interactions by micro-fluorimetry. Biochim Biophys Acta 1987;927(1):55–64.
65. Faraday N, Goldschmidt-Clermont P, Dise K, et al. Quantitation of soluble fibrinogen binding to platelets by fluorescence-activated flow cytometry. J Lab Clin Med 1994;123(5):728–40.
66. Heilmann E, Hynes LA, Burstein SA, et al. Fluorescein derivatization of fibrinogen for flow cytometric analysis of fibrinogen binding to platelets. Cytometry 1994;17(4):287–93.
67. Marwali MR, Hu CP, Mohandas B, et al. Modulation of ADP-induced platelet activation by aspirin and pravastatin: role of lectin-like oxidized low-density lipoprotein receptor-1, nitric oxide, oxidative stress, and inside-out integrin signaling. J Pharmacol Exp Therapeut 2007;322(3):1324–32.
68. Su X, Mi J, Yan J, et al. RGT, a synthetic peptide corresponding to the integrin beta 3 cytoplasmic C-terminal sequence, selectively inhibits outside-in signaling in human platelets by disrupting the interaction of integrin alpha IIb beta 3 with Src kinase. Blood 2008;112(3):592–602.
69. Shi X, Yang J, Cui X, et al. Functional effect of the mutations similar to the cleavage during platelet activation at integrin beta3 cytoplasmic tail when expressed in mouse platelets. PLoS One 2016;11(11):e0166136.
70. Canault M, Ghalloussi D, Grosdidier C, et al. Human CalDAG-GEFI gene (RASGRP2) mutation affects platelet function and causes severe bleeding. J Exp Med 2014;211(7):1349–62.

71. Zamarron C, Ginsberg MH, Plow EF. A receptor-induced binding site in fibrinogen elicited by its interaction with platelet membrane glycoprotein IIb-IIIa. J Biol Chem 1991;266(24):16193–9.
72. Gralnick HR, Williams SB, McKeown L, et al. Endogenous platelet fibrinogen: its modulation after surface expression is related to size-selective access to and conformational changes in the bound fibrinogen. Br J Haematol 1992;80(3):347–57.
73. Warkentin TE, Powling MJ, Hardisty RM. Measurement of fibrinogen binding to platelets in whole blood by flow cytometry: a micromethod for the detection of platelet activation. Br J Haematol 1990;76(3):387–94.
74. Perfetto SP, Ambrozak D, Nguyen R, et al. Quality assurance for polychromatic flow cytometry using a suite of calibration beads. Nat Protoc 2012;7(12):2067–79.
75. Huskens D, Sang Y, Konings J, et al. Standardization and reference ranges for whole blood platelet function measurements using a flow cytometric platelet activation test. PLoS One 2018;13(2):e0192079.
76. Pasalic L, Pennings GJ, Connor D, et al. Flow cytometry protocols for assessment of platelet function in whole blood. Methods Mol Biol 2017;1646:369–89.
77. O'Brien JR. Platelet aggregation: Part II Some results from a new method of study. J Clin Pathol 1962;15(5):452–5.
78. Born GV. Aggregation of blood platelets by adenosine diphosphate and its reversal. Nature 1962;194:927–9.
79. De Cuyper IM, Meinders M, van de Vijver E, et al. A novel flow cytometry-based platelet aggregation assay. Blood 2013;121(10):e70–80.
80. Vinholt PJ, Frederiksen H, Hvas AM, et al. Measurement of platelet aggregation, independently of patient platelet count: a flow-cytometric approach. J Thromb Haemost 2017;15(6):1191–202.
81. Larsen E, Celi A, Gilbert GE, et al. PADGEM protein: a receptor that mediates the interaction of activated platelets with neutrophils and monocytes. Cell 1989;59(2):305–12.
82. Hamburger SA, McEver RP. GMP-140 mediates adhesion of stimulated platelets to neutrophils. Blood 1990;75(3):550–4.
83. Furie B, Furie BC. The molecular basis of platelet and endothelial cell interaction with neutrophils and monocytes: role of P-selectin and the P-selectin ligand, PSGL-1. Thromb Haemostasis 1995;74(1):224–7.
84. Michelson AD, Barnard MR, Krueger LA, et al. Circulating monocyte-platelet aggregates are a more sensitive marker of in vivo platelet activation than platelet surface P-selectin: studies in baboons, human coronary intervention, and human acute myocardial infarction. Circulation 2001;104(13):1533–7.
85. Michelson AD, Barnard MR, Hechtman HB, et al. In vivo tracking of platelets: circulating degranulated platelets rapidly lose surface P-selectin but continue to circulate and function. Proc Natl Acad Sci USA 1996;93(21):11877–82.
86. Gerrits AJ, Frelinger AL 3rd, Michelson AD. Whole blood analysis of leukocyte-platelet aggregates. Current protocols in cytometry/editorial board, J Paul Robinson, managing editor [et al] 2016;78:6 15 1–6 15 10.
87. Blann AD, Nadar SK, Lip GY. The adhesion molecule P-selectin and cardiovascular disease. Eur Heart J 2003;24(24):2166–79.
88. Ridker PM, Buring JE, Rifai N. Soluble P-selectin and the risk of future cardiovascular events. Circulation 2001;103(4):491–5.
89. Sheremata WA, Jy W, Horstman LL, et al. Evidence of platelet activation in multiple sclerosis. J Neuroinflammation 2008;5:27.

90. Furman MI, Barnard MR, Krueger LA, et al. Circulating monocyte-platelet aggregates are an early marker of acute myocardial infarction. J Am Coll Cardiol 2001; 38(4):1002–6.

91. Hui H, Fuller KA, Erber WN, et al. Imaging flow cytometry in the assessment of leukocyte-platelet aggregates. Methods 2017;112:46–54.

92. Finsterbusch M, Schrottmaier WC, Kral-Pointner JB, et al. Measuring and interpreting platelet-leukocyte aggregates. Platelets 2018;29(7):677–85.

93. Allen N, Barrett TJ, Guo Y, et al. Circulating monocyte-platelet aggregates are a robust marker of platelet activity in cardiovascular disease. Atherosclerosis 2019;282:11–8.

94. Brunet JG, Iyer JK, Badin MS, et al. Electron microscopy examination of platelet whole mount preparations to quantitate platelet dense granule numbers: implications for diagnosing suspected platelet function disorders due to dense granule deficiency. Int J Lit Humanit 2018;40(4):400–7.

95. Cattaneo M. The platelet P2 receptors. In: Michelson AD, Cattaneo M, Frelinger III AL, et al, editors. Platelets. 4th edition. San Diego: Elsevier; 2019. p. 259–78, chap 14.

96. Dupuis A, Bordet JC, Eckly A, et al. Platelet delta-storage pool disease: an update. J Clin Med 2020;9(8). https://doi.org/10.3390/jcm9082508.

97. Gordon N, Thom J, Cole C, et al. Rapid detection of hereditary and acquired platelet storage pool deficiency by flow cytometry. Br J Haematol 1995;89(1): 117–23.

98. Hanby HA, Bao J, Noh JY, et al. Platelet dense granules begin to selectively accumulate mepacrine during proplatelet formation. Blood Adv 2017;1(19): 1478–90.

99. Cai H, Mullier F, Frotscher B, et al. Usefulness of flow cytometric mepacrine uptake/release combined with CD63 assay in diagnosis of patients with suspected platelet dense granule disorder. Semin Thromb Hemost 2016;42(3):282–91.

100. Wall JE, Buijs-Wilts M, Arnold JT, et al. A flow cytometric assay using mepacrine for study of uptake and release of platelet dense granule contents. Br J Haematol 1995;89(2):380–5.

101. Mumford AD, Frelinger AL, 3rd Gachet C, et al. A review of platelet secretion assays for the diagnosis of inherited platelet secretion disorders. Thromb Haemostasis 2015;114(1):14–25.

102. Jedlitschky G, Greinacher A, Kroemer HK. Transporters in human platelets: physiologic function and impact for pharmacotherapy. Blood 2012;119(15): 3394–402.

103. R S, Saharia GK, Patra S, et al. Flow cytometry based platelet activation markers and state of inflammation among subjects with type 2 diabetes with and without depression. Sci Rep 2022;12(1):10039.

104. Febbraio M, Silverstein RL. Identification and characterization of LAMP-1 as an activation-dependent platelet surface glycoprotein. J Biol Chem 1990;265(30): 18531–7.

105. Zhang J, Zeng W, Han Y, et al. Lysosomal LAMP proteins regulate lysosomal pH by direct inhibition of the TMEM175 channel. Mol Cell 2023;83(14): 2524–2539 e7.

106. Barbosa MD, Nguyen QA, Tchernev VT, et al. Identification of the homologous beige and Chediak-Higashi syndrome genes. Nature 1996;382(6588):262–5.

107. Tchernev VT, Mansfield TA, Giot L, et al. The Chediak-Higashi protein interacts with SNARE complex and signal transduction proteins. Mol Med 2002;8(1): 56–64.

108. Bryceson YT, Pende D, Maul-Pavicic A, et al. A prospective evaluation of degranulation assays in the rapid diagnosis of familial hemophagocytic syndromes. Blood 2012;119(12):2754–63.

109. Sodergren AL, Tynngard N, Berlin G, et al. Responsiveness of platelets during storage studied with flow cytometry–formation of platelet subpopulations and LAMP-1 as new markers for the platelet storage lesion. Vox Sang 2016; 110(2):116–25.

110. Lonati PA, Scavone M, Gerosa M, et al. Blood cell-bound C4d as a marker of complement activation in patients with the antiphospholipid syndrome. Front Immunol 2019;10:773.

111. Svenungsson E, Gustafsson JT, Grosso G, et al. Complement deposition, C4d, on platelets is associated with vascular events in systemic lupus erythematosus. Rheumatology (Oxford) 2020;59(11):3264–74.

112. Mehta N, Uchino K, Fakhran S, et al. Platelet C4d is associated with acute ischemic stroke and stroke severity. Stroke 2008;39(12):3236–41.

113. Peerschke EI, Yin W, Grigg SE, et al. Blood platelets activate the classical pathway of human complement. J Thromb Haemost 2006;4(9):2035–42.

114. Peerschke EI, Panicker S, Bussel J. Classical complement pathway activation in immune thrombocytopenia purpura: inhibition by a novel C1s inhibitor. Br J Haematol 2016;173(6):942–5.

115. Bruhns P, Iannascoli B, England P, et al. Specificity and affinity of human Fcgamma receptors and their polymorphic variants for human IgG subclasses. Blood 2009;113(16):3716–25.

116. Boylan B, Gao C, Rathore V, et al. Identification of FcgammaRIIa as the ITAM-bearing receptor mediating alphaIIbbeta3 outside-in integrin signaling in human platelets. Blood 2008;112(7):2780–6.

117. McMahon SR, Chava S, Taatjes-Sommer HS, et al. Variation in platelet expression of FcgammaRIIa after myocardial infarction. J Thromb Thrombolysis 2019;48(1):88–94.

118. Calverley DC, Brass E, Hacker MR, et al. Potential role of platelet FcgammaRIIA in collagen-mediated platelet activation associated with atherothrombosis. Atherosclerosis 2002;164(2):261–7.

119. Schneider DJ, McMahon SR, Chava S, et al. FcgammaRIIa: a new cardiovascular risk marker. J Am Coll Cardiol 2018;72(2):237–8.

120. Spurgeon BEJ, Frelinger AL 3rd. OMIP-097: high-parameter phenotyping of human platelets by spectral flow cytometry. Cytometry A 2023. https://doi.org/10.1002/cyto.a.24797.

121. Spurgeon BEJ, Frelinger AL 3rd. Platelet phenotyping by full spectrum flow cytometry. Curr Protoc 2023;3(2):e687.

122. Ault KA, Cannon CP, Mitchell J, et al. Platelet activation in patients after an acute coronary syndrome: results from the TIMI-12 trial. Thrombolysis in Myocardial Infarction. J Am Coll Cardiol 1999;33(3):634–9.

123. Gawaz M, Ruf A, Neumann FJ, et al. Effect of glycoprotein IIb-IIIa receptor antagonism on platelet membrane glycoproteins after coronary stent placement. Thromb Haemostasis 1998;80(6):994–1001.

124. Peter K, Kohler B, Straub A, et al. Flow cytometric monitoring of glycoprotein IIb/IIIa blockade and platelet function in patients with acute myocardial infarction receiving reteplase, abciximab, and ticlopidine: continuous platelet inhibition by the combination of abciximab and ticlopidine. Circulation 2000;102(13):1490–6.

125. Althaus K, Pelzl L, Hidiatov O, et al. Evaluation of a flow cytometer-based functional assay using platelet-rich plasma in the diagnosis of heparin-induced thrombocytopenia. Thromb Res 2019;180:55–61.

126. Runser A, Schaning C, Allemand F, et al. An optimized and standardized rapid flow cytometry functional method for heparin-induced thrombocytopenia. Biomedicines 2021;9(3). https://doi.org/10.3390/biomedicines9030296.

127. Gawaz M, Neumann FJ, Ott I, et al. Platelet activation and coronary stent implantation. Effect of antithrombotic therapy. Circulation 1996;94(3):279–85.

128. Michelson AD. Flow cytometric analysis of platelet surface glycoproteins: phenotypically distinct subpopulations of platelets in children with chronic myeloid leukemia. J Lab Clin Med 1987;110(3):346–54.

129. Cohn RJ, Sherman GG, Glencross DK. Flow cytometric analysis of platelet surface glycoproteins in the diagnosis of Bernard-Soulier syndrome. Pediatr Hematol Oncol Jan-Feb 1997;14(1):43–50.

130. Jennings LK, Ashmun RA, Wang WC, et al. Analysis of human platelet glycoproteins IIb-IIIa and Glanzmann's thrombasthenia in whole blood by flow cytometry. Blood 1986;68(1):173–9.

131. Giannini S, Cecchetti L, Mezzasoma AM, et al. Diagnosis of platelet-type von Willebrand disease by flow cytometry. Haematologica 2010;95(6):1021–4.

132. Huizing M, Malicdan MCV, Wang JA, et al. Hermansky-Pudlak syndrome: mutation update. Hum Mutat 2020;41(3):543–80.

133. Semple JW, Siminovitch KA, Mody M, et al. Flow cytometric analysis of platelets from children with the Wiskott-Aldrich syndrome reveals defects in platelet development, activation and structure. Br J Haematol 1997;97(4):747–54.

134. Albers CA, Paul DS, Schulze H, et al. Compound inheritance of a low-frequency regulatory SNP and a rare null mutation in exon-junction complex subunit RBM8A causes TAR syndrome. Nat Genet 2012;44(4):435–9. S1-2.

135. Smethurst PA, Onley DJ, Jarvis GE, et al. Structural basis for the platelet-collagen interaction: the smallest motif within collagen that recognizes and activates platelet Glycoprotein VI contains two glycine-proline-hydroxyproline triplets. J Biol Chem 2007;282(2):1296–304.

136. Vu TK, Hung DT, Wheaton VI, et al. Molecular cloning of a functional thrombin receptor reveals a novel proteolytic mechanism of receptor activation. Cell 1991;64(6):1057–68.

137. Xu WF, Andersen H, Whitmore TE, et al. Cloning and characterization of human protease-activated receptor 4. Proc Natl Acad Sci U S A 1998;95(12):6642–6.

138. Faruqi TR, Weiss EJ, Shapiro MJ, et al. Structure-function analysis of protease-activated receptor 4 tethered ligand peptides. Determinants of specificity and utility in assays of receptor function. J Biol Chem 2000;275(26):19728–34.

139. Yang J, Mapelli C, Wang Z, et al. An optimized agonist peptide of protease-activated receptor 4 and its use in a validated platelet-aggregation assay. Platelets 2022;1–8. https://doi.org/10.1080/09537104.2022.2053091.

140. Watson AA, Eble JA, O'Callaghan CA. Crystal structure of rhodocytin, a ligand for the platelet-activating receptor CLEC-2. Protein Sci 2008;17(9):1611–6.

Routine Coagulation

Emmanuel J. Favaloro, PhD, FFSc (RCPA)[a,b,c],*,
Leonardo Pasalic, FRCPA, FRACP, PhD[a,d]

KEYWORDS

- Routine coagulation • Activated partial thromboplastin time • Prothrombin time
- Thrombin time • Fibrinogen • D-dimer

KEY POINTS

- Routine coagulation typically comprises of assays performed in most hematology laboratories, often offered 24/7, and primarily the prothrombin time or international normalized ratio, activated partial thromboplastin time, fibrinogen, thrombin time, and D-dimer.
- Additional assays may selectively be performed in some routine coagulation laboratories, given increasing utility, advanced automation, and clinical need.
- Although almost all hemostasis assays can be performed on instruments available in routine coagulation laboratories, there are good reasons to not provide every available assay 24/7.
- This article reflects on increasing automation in the age of increasing artificial intelligence use, and tries to provide a balanced view on testing that could/should be offered in routine coagulation laboratories.

INTRODUCTION

The term 'routine coagulation' typically applies to hemostasis tests that are routinely performed in hematology laboratories. These tests are often available 24 hours a day, 7 days a week (ie, 24/7), and may also be ordered urgently ('STAT'). There is no mandatory requirements for test inclusion within the category of routine coagulation, but at a minimum; this category of tests should comprise of the prothrombin time (PT), the PT converted to an international normalized ratio (INR), and the activated partial thromboplastin time (APTT; often called partial thromboplastin time [PTT] in North

[a] Haematology, Sydney Centres for Thrombosis and Haemostasis, Institute of Clinical Pathology and Medical Research (ICPMR), NSW Health Pathology, Westmead Hospital, Westmead, NSW 2145, Australia; [b] School of Dentistry and Medical Sciences, Charles Sturt University, Wagga Wagga, New South Wales, Australia; [c] School of Medical Sciences, University of Sydney, Westmead Hospital, Westmead, New South Wales, Australia; [d] Westmead Clinical School, University of Sydney, Westmead, NSW, Australia
* Corresponding author. Haematology, Sydney Centres for Thrombosis and Haemostasis, Institute of Clinical Pathology and Medical Research (ICPMR), NSW Health Pathology, Westmead Hospital, Westmead, NSW 2145, Australia.
E-mail address: Emmanuel.Favaloro@health.nsw.gov.au

Clin Lab Med 44 (2024) 527–539
https://doi.org/10.1016/j.cll.2024.04.012 **labmed.theclinics.com**
0272-2712/24/Crown Copyright © 2024 Published by Elsevier Inc. All rights reserved.

Table 1
What constitutes 'routine coagulation assays'?

Test Abbreviation	Test	What the Test Measures	What the Test is Used for	What Else is the Test Sensitive to?	Available in Routine Coagulation Laboratories in Our Network?
A. Assays available in "all" routine coagulation laboratories					
PT	Prothrombin time	**Fig. 1A.** Test measures TF (also called extrinsic) pathway plus common coagulation pathway	Assessment of factor deficiency (I, II, V, VII, X). Monitoring of VKA (eg, warfarin) therapy (typically as the INR) Screen for disseminated intravascular coagulation (DIC)	Various anticoagulants (eg, UFH in excess to heparin neutralizer capacity, and DOACs)	Yes, all 60 laboratories (84 instruments)
INR	International normalized ratio	Same as PT, but reflective of a normalized ratio.	Used to monitor patients on VKA therapy	Same as PT	
APTT	Activated partial thromboplastin time	**Fig. 1A.** Test measures contact factor (also called intrinsic) pathway plus common coagulation pathway	Assessment of factor deficiency (I, II, V, VIII, IX, X, XI, XII). Monitoring of UFH therapy Screen for DIC	Various anticoagulants (eg, DOACs)	
B. Assays available in "most" routine coagulation laboratories					
TT	Thrombin Time	**Fig. 1A**	Screen for fibrinogen deficiency. Screen for UFH and other anti-II agents (eg, dabigatran) Screen for DIC	Various anticoagulants (eg, lepirudin, bivalirudin)	Yes, most but not all laboratories
D-D	D-dimer	The fibrin degradation product called D-D	Screen for venous thrombosis (eg, DVT; PE). Screen for DIC	Depending on antibody used in assay, potentially variously sensitive to other fibrin or fibrinogen degradation products	
FBN	Fibrinogen	FBN level (FBN is the major coagulation protein)	Assessment of congenital or acquired FBN deficiencies or abnormalities	Some assays may be affected by very high levels of some anticoagulants (eg, UFH, dabigatran)	

C. Assays potentially available in a few or "select" routine coagulation laboratories

AT	Antithrombin	AT level	Quantitation of AT activity	Depending on how assay is performed (ie, as based on anti-Xa or anti-IIa) may be sensitive to various anticoagulants (eg, DOACs)	No, but can be performed urgently in the larger diagnostic hemostasis laboratories
LA	Lupus anticoagulant	Presence or absence of LA	To exclude or identify LA as a cause of APTT prolongation. To help determine anticoagulant treatment for inpatient pending discharge	Various anticoagulants depending on assays or reagents employed	No, but can be performed urgently in the larger diagnostic hemostasis laboratories
Anti-Xa or anti-FXa	Anti-factor Xa	Level of various anticoagulants depending on test set up	To quantify levels of UFH, LMWH, direct and indirect anti-FXa agents (eg, apixaban, rivaroxaban, edoxaban, and fondaparinux)	Each 'specific' anti-Xa assay is variously sensitive to the other anti-FXa agents	Yes, but only at select (larger or central) laboratory sites
DTI or dTT	Direct thrombin inhibitor or dilute thrombin time	Level of various anticoagulants depending on test set up	To quantify levels of anti-IIa agents (eg, dabigatran)	Each 'specific' anti-IIa assay potentially sensitive to other anti-IIa agents	Yes, but only at select (larger or central) laboratory sites
FVIII, FIX (FXI, FXII)	Factors VIII and IX; potentially also XI and XII	Level of factor VIII and factor IX activity (possibly also XI and XII)	To quantify levels of these factors if urgently required	Variously sensitive to various anticoagulants	No, but can be performed urgently in the larger diagnostic hemostasis laboratories

American laboratories) (**Table 1**). Indeed, it would be rare that any of these tests would be omitted in any 'routine coagulation' laboratory around the world.

The other 'routine coagulation' tests available in most routine coagulation laboratories worldwide would be the thrombin time (TT), the D-dimer (D-D) assay, and fibrinogen (Fib or FBN) assays (**Table 1**). These tests may not be available in some smaller or remote laboratories because of costs associated to reagent wastage with low test numbers, and the difficulties maintaining staff skills and competencies for low volume tests.

Finally, some tests may or may not be included in some 'routine coagulation' test panels for a variety of reasons. In addition to reagent wastage and the difficulties maintaining staff skills and competencies for low volume tests, especially in small and intermediate sized laboratories, test make up will also be based on available instrumentation, the facilities being serviced by the laboratory, and the regulatory landscape. Some of the tests that may be available, particularly in larger routine coagulation laboratories, servicing tertiary teaching hospitals would be assays for antithrombin (AT), Lupus anticoagulant (LA), anti-factor Xa (anti-Xa or anti-FXa), and direct thrombin inhibitor (DTI) or dilute thrombin time (dTT) (**Table 1**).

This narrative article will describe these assays, what they are used for, why they may (or may not) be included in particular laboratories, as well as test interferences and limitations. The authors also identify usage in their large network of 60 laboratories housing 84 automated hemostasis analyzers as an example of their reasoning. The authors also provide a snapshot of the potential use of artificial intelligence (AI) in shaping the future landscape of hemostasis.

A SHORT DESCRIPTION OF A LONG HISTORY

The history of coagulation is rich and long. Several assays have been developed over time, with some morphing into the 'modern' tests the authors now describe, and some disappearing entirely from view. The term "prothrombin time" captures over 20,000 citations in PubMed. Interestingly, the first citation dates back to 1916.[1] However, the 'modern' PT as the authors know it, developed from the work of Armand J Quick and other early pioneers, and dates back to around 1935.[2–5] The discovery of various clotting factors in the 1940's and 1950's led to their assays, and the development of the PTT in the late 1950's lead to the development of the APTT in the 1960's.[5–11] TT was also developed in the 1940's and 1950's, as was the von Clauss FBN assay.[12–14]

The other assays have a more recent history. The presence of D-D as a fibrin degradation product (FDP) was first explored in the mid-1970's.[15–18] However, early laboratory assays performed by ELISA (enzyme linked immunosorbent assay) were migrated to latex agglutination assays (ie, more akin to current assays) in the 1980's and 1990's.[18–23] The earlier incarnations of the D-D assay were those of the 1960's measuring FDPs.[24–26] Because the FDP assays measured both fibrinogen degradation products and FDPs, they were less useful for exclusion of venous thrombosis. The INR was developed in the 1980's because of the problems evident with use of the PT to monitor vitamin K antagonist (VKA) therapy, such as warfarin.[27–29] In brief, quite variable PT values will be obtained for the same plasma tested using different reagents and instruments, and the INR 'corrects' for the influence of the different reagents and instruments using a normalization procedure.

UTILITY AND LIMITATIONS OF THE MOST COMMON ROUTINE COAGULATION ASSAYS

All laboratory assays can be considered to have some utility, as well as limitations that constrain this utility, with routine coagulation assays being no exception. The PT measures the tissue factor (TF; also called the extrinsic) pathway of coagulation plus the 'common pathway' (**Table 1** and **Fig. 1**). The PT is thus sensitive to several coagulation factors in the coagulation cascade, and namely factors I (FBN), II (prothrombin), V, VII and X. The test can therefore be used to assess for deficiencies or defects in these factors, both acquired and congenital. The PT is also used as a screen for disseminated intravascular coagulation (DIC).[30] The INR is sensitive to the same factor deficiencies, but is primarily used for measuring the anticoagulant status of patients on vitamin K antagonists (VKAs), such as warfarin.[31] The APTT measures the contact factor (also called intrinsic) pathway of coagulation plus common coagulation pathway (**Table 1** and **Fig. 1**). The APTT is thus sensitive to several coagulation factors in the coagulation cascade, and namely factors I, II, V, VIII, IX, X, XI and XII. This test can therefore be used to assess for deficiencies or defects in these factors, both acquired and congenital. The APTT is also used as a screen for DIC, and also to monitor patients on unfractionated heparin (UFH) therapy.[30,32] The TT is a simple test performed by adding a 'low' concentration of thrombin to plasma, and reflects the conversion of FBN to fibrin, and is thus sensitive to and used as a screen for, FBN deficiency.[33] The TT is also very sensitive to thrombin inhibitors, and thus can be used as a screen for the presence of both UFH and the direct oral anticoagulant (DOAC) dabigatran.

The D-D assay reflects a 'specific' FDP, and so is primarily used to exclude the presence of venous thrombosis, including deep vein thrombosis (DVT) and pulmonary thrombosis (PE).[34] The D-D assay is also useful as a screen for DIC.[30] Fibrinogen represents the major clotting protein in plasma, and thus its measurement is useful for assessing for deficiencies or defects in FBN, either congenital or acquired (eg, DIC).[30,33]

Although clinically useful, none of these assays is specific for any disorder, and so they all have limitations. The PT, and by extension the INR, is not solely sensitive to factor deficiencies or VKA therapy. Both are also affected by the presence of other anticoagulants, including the DOACs,[35,36] and UFH if in excess to the reagent heparin-neutralizing ability (**Fig. 1, Table 1**). Similarly, the APTT is not solely sensitive to factor deficiency and UFH; it is also affected by the presence of other anticoagulants, including the DOACs.[35,36] Although the D-D reflects a 'specific' assay measuring FDPs, there are a large number of different reagents in use, and there is some potential cross reactivity with other fibrinogen degradation products or FDPs.[37] Also, D-D levels can rise in a variety of conditions other than thrombosis.[34] Finally, the FBN assay is made fairly specific to FBN detection because of the assay design, but excess levels of anticoagulants, especially dabigatran, may affect test results.[35]

UTILITY AND LIMITATIONS OF LESS COMMON 'ROUTINE COAGULATION ASSAYS'

Table 1 includes other tests that are not commonly employed in most routine coagulation laboratories, but which may be found in some routine coagulation laboratories, perhaps increasingly in times to come.

AT represents one of the natural anticoagulants. Congenital deficiencies of AT are rare, and thus 'urgent' testing of congenital deficiencies is largely unwarranted. However, 'urgent' testing may be warranted in assessing for an acquired AT deficiency, for example, as associated with PEG L-asparaginase treatment of acute lymphoblastic leukemia, which can reduce levels of AT and cause thrombosis. Although AT assays are fairly specific for AT, the most common assays measure AT activity using either an anti-Xa or anti-IIa based chromogenic assay. Therefore, AT assays may yield unreliable test results in patients on DOACs (apixaban, rivaroxaban, and edoxaban if using an anti-Xa assay or dabigatran if using an anti-IIa assay). Because anti-Xa DOACs are

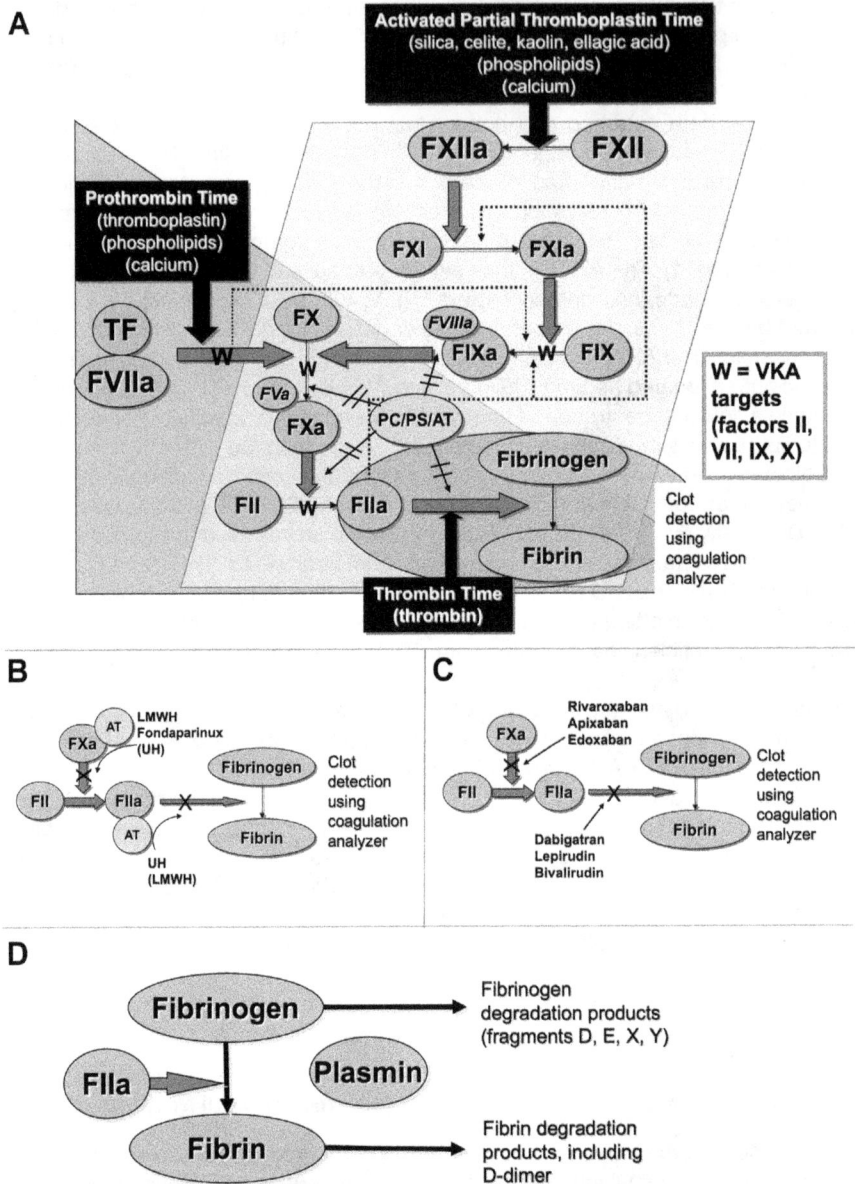

Fig. 1. A pictorial representation of the main laboratory tests performed in routine coagulation laboratories. The figure also summarizes inhibition points for various anticoagulants. (*A*) A pictorial representation of the PT (prothrombin time), APTT (activated partial thromboplastin time) and TT (thrombin time) assays, identifying regions of these pathways affected by VKAs (vitamin K antagonists), such as warfarin (W), which inhibits production of fully functional factors II, VII, IX and X. Inhibition sites for antithrombin (AT), protein C (PC) and protein S (PS) shown for comparison. (*B*) A pictorial representation of the terminal stages of the common pathway of coagulation (eg, from **Fig. 1**A) identifying the regions inhibited by low molecular weight heparin (LMWH), unfractionated heparin (UFH) and fondaparinux. LMWH mainly inhibits factor Xa, and UFH mainly inhibits factor IIa (ie, thrombin). These effects are indirect and require antithrombin (AT) as a cofactor. (*C*) A pictorial

more frequently prescribed than dabigatran,[38] the authors' laboratory network opted to harmonize on an anti-IIa method.[39] Still, the authors' laboratory network does not have this test available within the routine coagulation laboratory, although all laboratories have instruments capable of performing urgent AT tests. Indeed, all 60 laboratories in the authors' laboratory network, for a total of 84 instruments, have automated hemostasis instruments capable of performing most tests of hemostasis.[40] However, theoretic feasibility is not the same as practical reality. To enable testing of hemostasis tests in all the routine coagulation laboratories, AT included, the authors would need to train well over 200 staff, and maintain their skills using ongoing competency assessments, for an infrequently performed assay, as well as enrolling each laboratory in an external quality assessment (EQA) module, and include these tests in an accreditation process. There would also be extra costs associated with performance of internal quality control (QC). Because these tests would be infrequent in these settings, most of the assay kit would be wasted and discarded because 'use by dates' would be exceeded. In any case, the limited indications would likely only be applicable to larger or central sites. In the Westmead laboratory, AT is performed in the diagnostic hemostasis laboratory, and performed urgently if appropriately clinically justified. This laboratory only operates 5 days a week during normal hours (8am-5pm), but this likely aligns to times of clinical treatment (ie, when patients are undergoing treatment and being monitored), and thus, test need.

Lupus anticoagulant (LA) represents a risk factor for thrombosis and pregnancy or fetal morbidity.[41] Urgent testing is rarely required, but there may be situations where it can be justified. For example, the identification of an unexpectedly prolonged APTT ahead of imminent surgery may require urgent testing for LA or factor assays to explain the prolongation, and thus, avoid surgical cancellation. It can be noted that LA is a common finding explaining isolated unexpected elevated APTTs. Another potential reason for 'urgent' LA testing may be in a patient about to be discharged on anticoagulant therapy after a thrombotic event, and where testing for antiphospholipid antibodies (aPL) was found to be previously positive. Here, the clinicians may prefer to avoid rivaroxaban or apixaban therapy in the case of LA (or triple aPL) positivity. As for the case for AT, the authors' network does not include LA testing in the routine coagulation laboratories, nor is it available in the routine coagulation laboratory at Westmead, and for essentially the same reasons identified for AT. LA testing is performed in the diagnostic hemostasis laboratory, and performed urgently if appropriately clinically justified. Other options to avoid the aforementioned scenarios are: (i) to avoid identification of 'asymptomatic LA' carriers- (a) select a relatively LA insensitive APTT reagent for general APTT screening, in line with the LA guidelines[42-44], (b) educate proceduralists to not order APTT assays as a routine screen for bleeding risk because the APTT is a poor predictor of same[45]; (ii) to avoid urgent requests on patients about to be discharged and educate clinicians to use pathology wisely, including earlier (rather than last minute) LA investigations as necessary.

Anti-factor Xa (anti-Xa or anti-FXa) assays are used to measure the level of anti-Xa agents. Historically, this was for low molecular weight heparin (LMWH), and occasionally

---

representation of the terminal stages of the common pathway of coagulation (eg, from **Fig. 1**A) identifying the regions inhibited by direct inhibitors of factor Xa (eg, the direct oral anticoagulants (DOACs) rivaroxaban, apixaban, edoxaban), and factor IIa (eg, the DOAC dabigatran, and the parenteral agents lepirudin and bivalirudin). (*D*) A pictorial representation of the formation of fibrinogen degradation products and fibrin degradation products, the latter including D-dimer.

for UFH (eg, in LA positive or FXII deficient patient).[46] However, the test is increasingly becoming available for measuring the anti-Xa DOACs (apixaban, rivaroxaban, and edoxaban).[47] Again, the authors do not include anti-Xa testing in the test repertoire of most routine coagulation laboratories in their network, despite it being technically feasible (kits are available and all instruments are capable), and for essentially the same reasons identified for AT and LA as mentioned before. However, the tests are available in the routine coagulation laboratory at Westmead (thus available 24/7), and also available for LMWH/UFH monitoring at some select central sites in the network. Similarly, DTI testing is also available in the routine coagulation laboratory at Westmead (thus available 24/7) for the anti-IIa DOAC dabigatran, as performed as a dTT assay.

Finally, urgent factor testing may also be required for similar reasons to those for LA (eg, unexpectedly raised APTT ahead of planned surgery), as well as for other reasons (eg, actively bleeding patient). Here, there may be a preference to restrict urgent factor testing to FVIII and FIX because these are the most common deficiencies associated with bleeding risk. However, exclusion of FXII may risk missing FXII deficiency, which is a common cause of APTT prolongation, and not associated with bleeding. Finally, if a laboratory is performing urgent testing for FVIII, FIX and FXII, it may as well include FXI to complete the panel. The authors do not include this testing in the test repertoire of routine coagulation laboratories in the authors' network, despite it being technically feasible (kits are available and all instruments are capable), and for essentially the same reasons identified for AT and LA aforementioned. Urgent testing for these factors is available in the larger hemostasis laboratories in the authors network, which also more likely aligns to urgent clinical requests (eg, surgical and obstetric). As for LA, a strategy to avoid urgent factor requests on patients headed to surgery is to educate clinicians to wise use of pathology, including earlier investigations of prolonged APTTs as necessary, as well as to not order APTT screens for assessment of bleeding risk ahead of surgery.[45]

USE OF ARTIFICIAL INTELLIGENCE FOR HEMOSTASIS TESTING

The authors believe it is worthwhile to undertake a short analysis of the use of AI in hemostasis testing, especially as it pertains to routine coagulation. The concept of AI, as currently expressed in the scientific literature, involving 'machine learning' and refinement is not really our focus because this process is in its infancy.[48] What the authors mean here is the use of AI to leverage computers and machines (ie, instruments) to mimic the problem-solving and decision-making capabilities of the human mind, thus, including computers, laboratory information systems, electronic ordering systems, laboratory middle ware, and hemostasis instrumentation, to streamline test ordering, assay performance, and reporting. The power of AI here is enormous, saving time, improving test selection and accuracy, and standardizing post-analytical reporting. Again, the authors will largely draw on their own experience here.

Hemostasis testing, including routine coagulation, can be seen within three phases – pre-analytical, analytical, and post-analytical. The pre-analytical phase reflects what happens before laboratory testing, from clinical ordering, blood collection, and blood processing. Clinicians do not always make wise decisions. There are several strategies to help control inappropriate test utilization, including the various "Choosing wisely' campaigns to educate on wise choices for pathology testing.[49] Several recommendations related to hemostasis appear in various "choose wisely" lists, including "Do not measure the INR in patients who are taking an anti-Xa inhibitor" and "Don't employ a specific DOAC reversal agent without identifying the DOAC and estimating its plasma concentration." One of the authors own recommendations related to routine coagulation would be for clinicians to not order routine coagulation tests in patients taking anticoagulants other than VKAs and heparin, therefore, including DOACs, and then request follow-up factor assays or LA testing to explain any 'unexpected' prolongations. To facilitate wise test selection, electronic ordering systems can be designed to either put stops on unnecessary testing or to gather important clinical information to help explain downstream test results. Some examples: (a) querying the need for routine coagulation tests, or other hemostasis tests, when an order for that test has already (or recently) been made (to avoid duplicate orders), (b) requesting information about patient anticoagulation (all possibilities), (c) requesting completion of a 4T score ahead of ordering heparin induced thrombocytopenia testing or a PLAS-MIC score ahead of ADAMTS13 testing. In the authors' local network of 27 laboratories, they developed such initiatives in their electronic ordering systems, which were supplemented by an expert rule set that analyzed routine coagulation test results in view of this information, and then reflexed to additional testing as necessary (eg, mixing tests, TTs or FBN assays), as well as automating verification and harmonized test comments.[50]

Additional strategies to facilitate improved test performance (pre-analytical and analytical phases) include instrument capacity to test for underfilling of primary citrate blood collection tubes, presence of clots in these tubes, and presence of hemolysis, jaundice and lipemia in plasma.[51] The outcome of these checks may be to produce an error alert, or to switch instrument wavelengths used for clot detection to provide more accurate test results.

Finally, harmonization of associated test comments provides opportunities to improve test reporting and avoid ambiguous or variable or potentially erroneous comments in the post-analytical phase.[50,52]

DISCUSSION

In this article, the authors have identified those tests commonly performed in routine coagulation laboratories, as well as those tests performed selectively in such laboratories. It is without doubt that there is technical feasibility to perform most tests of hemostasis in routine coagulation laboratories because all modern hemostasis instruments have similar test feasibility. This is certainly true of the 84 instruments housed in the 60 laboratories in the authors' large extended network, which comprise of ACL TOP 350s, 550s, or 750s.[53] The differences in the instruments are primarily related to throughput, with this increasing from 350 to 550 to 750. The technically feasible test menus are the same across all instruments. However, technical feasibility does not equate to practical application. To perform a particular test on an instrument, the technicians have to be appropriately trained and their competencies (ie, skills in test performance) maintained through regular assessments. This process needs to be manageable, and its application costed (ie, technician training time and supervisor trainer time). The tests applied at each site also need to be accredited at that site, meaning greater accreditation oversight for each laboratory. This will also need each test site to undergo regular EQA assessments. Additional accreditation oversight and EQA assessments are costly, and thus, also need to be considered. Every time a test is performed urgently, a technician is removed from their routine workflow, and then also needs to perform QC testing for the urgent test ahead of patient test performance. This also entails additional test reagent costs. These infrequently performed tests comprise of assay kits that may need to be removed from instruments and placed under refrigeration to maximize shelf life. Thus, test performance in the routine coagulation laboratory means increased technician time requirements and disruption to routine workflow, potentially extending test turnaround times for the more typical routine coagulation tests. These rarely performed tests will also lead to high test reagent wastage because most of the test kit will not be used up before its expiry date. In total, from a cost perspective, a test such as AT that may cost $5 per test to perform as a batch in a specialized laboratory, may end up costing as much as $500 per test in a routine coagulation laboratory when all costs of test implementation and service maintenance are considered.

Put simply, there are clear economies of scale, and costs need to be recovered. Testing of all hemostasis tests in the routine coagulation laboratory is technically feasible, but it is unlikely that hospitals would be willing to pay all the costs associated with urgent or rare testing in a routine coagulation laboratory.

SUMMARY

The modern hemostasis laboratory has at its disposal modern equipment capable of high throughput and wide test selection. However, although the same hemostasis tests performed in specialized laboratories are also technically feasible in routine coagulation laboratories; this does not mean that all routine laboratories should be enabled to perform all such hemostasis tests. Most hemostasis tests performed in specialized hemostasis laboratories are batched to increase cost effectiveness, which in the end translates to the most cost-effective service for the authors' health care partners – mostly public funded hospitals. It is unlikely these hospitals would be happy to fund the cost of services when these are performed in an inefficient manner. The difference in costs can be huge and would need to include not only the direct costs of the instruments, test reagents, and control material, but also the indirect costs of training, maintaining competencies, EQA, and maintaining accreditation.

CLINICS CARE POINTS

- All modern hemostasis instrumentation can perform most tests of hemostasis, even those normally restricted to specialised centers.
- Such tests could feasibly be run in routine coagulation laboratories, but costs, lack of expertise, and the ongoing needs of accreditation, training and maintaining competence usually prevents them from inclusion in routine laboratory test panels.

DISCLOSURE

The authors have no conflicts of interest to disclose.

ACKNOWLEDGMENTS/SOURCES OF FUNDING

The views expressed herein are those of the authors and are not necessarily those of NSW Health Pathology or other affiliated institutions.

REFERENCES

1. Minot GR. The effect of temperature upon the clotting time (prothrombin time) of oxalated plasma with calcium. J Media Res 1916;33(3):503–6.
2. Quick AJ. The one-stage prothrombin time determination. Its history and interpretation. Chemotherapia 1961;3:313–20.

3. Biggs R. Editorial: Forty years of the one-stage prothrombin time. Thrombosis Diath Haemorrh 1975 30;33(2):139–40.
4. Dirckx JH, Armand J. Quick: pioneer and prophet of coagulation research. Ann Intern Med 1980;92(4):553–8.
5. Owen CA Jr. Historical account of tests of hemostasis. Am J Clin Pathol 1990;93(4 Suppl 1):S3–8.
6. Rodman NF Jr, Barrow EM, Graham JB. Diagnosis and control of the hemophilioid states with the partial thromboplastin time (PTT) test. Am J Clin Pathol 1958;29(6): 525–38.
7. Proctor RR, Rapaport SI. The partial thromboplastin time with kaolin. A simple screening test for first stage plasma clotting factor deficiencies. Am J Clin Pathol 1961;36:212–9.
8. Struver GP, Bittner DL, Wall CA. The use of the cephalin time (partial thromboplastin time) in anticoagulation therapy with heparin. Surg Forum 1962;13:127–9.
9. Weiss DL, Reiner M, Ibanez R. The partial thromboplastin time (P.T.T.) as a screening procedure. Preliminary report. Med Ann Dist Columbia 1962;31:140–2.
10. Lenahan JG, Phillips GE. Some variables which influence the activated partial thromboplastin time assay. Clin Chem 1966;12(5):269–73.
11. Lenaham JG, Frye S Jr, Phillips GE. Use of the activated partial thromboplastin time in the control of heparin administration. Clin Chem 1966;12(5):263–8.
12. Honorato R. A simple means to determine exact moment of clotting in prothrombin or thrombin time determination. Proc Soc Exp Biol Med 1947;65(1):41.
13. Shinowara GY, Rosenfeld L. Enzyme studies on human blood. VIII. The effect of fibrinogen concentration on the thrombin clotting time. J Lab Clin Med 1951; 37(2):303–10.
14. Clauss VA. Gerinnungsphysiologische Schnellmethode zur Bestimmung des Fibrinogens. Ada Haematol 1957;17:237–46.
15. Gaffney PJ, Lane DA, Kakkar VV, et al. Characterisation of a soluble D dimer-E complex in crosslinked fibrin digests. Thromb Res 1975;7(1):89–99.
16. Gaffney PJ, Lane DA, Brasher M. Soluble high-molecular-weight E fragments in the plasmin-induced degradation products of cross-linked human fibrin. Clin Sci Mol Med 1975;49(2):149–56.
17. Ferguson EW, Fretto LJ, McKee PA. A re-examination of the cleavage of fibrinogen and fibrin by plasmin. J Biol Chem 1975 25;250(18):7210–8.
18. Gaffney PJ. Distinction between fibrinogen and fibrin degradation products in plasma. Clin Chim Acta 1975 15;65(1):109–15.
19. Rowbotham BJ, Carroll P, Whitaker AN, et al. Measurement of crosslinked fibrin derivatives–use in the diagnosis of venous thrombosis. Thromb Haemostasis 1987 3;57(1):59–61.
20. Heaton DC, Billings JD, Hickton CM. Assessment of D dimer assays for the diagnosis of deep vein thrombosis. J Lab Clin Med 1987;110(5):588–91.
21. Chapman CS, Akhtar N, Campbell S, et al. The use of D-Dimer assay by enzyme immunoassay and latex agglutination techniques in the diagnosis of deep vein thrombosis. Clin Lab Haematol 1990;12(1):37–42.
22. Bick RL, Baker WF. Diagnostic efficacy of the D-dimer assay in disseminated intravascular coagulation (DIC). Thromb Res 1992 15;65(6):785–90.
23. Brenner B, Pery M, Lanir N, et al. Application of a bedside whole blood D-dimer assay in the diagnosis of deep vein thrombosis. Blood Coagul Fibrinolysis 1995; 6(3):219–22.

24. Ferreira HC, Murat LG. An immunological method for demonstrating fibrin degradation products in serum and its use in the diagnosis of fibrinolytic states. Br J Haematol 1963;9:299–310.

25. Lewis JH, Wilson JH. Fibrinogen breakdown products. Am J Physiol 1964;207: 1053–7.

26. Niléhn JE, Robertson B. On the degradation products of fibrinogen or fibrin after infusion of streptokinase in patients with venous thrombosis. Scand J Haematol 1965;2(4):267–76.

27. van den Besselaar AM, Evatt BL, Brogan DR, et al. Proficiency testing and standardization of prothrombin time: effect of thromboplastin, instrumentation, and plasma. Am J Clin Pathol 1984;82(6):688–99.

28. van den Besselaar AM. Standardization of the prothrombin time in oral anticoagulant control. Haemostasis 1985;15(4):271–7.

29. Loeliger EA, van den Besselaar AM, Lewis SM. Reliability and clinical impact of the normalization of the prothrombin times in oral anticoagulant control. Thromb Haemostasis 1985;53(1):148–54.

30. Favaloro EJ. Laboratory testing in disseminated intravascular coagulation. Semin Thromb Hemost 2010;36(4):458–67.

31. Favaloro EJ. How to generate a more accurate laboratory-based international normalized ratio: solutions to obtaining or verifying the mean normal prothrombin time and international sensitivity index. Semin Thromb Hemost 2019;45(1):10–21.

32. Favaloro EJ, Kershaw G, Mohammed S, et al. How to optimize activated partial thromboplastin time (APTT) testing: solutions to establishing and verifying normal reference intervals and assessing APTT reagents for sensitivity to heparin, lupus anticoagulant, and clotting factors. Semin Thromb Hemost 2019;45(1):22–35.

33. Undas A. Determination of fibrinogen and thrombin time (TT). Methods Mol Biol 2017;1646:105–10.

34. Thachil J, Favaloro EJ, Lippi G. D-dimers-"Normal" levels versus elevated levels due to a range of conditions, including "D-dimeritis," inflammation, thromboembolism, disseminated intravascular coagulation, and COVID-19. Semin Thromb Hemost 2022;48(6):672–9.

35. Bonar R, Favaloro EJ, Mohammed S, et al. The effect of dabigatran on haemostasis tests: a comprehensive assessment using in-vitro and ex-vivo samples. Pathology 2015;47(4):355–64.

36. Bonar R, Favaloro EJ, Mohammed S, et al. The effect of the direct factor Xa inhibitors apixaban and rivaroxaban on haemostasis tests: a comprehensive assessment using in vitro and ex vivo samples. Pathology 2016;48(1):60–71.

37. Longstaff C, Adcock D, Olson JD, et al. Harmonisation of D-dimer - a call for action. Thromb Res 2016;137:219–20.

38. Favaloro EJ, Pasalic L, Lippi G. Oral anticoagulation therapy: an update on usage, costs and associated risks. Pathology 2020;52(6):736–41.

39. Favaloro EJ, Mohammed S, Vong R, et al. A multi-laboratory assessment of congenital thrombophilia assays performed on the ACL Top 50 family for harmonisation of thrombophilia testing in a large laboratory network. Clin Chem Lab Med 2021 14;59(10):1709–18.

40. Favaloro EJ, Mohammed S, Vong R, et al. Verification of the ACL Top 50 family (350, 550 and 750) for harmonization of routine coagulation assays in a large network of 60 laboratories. Am J Clin Pathol 2021;156(4):661–78.

41. Miyakis S, Lockshin MD, Atsumi T, et al. International consensus statement on an update of the classification criteria for definite antiphospholipid syndrome (APS). J Thromb Haemostasis 2006;4(2):295–306.

42. Devreese KMJ, de Groot PG, de Laat B, et al. Guidance from the Scientific and Standardization Committee for lupus anticoagulant/antiphospholipid antibodies of the International Society on Thrombosis and Haemostasis: update of the guidelines for lupus anticoagulant detection and interpretation. J Thromb Haemostasis 2020;18(11):2828–39.

43. Pengo V, Tripodi A, Reber G, et al. Subcommittee on lupus anticoagulant/antiphospholipid antibody of the scientific and standardisation committee of the international Society on thrombosis and haemostasis. Update of the guidelines for lupus anticoagulant detection. Subcommittee on lupus anticoagulant/antiphospholipid antibody of the scientific and standardisation Committee of the International Society on Thrombosis and Haemostasis. J Thromb Haemostasis 2009;7(10):1737–40.

44. Clinical and Laboratory Standards Institute (CLSI). Laboratory testing for the Lupus anticoagulant; approved guideline. CLSI document H60-A. Wayne, PA: CLSI; 2014.

45. Larsen JB, Hvas AM. Predictive value of whole blood and plasma coagulation tests for intra- and postoperative bleeding risk: a systematic review. Semin Thromb Hemost 2017;43(7):772–805.

46. Dean CL. An overview of heparin monitoring with the anti-xa assay. Methods Mol Biol 2023;2663:343–53.

47. Gosselin RC, Adcock DM, Bates SM, et al. International Council for standardization in Haematology (ICSH) recommendations for laboratory measurement of direct oral anticoagulants. Thromb Haemostasis 2018;118(3):437–50.

48. Favaloro EJ, Negrini D, Negrini D. Machine learning and coagulation testing: the next big thing in hemostasis investigations? Clin Chem Lab Med 2021;59(7):1177–9.

49. About choosing wisely. Available at: https://www.ascp.org/content/get-involved/choosing-wisely. [Accessed 6 September 2023].

50. Mohammed S, Ule Priebbenow V, Pasalic L, et al. Development and implementation of an expert rule set for automated reflex testing and validation of routine coagulation tests in a large pathology network. Int J Lab Hematol 2019;41(5):642–9.

51. Lippi G, Mattiuzzi C, Favaloro EJ. Artificial Intelligence in the pre-analytical phase: state-of-the art and future perspectives. J Med Biochem 2023;42:1–10.

52. Favaloro EJ, Gosselin RC, Pasalic L, et al. Post-analytical issues in hemostasis and thrombosis testing: an update. Methods Mol Biol 2023;2663:787–811.

53. Favaloro EJ, Mohammed S, Vong R, et al. Harmonization of hemostasis testing across a large laboratory network: an example from Australia. Methods Mol Biol 2023;2663:71–91.

Heparin Induced Thrombocytopenia Testing

Daniel C. Dees, DCLS, MLS(ASCP)*

KEYWORDS

- Heparin induced thrombocytopenia • Automation • Hematology • Coagulation

KEY POINTS

- Heparin induced thrombocytopenia (HIT) can be a difficult condition to recognize and diagnosis.
- Accurate diagnosis is dependent on screening and confirmatory laboratory tests.
- Automation has increased the efficiency and turnaround for HIT values.

INTRODUCTION

Heparin is a commonly used anticoagulant discovered in 1916 that remains extremely relevant in both inpatient and outpatient settings. Heparin-induced thrombocytopenia (HIT) is a potentially life-threatening immune-mediated reaction that occurs in response to heparin administration and involves the formation of antibodies targeting complexes of platelet factor 4 (PF4) and heparin.[1] HIT manifests as a paradoxic phenomenon of thrombocytopenia, a significant reduction in platelet count, occurring concurrently with an increased risk of thrombosis. This typically occurs within 5 to 10 days of heparin exposure and causes an unanticipated drop in the platelet count. Two distinct clinical variants of this reaction are recognized: HIT Type I: a non-Immune-mediated mild form characterized by a transient, modest decrease in platelet count, which does not routinely require treatment, and HIT Type II: an immune-mediated, severe form associated with a higher risk of thrombotic complications requiring immediate treatment.[2]

While HIT remains infrequent, it poses substantial risks in clinical settings utilizing heparin for anticoagulation. The reported incidence varies among patient populations with estimates suggesting a prevalence ranging from 0.1% to 5%, and individuals receiving unfractionated heparin showing a higher incidence rate then seen in patients treated with low-molecular-weight heparin (LMWH).[3] Certain factors, such as duration of heparin exposure, type of heparin used, and gender can increase risk for the more severe Type II variation of HIT.[3] Despite its relatively low frequency, HIT remains a

Clinical Hematology, Brigham and Women's Hospital, Boston, MA, USA
* Corresponding author. 75 Francis Street, Boston, MA 02125.
E-mail address: ddees@bwh.harvard.edu

Clin Lab Med 44 (2024) 541–550
https://doi.org/10.1016/j.cll.2024.04.013
0272-2712/24/© 2024 Elsevier Inc. All rights reserved.

critical concern because of its potential to induce catastrophic thrombotic events, resulting in increased morbidity and mortality if left unrecognized and untreated. Understanding the epidemiologic landscape and recognizing the clinical manifestations assists clinicians in early suspicion, prompt diagnosis, and appropriate management of HIT, thereby mitigating the associated thrombotic complications and optimizing patient outcomes.

HISTORY OF HEPARIN-INDUCED THROMBOCYTOPENIA

HIT was first recognized in the 1950s approximately 30 years after the discovery of heparin. Initially, the drop in platelet counts observed in some patients receiving heparin therapy was thought to be a benign side effect of the anticoagulant. However, it eventually became apparent that this condition could lead to potentially fatal thrombotic complications. This response from some patients sparked significant interest and research into the condition. In 1957, at a meeting of the International Society of Angiology in New York the relationship between heparin and new thrombosis in patients was described by an assistant professor of clinical surgery at Dartmouth medical school, Dr Rodger Weismann, and his surgical resident, Dr Richard Tobin.[4] Over the following decades, the understanding of HIT pathogenesis increased and a paper in 1973 helped to establish HIT as an immune-mediated response by noting an increase in bone marrow megakaryocytes and the rapid drop in platelet counts upon repeat exposure to heparin.[4] The subsequent development of laboratory tests for HIT and the establishment of clinical scoring systems have further refined the diagnosis and management of this complex condition. Today, HIT stands as a well-characterized and critical consideration in patients receiving heparin therapy, representing a significant chapter in hematology and pharmacology.

CLINICAL PRESENTATION OF HEPARIN-INDUCED THROMBOCYTOPENIA

HIT commonly presents clinically with a distinctive pattern, characterized by a significant and abrupt decrease in platelet count by 50% or more from the patient's baseline values. HIT can also manifest with new or worsening thrombosis in the form of venous or arterial thromboembolism leading to severe complications such as limb ischemia, stroke, or myocardial infarction.[5] Less common manifestations can include localized reactions around the heparin injection site such as erythema, pain, or skin necrosis. The clinical presentation of HIT can be challenging for primary clinicians because of the numerous other potential pathologic causes of both thrombocytopenia and thrombosis. Clinical symptom scoring systems assist providers in determining the pre-test probability of HIT in patients and serves as a valuable tool when interpreting diagnostic laboratory testing. The most well-known of these scoring systems is the 4T score, which evaluates the following: *T*hrombocytopenia, *T*iming of platelet fall, *T*hrombosis, and o*T*her clinically overlapping thrombocytopenic conditions.[6]

LABORATORY DIAGNOSIS OF HEPARIN-INDUCED THROMBOCYTOPENIA

Accurate and timely laboratory diagnosis of HIT plays a pivotal role in guiding clinical management decisions and mitigating the risk of thrombotic complications associated with this condition. Given the complexity and varying presentations of HIT, a comprehensive and researched approach to laboratory testing is essential. Laboratory testing for HIT most often involves a combination of serologic assays for screening and functional assays for confirmation. A comparison of these assays is shown in **Table 1**.

Table 1
Heparin induced thrombocytopenia assay comparison

Feature	Serologic Assays	Functional Assays
Principle	Detect antibodies that bind to platelet factor 4/heparin complexes	Measure the ability of patient serum to activate platelets in the presence of heparin
Examples	ELISA (Enzyme-Linked Immunosorbent Assay), Particle Immunoassay, Chemiluminescence	Serotonin Release Assay (SRA), Heparin-Induced Platelet Activation (HIPA) test
Sensitivity	High sensitivity, can detect low levels of HIT antibodies	Less sensitive compared to serologic assays
Specificity	Lower specificity, can have false positives	High specificity, more accurate in confirming HIT diagnosis
Time to Results	Relatively quicker, results available within a few hours if not batched	Time-consuming, often taking several hours to a day
Cost	Generally, less expensive	More expensive because of labor-intensive processes
Availability	Widely available in most laboratories	Limited to specialized laboratories

SEROLOGIC ASSAYS

Serologic assays serve as fundamental tools in the initial assessment and screening for HIT because of the quicker turnaround times, lower cost, and the high sensitivity of these assays. These assays aim to detect the presence of anti-PF4 or heparin antibodies in patient serum, providing valuable insight into the immune response triggered by heparin administration. Examples of serologic assays include enzyme-linked immunosorbent assays (ELISAs) and particle agglutination, both detects these PF4 or heparin complex antibodies. ELISAs involve immobilizing PF4 or heparin complexes on a solid phase and detecting patient antibodies binding to these complexes.[7] Particle agglutination assays measure the ability of patient antibodies to cause agglutination of particles coated with PF4 or heparin complexes.[7]

Despite their widespread use and high sensitivity, serologic assays are subject to several limitations that impact clinical utility. One of the primary drawbacks is lower specificity, which can potentially lead to a higher rate of false-positive results. This limitation arises because these tests detect antibodies that bind to PF4 or heparin complexes, but not all of these antibodies are capable of causing platelet activation, which is essential for the development of clinically relevant HIT.[7] Consequently, positive serologic test results may not always indicate true HIT, leading to potential overdiagnosis and unnecessary treatment. Furthermore, the manual ELISA assays are often labor intensive and time consuming leading to them being performed in batches, which severely limits clinically useful turnaround for results. While a negative serologic assay result decreases the probability of HIT, subsequent testing with confirmatory functional assays may be required, especially in cases with strong clinical suspicion.

PLATELET ACTIVATION ASSAYS

While serologic assays are valuable for initial screening, they lack the ability to differentiate between HIT Type 1 (non-immune-mediated), HIT Type 2 (immune-mediated), and other potential causes of thrombocytopenia. This was first described as the "iceberg model" by Warkentin and colleagues in 2003.[8] Platelet activation assays act as confirmatory tests by directly assessing the ability of the anti-PF4 or heparin antibodies to induce platelet activation. A positive result in a platelet activation assay indicates the functional capacity of patient antibodies to induce platelet activation, supporting the diagnosis of HIT Type 2.[7] The most common platelet activation assays include the serotonin-release assay (SRA) and the heparin-induced platelet activation (HIPA) assay. In the SRA, patient serum is incubated with donor platelets in the presence of heparin. The extent of serotonin release is then measured, reflecting the ability of patient antibodies to activate platelets.[9] The HIPA assay assesses platelet activation by flow cytometry, measuring the expression of activation markers, such as P-selectin and activated GPIIb/IIIa, on platelet surfaces.[9]

Platelet activation assays, while highly specific for diagnosing HIT do have limitations that can impact their clinical application. One significant constraint is their limited availability; these tests are typically performed in specialized laboratories, which can lead to delays in obtaining results. This delay is critical in the context of HIT, where timely diagnosis and management are essential. Another challenge is the technical complexity and expertize required to perform and interpret these assays accurately. For example, the SRA is considered the gold standard for HIT testing, but requires live platelets and radioisotopes, making them labor-intensive and not feasible for many clinical laboratories.[9] Additionally, these assays can be affected by the presence of other drugs or disorders that may influence platelet reactivity, potentially leading to false-negative or inconsistent results. These tests are costlier compared with serologic assays, making them less accessible in some health care settings. These limitations necessitate a balanced approach to HIT diagnosis, often involving an initial screening with serologic assays followed by confirmation with functional assays only when necessary.

QUALITY CONTROL AND ASSURANCE IN HEPARIN-INDUCED THROMBOCYTOPENIADIAGNOSTICS

Quality control (QC) and quality assurance measures are integral components of any laboratory testing and testing for HIT is no exception. A robust quality management plan is required for ensuring the accuracy, reliability, and consistency of diagnostic assays. The quality management plan should include initial validation studies, internal or external QC, proficiency testing, calibrations, maintenance, and a complete competency assessment plan. These are essential to minimize errors, maintain assay performance, and uphold the credibility of test results.

Validation studies for HIT assays involve rigorous testing to establish assay sensitivity, specificity, precision, accuracy, and analytical performance characteristics. These validations ensure that assays meet predefined criteria for clinical use. QCs, both internal and external, ensure frequent monitoring of assay performance using control materials with known values. These QC results can be charted out over time to enable laboratories to detect trends or shifts in assay performance, triggering investigations, and corrective actions proactively as required.

Participation in proficiency testing programs is also vital for laboratories conducting HIT diagnostics. These programs involve receiving blinded samples from external agencies for independent assessment, allowing laboratories to benchmark their performance against peers. This provides an external validation of laboratory accuracy, identifying potential areas for improvement, and ensuring alignment with standardized practices.

Regular maintenance and calibration of instruments used in HIT assays is imperative to maintain accuracy. Calibration involves verifying and adjusting instrument settings to ensure accurate measurements while scheduled maintenance and servicing of laboratory equipment helps to prevent downtime and can help extend the life of laboratory equipment. The calibration and maintenance should always adhere to manufacturer recommendations for best results.

Continuous training and education of laboratory staff on updated protocols, modern technologies, and best practices contribute to maintaining high-quality standards. This is most often accomplished through the Clinical Laboratory Improvement Amendments requirement for initial, 6-month, and annual competency of staff performing testing.[10] Comprehensive documentation of this training should be kept in personnel folders and readily available, if requested. Accurate record-keeping allows for traceability and retrospective analysis if discrepancies arise.

AUTOMATION IN HEPARIN-INDUCED THROMBOCYTOPENIA DIAGNOSTIC TESTING

The implementation of automation in clinical laboratory testing marks a revolutionary stride in medical diagnostics, fundamentally transforming the landscape of how tests are conducted and interpreted. This paradigm shift began in the late 20th century in response to the increasing need for faster, more accurate, and high-throughput methodologies amidst an increasingly complex health care landscape. Automation in the laboratory ranges from simple mechanization of repetitive tasks, such as fluid handling, to the incorporation of sophisticated artificial intelligence (AI) and machine learning models for data analysis and interpretation. Automation has also bolstered QC and assurance measures in the clinical laboratory. Automated systems incorporate built-in QC checks, calibration protocols, and continuous monitoring functionalities, ensuring the reliability and accuracy of test results.[11] This shift allows laboratories to streamline workflows, decrease human errors, significantly increases turnaround times, and helps to alleviate the burden of the chronically undermanned field.

The history of diagnostic testing for HIT mirrors this broader trend in laboratory medicine and adequately represents significant shift from manual to automated methods. Manual testing methods, such as the ELISA serologic assay and the SRA platelet activation assay, remain labor-intensive, time-consuming, and require a high degree of technical expertise to complete and troubleshoot. The shift to automated assays, such as chemiluminescent assays, have emerged offering a more standardized approach with minimal hands-on time and turnaround time drops from 24 to 48 hours to as quickly as 30 minutes after receiving the sample in the laboratory.[12] Integration of robotic sample-handling systems in laboratories enhances the consistency and accuracy of sample handling, thereby minimizing pre-analytical variability and contributing to the reliability of test results.

Improvements in laboratory information systems (LIS) have helped advanced data management and result reporting in HIT diagnostics as well. These systems are capable of seamlessly integrating with automated platforms, facilitating real-time data capture, result interpretation, and report generation. An automated LIS also enables efficient tracking of sample processing, QC metrics, and interpretation of assay results. They also support interfacing with electronic health records, and clinical decision support systems enhancing accessibility and integration of laboratory data into patient care workflows.[13]

Advancements in automation have significantly transformed the landscape of HIT diagnostics, offering laboratories sophisticated tools and platforms to enhance efficiency, accuracy, and standardization of testing methodologies. These innovations play a pivotal role in improving diagnostic accuracy, reducing turnaround times, and optimizing HIT management to improve patient outcomes.

CHALLENGES IN DIAGNOSING HEPARIN-INDUCED THROMBOCYTOPENIA

Accurate diagnosis of HIT poses challenges because of overlapping clinical presentations with other conditions causing thrombocytopenia and thrombotic events. Differential diagnosis involves distinguishing HIT from various conditions presenting similar clinical features, requiring astute clinical judgment and comprehensive laboratory evaluation. Causes other than HIT for thrombocytopenia include, immune thrombocytopenic purpura (ITP), thrombotic thrombocytopenic purpura, drug-induced thrombocytopenia, and disseminated intravascular coagulation.[14] In addition, conditions like deep vein thrombosis, pulmonary embolism, or arterial thrombosis (eg, stroke or myocardial infarction) may present with thrombocytopenia, necessitating differentiation from HIT-associated thrombotic complications.[14] Timing of symptoms in HIT can also pose an issue for accurate diagnosis. Symptoms can manifest several days after initial heparin exposure, making it challenging to establish a direct temporal relationship between heparin administration and the onset of symptoms, and negatively impacting the sensitivity of the clinical scoring system used.[15]

Interpretation of laboratory results in HIT diagnosis requires careful consideration. Patients with underlying medical conditions or receiving multiple medications may present with complex clinical profiles, confounding the identification of HIT. Concurrent infections, inflammatory states, or other medications can influence platelet counts and mimic HIT symptoms. Serologic assays may yield false-positive results in these conditions, necessitating further confirmation through functional assays for accurate diagnosis. A multidisciplinary approach involving primary clinicians, hematologists, and clinical laboratory professionals is crucial in navigating the challenges of differential diagnosis in HIT. Collaboration allows for comprehensive evaluation, incorporating clinical history, laboratory findings, and imaging studies. Comprehensive evaluation involves assessing the clinical context, temporal relationship with heparin exposure, evaluating alternative diagnoses, and performing confirmatory assays for HIT when indicated.

MANAGEMENT STRATEGIES IN HEPARIN-INDUCED THROMBOCYTOPENIA

As previously discussed, HIT represents a clinical challenge because of its potential for severe thrombotic complications and the need for prompt intervention. The onset of clinical implications of HIT can be rapid and unpredictable. Recognizing them quickly and implementing appropriate management strategies are crucial in mitigating adverse outcomes associated with this condition. The management of patients with HIT is critical and requires immediate and specific interventions. The management steps can be seen outlined in **Table 2**. The cornerstone of HIT management is the prompt cessation of all heparin products, including both unfractionated and LMWH.[16] To ensure the patient remains therapeutically anticoagulated and avoids thrombotic complications, an alternative anticoagulant should be implemented. Alternatives such as argatroban, bivalirudin, fondaparinux, or direct thrombin inhibitors are preferred according to current guidelines.[17] The choice of alternative anticoagulant is dependent on several factors including severity of thrombocytopenia, renal function, and the active presence of thrombosis.[17] In specific populations, such as pregnant women or those with comorbidities, tailored management approaches are necessary, balancing the risks and benefits of alternative anticoagulants. Platelet transfusions are generally avoided in HIT patients unless there is active or a high risk for bleeding as they may further increase the risk for thrombosis. Cooperation among primary clinicians, hematologists, pharmacists, clinical laboratory professionals, and other specialists is imperative in managing HIT cases, particularly in complex scenarios or when considering surgical interventions requiring anticoagulation.

Table 2
Heparin induced thrombocytopenia management strategies

Management Strategies	Key Steps
1. Immediate withdrawal of heparin	• Cease all heparin formulations (unfractionated or low-molecular-weight heparin) immediately upon suspicion or diagnosis of HIT
2. Laboratory confirmation and risk assessment	• Confirm HIT diagnosis through appropriate serologic and functional assays. • Assess thrombotic risk based on clinical presentation, comorbidities, and prior thrombotic history.
3. Alternative anticoagulation	• Initiate non-heparin anticoagulants: Direct thrombin inhibitors (eg, argatroban, bivalirudin), Factor Xa inhibitors (eg, fondaparinux, direct oral anticoagulants)
4. Monitoring and dose adjustment	• Monitor anticoagulant effects using appropriate laboratory tests (eg, activated partial thromboplastin time [aPTT], anti-Xa levels). • Adjust doses based on patient response.
5. Thrombosis prevention and management	• Implement thromboprophylaxis strategies tailored to individual patient risk factors. • Manage thrombotic events promptly with appropriate therapies.
6. Consideration for surgical/invasive procedures	• Assess risk-benefit ratio before performing procedures requiring anticoagulation, considering alternative agents and reversal strategies.
7. Consultation and multidisciplinary care	• Involve hematology, cardiology, or relevant specialists for guidance in managing HIT cases, especially in complex or high-risk situations.
8. Patient education and follow-up	• Educate patients and caregivers regarding HIT, anticoagulant therapy, and signs of thrombotic complications. • Ensure regular follow-up and monitoring for efficacy and safety.

Note: Specific management may vary based on individual patient factors, and this table serves as a general guide based on latest clinical guidelines.[17]

A patient diagnosed with HIT should have it well-documented in the clinical history to prevent future exposure to heparin. Long-term patient education regarding HIT, the importance of alternative anticoagulation, and recognition of signs of thrombotic complications is crucial.[17] Regular follow-ups ensure adequate monitoring and adjustment of therapeutic strategies. Continuous monitoring of laboratory parameters, including platelet counts and anticoagulant therapeutic range, will help guide therapeutic interventions and aid in assessing treatment efficacy and safety.

FUTURE PERSPECTIVES AND EMERGING TECHNOLOGIES IN HEPARIN-INDUCED THROMBOCYTOPENIA

The landscape of HIT diagnostics and management continues to evolve, driven by ongoing research, technological advancements, and the need for more precise and efficient diagnostic tools. Several future perspectives and emerging technologies hold promise in further enhancing our understanding and approach to HIT.

Biomarker Identification and Validation

Ongoing research focuses on identifying novel biomarkers or combinations of bio-markers that could aid in the rapid diagnosis of conditions such as ITP, which show clinical overlap with HIT. These efforts aim to enhance the turnaround time, specificity, and sensitivity of diagnostic assays for these confounding conditions.[18] Eliminating these additional conditions from the differential diagnosis early could help further expedite a rule in or out for HIT diagnosis.

Advancements in Assay Sensitivity and Specificity

Continuous refinement and optimization of serologic and functional assays aim to improve their sensitivity, specificity, and accuracy in detecting both anti-PF4 and anti-PF4 or heparin antibodies. It is currently theorized that combination of these 2 results could enhance diagnostic sensitivity while simultaneously detecting anti-PF4 only antibodies associated with autoimmune thrombocytopenia and vaccine induced thrombocytopenia.[19,20] This enhanced assay performance is crucial in reducing erroneous results and increasing diagnostic reliability.

Use of Artificial Intelligence and Machine Learning

The use of AI and machine learning facilitates the analysis of large data sets of predictor variables such as patient histories, diagnostic laboratory results, and clinical scoring systems to identify patterns that may elude human analysis. Integration of AI and machine learning algorithms in HIT diagnostics holds promise in increasing the sensitivity and specificity of the current diagnostic algorithms. These models can also potentially be trained to successfully differentiate between HIT and other thrombocytopenic conditions thus improving patient outcomes by ensuring quick and appropriate management.[21]

Development of Targeted Therapies

Novel research is currently focused on developing targeted therapies that modulate the immune response underlying HIT without compromising anticoagulation. As understanding of the underlying pathogenesis of HIT improves, new potential targets for non-anticoagulant treatments for HIT are discovered. Some of the more promising therapies that have the potential to disable the platelet activation that increases thrombotic activity include Immunoglobulin G degradation and Syk Kinase inhibition.[22] There is also promising research in the pharmacologic effects of PF4 itself that has the potential to further expand this research field.[23] These targeted therapies not only aim to provide safer and more effective treatment options for patients with HIT but also offer the potential for personalized medicine approaches, tailoring treatments based on individual patient profiles, and specific disease characteristics.

Microfluidics and Nanotechnology

Emerging microfluidics and nanotechnology are playing a transformative role in the diagnosis of HIT. Microfluidic devices not only offer the ability to manipulate small volumes of blood and create a more efficient and sensitive approach to detecting the antibodies responsible for HIT but also serve as effective platforms for researchers evaluating nanoparticle behavior in an environment that can be linked to their biologic performance.[24]

The future of HIT diagnostics and management is poised for transformation through interdisciplinary collaborations, technological innovations, and a deeper understanding of the intricate immunologic mechanisms underlying HIT. These evolving perspectives and technologies hold promise in advancing diagnostic accuracy, therapeutic interventions, and improving patient outcomes in HIT.

SUMMARY

HIT remains a challenging diagnosis that requires interdisciplinary collaboration to effectively recognize, manage, and monitor. Though the current methodologies have substantial limitations, there have been significant strides toward improving patient outcomes with this condition. Rapid advancements in automation, AI and machine offer a hopeful future for the rapid and effective treatment of HIT.

CLINICS CARE POINTS

- HIT commonly presents clinically with a distinctive pattern, characterized by a significant and abrupt decrease in platelet count by 50% or more from the patient's baseline values, and can also manifest with new or worsening thrombosis in the form of venous or arterial thromboembolism leading to severe complications such as limb ischemia, stroke, or myocardial infarction.[5]

- Serologic assays detect antibodies that bind to PF-4 or heparin complexes, but not all these antibodies are capable of causing platelet activation, which is essential for the development of clinically relevant HIT.[7]

- A positive result in a platelet activation assay indicates the functional capacity of patient antibodies to induce platelet activation, supporting the diagnosis of HIT Type 2.[7]

- Automated testing platforms have the capability to decrease turnaround time from 24 to 48 hours to as quickly as 30 minutes after receiving the sample in the laboratory.[12]

- Once diagnosed the most critical task for HIT management is the prompt cessation of all heparin products, including both unfractionated and LMWH.[16]

DISCLOSURE

The authors have nothing to disclose including funding.

REFERENCES

1. Hogan M, Berger JS. Heparin-induced thrombocytopenia (HIT): review of incidence, diagnosis, and management. Vasc Med 2020;25(2):160–73.
2. Favaloro EJ, Pasalic L, Lippi G. Antibodies against platelet factor 4 and their associated pathologies: from HIT/HITT to spontaneous HIT-like syndrome to COVID-19 to VITT/TTS. Antibodies 2022;11(1):7.
3. Dhakal B, Kreuziger LB, Kleman A, et al. Disease burden, complication rates, and health-care costs of heparin-induced thrombocytopenia in the USA: a population-based study. Lancet Haematol 2018;5(5):e220–31.
4. Kelton JG, Warkentin TE. Heparin-induced thrombocytopenia: a historical perspective. Blood 2008;112(7):2607–16.
5. Favaloro EJ, McCaughan G, Pasalic L. Clinical and laboratory diagnosis of heparin-induced thrombocytopenia: an update. Pathology 2017;49(4):346–55.
6. Warkentin TE. Heparin-induced thrombocytopenia. Hematol Oncol Clin North Am 2007;21(4):589–607.
7. Warkentin TE. Laboratory diagnosis of heparin-induced thrombocytopenia. Int J Lab Hematol 2019;41(Suppl. 1):15–25.

8. Gupta S, Tiruvoipati R, Green C, et al. Heparin induced thrombocytopenia in critically ill: diagnostic dilemmas and management conundrums. World J Crit Care Med 2015;4(3):202–12.

9. Minet V, Dogné JM, Mullier F. Functional assays in the diagnosis of heparin-induced thrombocytopenia: a review. Molecules 2017;22(4):617.

10. Centers for Medicare & Medicaid Services. 42 CFR ch. IV (10–1–22 edition) Part 493—laboratory requirements. Baltimore, MD: US Government Printing Office; 2022.

11. Lippi G, Da Rin G. Advantages and limitations of total laboratory automation: a personal overview. Clin Chem Lab Med 2019;57(6):802–11.

12. Warkentin TE, Sheppard JI, Smith JW, et al. Combination of two complementary automated rapid assays for diagnosis of heparin-induced thrombocytopenia (HIT). J Thromb Haemostasis 2020;18(6):1435–46.

13. Kwan JL, Lo L, Ferguson J, et al. Computerised clinical decision support systems and absolute improvements in care: meta-analysis of controlled clinical trials. BMJ 2020;370:m3216.

14. McCrae KR, Bussel JB, Mannucci PM, et al. Platelets: an update on diagnosis and management of thrombocytopenic disorders. Hematology 2001;1(282). https://doi.org/10.1182/asheducation-2001.1.282.

15. Warkentin TE, Sheppard JI, Smith JW, et al. Timeline of heparin-induced thrombocytopenia seroconversion in serial plasma samples tested using an automated latex immunoturbidimetric assay. Int J Lab Hematol 2019;41:493–502.

16. Koster A, Nagler M, Erdoes G, et al. Heparin-induced thrombocytopenia: perioperative diagnosis and management. Anesthesiology 2022;136:336–44.

17. Cuker A, Arepally GM, Chong BH, et al. American Society of Hematology 2018 guidelines for management of venous thromboembolism: heparin-induced thrombocytopenia. Blood Adv 2018;2(22):3360–92.

18. Allegra A, Cicero N, Mirabile G, et al. Novel biomarkers for diagnosis and monitoring of immune thrombocytopenia. Int J Mol Sci 2023;24(5):4438.

19. Warkentin TE. Autoimmune heparin-induced thrombocytopenia. J Clin Med 2023; 12(6921). https://doi.org/10.3390/jcm12216921.

20. Warkentin TE, Greinacher A. Laboratory testing for heparin-induced thrombocytopenia and vaccine-induced immune thrombotic thrombocytopenia: a narrative review. Semin Thromb Hemost 2023;49:621–33.

21. Nilius H, Cuker A, Haug S, et al. A machine-learning model for reducing misdiagnosis in heparin-induced thrombocytopenia: a prospective multicenter observational study. EClinicalMedicine 2023;55:101745.

22. Mongirdiene A, Liuize A, Kasauskas A. Novel knowledge about molecular mechanisms of heparin-induced thrombocytopenia type II and treatment targets. Int J Mol Sci 2023;24(9):8217.

23. Liu Z, Li L, Zhang H, et al. Platelet factor 4 (PF4) and its multiple roles in diseases. Blood Rev 2023. https://doi.org/10.1016/j.blre.2023.101155.

24. Shirejini SZ, Carberry J, Alt K, et al. Shear-responsive drug delivery systems in medical devices: focus on thrombosis and bleeding. Adv Funct Mater 2023; 33(12):2303717.

Assessing Direct Oral Anticoagulants in the Clinical Laboratory

Robert C. Gosselin, CLS[a],*, Adam Cuker, MD, MS[b]

KEYWORDS

- Direct oral anticoagulants (DOACs) • Dabigatran • Rivaroxaban • Apixaban
- Edoxaban • Laboratory • Anti-Xa

KEY POINTS

- Traditional screening tests such as the prothrombin time and activated partial thrombo-plastin time are insufficient for detecting *"on-therapy"* concentration of direct oral antico-agulants (DOACs).
- Thrombin clotting time and heparin calibrated anti-Xa assays are sensitive to screen for significant concentration ($\geq$30 ng/mL) of dabigatran and oral factor Xa inhibitors, respectively.
- Drug calibrated dilute thrombin time, ecarin-based assays, and chromogenic factor anti-IIa are rapid assays that can be used to quantify dabigatran.
- Heparin or a DOAC calibrated anti-Xa test is a rapid method that can be used to estimate or quantify factor Xa DOACs, respectively.
- At the time of writing, there are limited Food and Drug Administration-cleared methods for screening, quantifying, or neutralizing DOACs.

BACKGROUND

In 2010, the first direct oral anticoagulant (DOAC), dabigatran a direct thrombin (FIIa) inhibitor, was approved for use in the United States for stroke prevention in patients with non-valvular atrial fibrillation (NVAF)[1] and subsequently for prevention and treatment of venous thromboembolism (VTE). Soon thereafter, direct inhibitors of factor Xa (FXa), including rivaroxaban, apixaban, and edoxaban became available for prophy-laxis in NVAF, and for treatment and prophylaxis of VTE.[2,3] A fourth FXa DOAC,

[a] Thrombosis and Hemostasis Center, University of California, Davis Health System, Sacra-mento, CA 95817, USA; [b] Department of Medicine and Department of Pathology & Laboratory Medicine, Perelman School of Medicine, University of Pennsylvania Hospital of the University of Pennsylvania, Philadelphia, PA 19104, USA
* Corresponding author. UC Davis Hemostasis and Thrombosis Center, 2000 Stockton Boule-vard, Suite 202, Sacramento, CA 95817.
E-mail address: rcgosselin@outlook.com

Clin Lab Med 44 (2024) 551–562
https://doi.org/10.1016/j.cll.2024.04.014
0272-2712/24/© 2024 Elsevier Inc. All rights reserved.

betrixaban, was approved for use in the United States for VTE prophylaxis but was later pulled from the market for business reasons.[4] DOACs have several advantages compared with vitamin K antagonists (VKAs) including (1) fewer bleeding events; (2) fixed doses (based on indication); (3) predictable pharmacokinetics with a wide "on-therapy" range reflecting the lowest peak and highest trough concentrations for a given agent; and (4) the lack of need for routine drug monitoring.[5]

Prior to 2010, laboratory screening tests such as the prothrombin time (PT) and activated partial thromboplastin time (APTT) long served as reliable beacons for assessing the pharmacodynamic (PD) effect of oral and parenteral anticoagulation, respectively. However, the reliability of these same tests for assessing the DOAC PD effect has proved to be unsuitable. While "monitoring" DOACs in the same manner as VKAs or heparin is not required, we recommend that clinical laboratories have a testing algorithm in place to assist providers in determining DOAC presence, and when confirmed, quantifying drug concentration. This information may be a valuable tool in providing safe and effective management, including consideration of reversal, for patients with trauma, major bleeding, acute stroke requiring thrombolysis, or those in need of an emergent invasive procedure.[6] The purpose of this document is to describe laboratory assays that may be suitable for determining the PD or pharmacokinetic (PK) effect of DOACs.

MONITORING VERSUS MEASURING DIRECT ORAL ANTICOAGULANT EFFECT

A main feature of DOACs is the lack of need for routine laboratory "monitoring." "Monitoring" has long been used for measuring the PD effect of anticoagulation. For VKAs, the PD effect was initially monitored with the PT. Subsequently, the International Normalized Ratio was adopted to provide a more standard approach to monitoring.[7]

While DOACs are not intended to be monitored in the same manner as VKAs, measurement of DOACs may be important, especially in special situations such as trauma, acute stroke, need for emergent surgery, or bleeding. The ability to measure DOACs in the clinical laboratory, whether to determine drug presence or drug concentration, has been limited by lack of suitable assays, but also by the absence of assays with regulatory approval for this purpose.

In the acute setting, there are usually 2 clinical questions relating to DOAC exposure.[8] The first question is whether and which DOAC the patient is taking. This question can usually be answered from medical history and/or medical record but may not be ascertainable in patients with altered mental status. In patients with confirmed DOAC exposure, the second question is whether the DOAC concentration is sufficiently high to contribute to bleeding or bleeding risk. Recent approval of dabigatran and rivaroxaban in the pediatric population may result in increased interest in measuring drug concentrations in a similar manner that was observed when this population was treated with low molecular weight heparin, another anticoagulant that was Food and Drug Administration (FDA)-approved without the requirement for routine monitoring.

To address clinical needs, the laboratory should ideally provide tests that can rapidly and reliably determine DOAC exposure, whether the exposure is a FIIa or FXa DOAC, and provide a method to quantitate DOAC if exposure has been confirmed by screening tests or patient history. In the absence of quantifying concentrations, estimations of FXa DOAC exposure have also been described.[9–11]

While describing the use of commercially available laboratory tests in this study, the authors acknowledge that these assays have not been cleared by the FDA for DOAC assessment. In most circumstances, local use outside the manufacturer's instructions for use would suggest an off-label use, device remanufacture, or laboratory developed test (LDT), depending on the degree of changes made to the assay. Ironically, the FDA issued prescribing information for DOACs, which refers to tests (eg, ecarin-based assays, endogenous thrombin potential, anti-Xa) or expected drug concentrations (in the case of pediatric dabigatran use) despite the lack of FDA-cleared methods.[12] Conversely, outside the United States, prescribing information in some jurisdictions includes laboratory values and associated bleeding risks or expected drug concentrations for a given dose.[13] As the FDA is proposing rule changes to LDT use and oversight,[14] readers are advised to consult local, accrediting, and regulatory agencies for additional guidance.

SCREENING FOR DIRECT ORAL ANTICOAGULANT EXPOSURE

The PT and APTT are not sensitive enough for ascertaining drug exposure.[15,16] While some reagents are more sensitive than others, providers may be unaware of which reagent is being used in their clinical laboratory, and reagent sources can change over time. Therefore, a normal PT or APTT value cannot be assumed to rule out DOAC presence, including "on-therapy" concentrations.[15] Local determination of PT or APTT sensitivity to DOAC concentrations using DOAC treated patient samples in the range of 20 to 100 ng/mL (for each DOAC) is recommended; kit calibrators and controls should be avoided because their use may overestimate sensitivity of laboratory methods.[17,18] A prolonged PT or APTT in the setting of unknown DOAC exposure patient may lead to reflex testing, including mixing studies to differentiate whether test prolongation is secondary to factor deficiency(ies) or an inhibitor. Mixing study "correction" suggests a factor deficiency, whereas "non-correction" suggests the presence of an inhibitor. All DOACs should mimic an inhibitor effect (non-correction) on mixing studies, although the method used for determining "non-correction" has varying degrees of misprediction (false negative for DOAC presence).[19] As such, mixing studies should be interpreted with caution in patients with unknown clinical history. However, it is recommended that any PT or APTT prolongation in a patient with *known* DOAC exposure be considered secondary to drug effect until proven otherwise. Viscoelastic tests (VETs) such as thromboelastography or thromboelastometry are used In acute clinical settings and these methods have demonstrated variable sensitivity to DOAC exposure.[20] While some publications have suggested their use, data were based on drug naïve and post-drug exposure sampling and, although significant differences were noted between the 2 measurement periods, VET parameters were within the expected reference interval or normal range.[21]

The traditional thrombin clotting time (TCT) test is exquisitely sensitive for the FIIa DOAC, dabigatran. A normal TCT generally excludes significant concentrations of dabigatran. This test should not be confused with the dilute thrombin time (dTT), a modification made to increase the sensitivity to monitor parenteral direct thrombin inhibitors (ie, bivalirudin, argatroban). The TCT does not detect FXa DOAC exposure.

Coagulation instruments have the capacity to perform anti-Xa testing, which is used for monitoring/measurement of heparins, including unfractionated or low molecular weight heparin and fondaparinux. The anti-Xa kits associated with the instrumentation have the intended use for quantifying this class of anticoagulants. There is a linear relationship between heparin calibrated anti-Xa and FXa DOAC exposure, making this method a suitable test to both indicate presence of drug and estimate drug concentration. The suitability for drug presence is highly variable, and dependent on the reagent platform and calibrator material. Unlike the PT and APTT, local determination of sensitivity of the anti-Xa assay to FXa DOACs can be achieved using commercial calibrators and controls, as well as patient samples with known DOAC concentrations. Anti-Xa methods that supplement antithrombin in the assay should not be used for quantifying DOACs.[22,23] The heparin lower limit of quantitation (LLOQ) and corresponding FXa DOAC concentrations must be assessed to determine the lowest FXa DOAC concentration associated with the LLOQ. For laboratory tests that have dual heparin calibrations (unfractionated heparin, UFH and low molecular weight heparin, LMWH), the LLOQ may have different corresponding FXa DOAC thresholds, although typically the LMWH calibrated curve is more sensitive to FXa DOAC concentrations. An LMWH anti-Xa concentration below the LLOQ generally excludes the presence of clinically relevant ($\geq$30 ng/mL) FXa DOAC concentrations.[24] Use of published anti-Xa thresholds without local verification should not be used, given the discrepancies between different anti-Xa reagent and calibrator manufacturers to DOAC concentrations.[25] It should also be emphasized that anti-Xa assays cannot distinguish between FXa DOACs and heparins nor can they discriminate among different FXa DOACs. Anti-Xa assays are also unable to detect dabigatran.

SCREENING FOR DIRECT ORAL ANTICOAGULANT EXPOSURE—ALGORITHM

With local verification, the authors propose that laboratories that evaluate DOAC-treated populations consider the following algorithm for use in acutely ill patients with known DOAC exposure to determine DOAC presence or estimate concentration (**Fig. 1**). In patients with unknown clinical history, additional coagulation testing should be considered, such as PT, APTT, and D-dimer testing to rule out other coagulopathies or drug effect (warfarin). Due to variability of anti-Xa kit and LMWH calibrator performance, local verification of LMWH LLOQ to corresponding FXa DOAC concentration is necessary to ensure the reliability of excluding significant concentrations ($\geq$30 ng/mL) of each FXa DOAC.

QUANTIFYING DIRECT ORAL ANTICOAGULANT EXPOSURE

The gold standard method for measuring any DOAC is tandem liquid chromatography–mass spectrometry (LC-MS/MS).[20] This method has an extremely

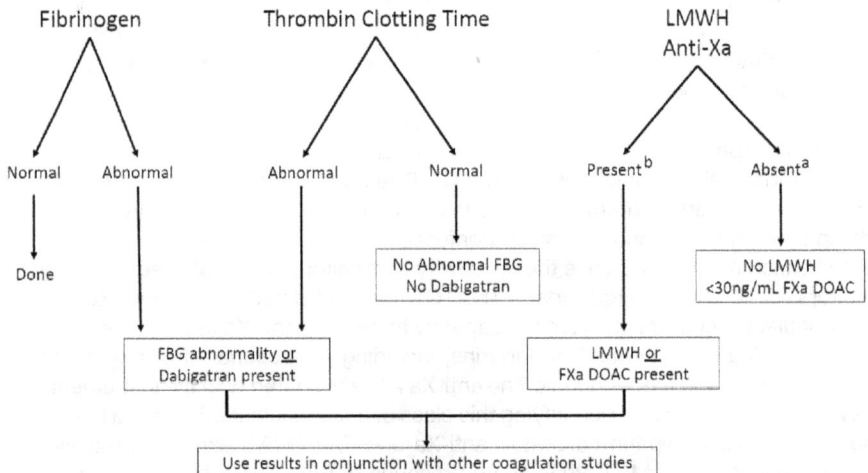

Fig. 1. Provisional algorithm for screening for clinically significant concentrations of direct oral anticoagulants. FBG, fibrinogen; LLOQ, lower limit of quantitation; LMWH, low molecular weight heparin. [a]<LLOQ, [b]$\geq$LLOQ

low LLOQ (~3 ng/mL) and can differentiate between different DOACs when appropriate standards are used. The limitations for routine use of this method include specialized equipment and relatively slow turn-around time (TAT), which are not suitable in emergent situations. Alternatively, there have been several rapid methods (analytical TAT <10 minutes) demonstrating equivalence to results generated by LC-MS/MS for both FIIa and FXa DOACs.[26]

Dabigatran

There are several methods that are available to quantify dabigatran concentrations with dabigatran calibrators, including dTT, ecarin-based assays (chromogenic and chronometric), and chromogenic anti-FIIa methods.[26–28] The specific details and performance of these tests have been described elsewhere[29,30] and all have demonstrated a linear relationship with plasma dabigatran concentration. Commercial kits are available, although no kits have been FDA cleared for use in the United States. Commercial kits suggest a minimum 3 point calibration curve, although 5 point calibrators are available. The reported LLOQ varies between 15 and 40 ng/mL, with samples requiring dilution and repeat testing if the concentrations exceed the upper limit of the calibration range (approximately >400–500 ng/mL). All assays can be adapted to "open" coagulation analyzers, which permit the creation of test protocols using external or third-party reagents, but a robust validation of test performance is required.[13] These assays are affected by parenteral and oral direct thrombin inhibitors (DTIs) and none can distinguish among DTIs unless sample manipulation is performed. Polybrene or protamine sulfate may be added to a plasma sample to mitigate heparin effect on some of these assays. Commercial products for neutralizing DOACs in plasma samples have also been described later in this document. Hyperbilirubinemia may interfere with any chromogenic assay and these samples will require alternative testing methods to quantitate dabigatran. Principles of these assays are as follows:

- dTT: A thrombin time test that has been modified by diluting the patient sample with normal saline, buffer, or pooled plasma at a 1:4 or 1:8 ratio. If pooled plasma is used, there are no interferences due to low prothrombin of fibrinogen concentrations.
- Ecarin assays: Based on cleavage of prothrombin by the venom (ecarin) from *Echis carinatus*, which primarily generates an intermediate called meizothrombin. For ecarin clotting time (ECT) assays, the degree of prolongation of the clotting time has a linear relationship to dabigatran concentration. ECT assays may be influenced by either prothrombin or fibrinogen deficiency. For ecarin chromogenic assay (ECA), the meizothrombin generated by ecarin will cleave a chromogenic substrate liberating para-nitroaniline (pNA), producing a yellow color. There is an inverse linear relationship between dabigatran concentration and pNA release. With the ECA method, the sample is added to a prothrombin buffer, thereby eliminating any interference from prothrombin deficiency. Both ecarin methods have been used in the past for monitoring parenteral direct thrombin inhibitors and are also able to differentiate prolongation of clotting times due to heparin, as meizothrombin is not neutralized by heparin.
- Chromogenic FIIa assay: Based on dabigatran's inhibition of thrombin added to plasma. Unbound thrombin hydrolyzes a thrombin-specific chromogenic substrate, releasing pNA, producing a yellow color. As with the ECA, there is an inverse relationship between dabigatran concentration and pNA release. Specific sample dilutions have been described to create both low and high dabigatran

calibration curves that measure drug concentrations between ~ 10 to 100 ng/mL and ~ 50 ng/mL to 500 ng/mL, respectively.

Apixaban, Edoxaban, and Rivaroxaban

The simplest, most rapid testing to quantify FXa DOACs is modification of an existing heparin anti-Xa assay by using apixaban, edoxaban, and rivaroxaban calibrators. While use of drug-specific calibrators will accurately quantify the drug of interest, the assay is not able to differentiate among FXa DOACs or other FXa-inhibiting drugs such as heparin. With anti-FXa testing, excess factor X is added to the sample, which will be complexed by any anti-FXa drug. Any residual FXa will cleave a FXa-specific chromogenic substrate, releasing pNA and producing yellow color. As noted with dabigatran chromogenic assays, there is an inverse relationship between FXa DOAC concentration and pNA release. As previously noted, anti-Xa methods that supplement antithrombin in the assay should not be used for quantifying DOACs.[22,23] In one author's (RCG) experience, the instrument protocol used for heparin testing was exactly duplicated for each respective FXa DOAC, which provided suitable quantitation of these drugs, based on comparison to gold standard testing (LC-MS/MS)[11] and peer comparison assessment (external quality control programs).

There is one FDA-cleared method for quantifying apixaban (HemosIL Liquid Anti-Xa, Werfen, Bedford MA), but it is limited to certain instruments with intended use approved for drug determination in a bleeding patient or patient at risk for bleeding.[31] Any use of this kit on other instruments or for other indications would likely constitute an off-label use, a local device re-manufacture, or an LDT.

UNINTENDED EFFECTS OF DIRECT ORAL ANTICOAGULANT ANTICOAGULATION

One of the unintended consequences, although not unexpected, is the effect DOACs have on other coagulation assays. DOACs affect (to varying degrees) other clot-based assays such as protein C, protein S, lupus anticoagulant methods using snake venoms, factor assays and others. Assays that incorporate reagents containing (or test methods generating) thrombin or FXa will be affected by dabigatran or FXa DOAC, respectively. Molecular and immunoassays are not influenced by DOAC presence.

While trough DOAC concentrations represent the low drug exposure in a treated patient, those DOAC concentrations may be sufficient to alter results of select coagulation assays, which may lead to factitiously abnormal or false-negative results.[32] Of particular importance is the effect of DOACs on lupus anticoagulant testing, as DOACs are contraindicated in patients with antiphospholipid syndrome.[33] Methods to neutralize DOAC effect using activated charcoal or filters (**Table 1**) have demonstrated effective removal of DOAC interference with minimal-to-no effect on the test itself.[34] However, these DOAC neutralizing products are currently not FDA cleared for clinical use.

A second challenge is for DOAC-treated patients that require transition to heparin anticoagulation. For patients who have recently taken dabigatran, the APTT may be prolonged. As such, monitoring heparin anticoagulation using heparin or hybrid calibrated anti-Xa testing is recommended. For patients who have recently taken a FXa DOAC, the APTT may or may not be prolonged, but the heparin calibrated anti-Xa test will have "therapeutic" heparin concentrations (0.3–0.7 IU/mL) due to FXa DOAC alone (**Fig. 2**).

If the baseline APTT is prolonged and therefore cannot be used, alternatives for monitoring UFH anticoagulation in patients with circulating FXa DOAC include

Table 1
Characteristics of direct oral anticoagulation neutralizing products

	DOAC-Stop	DOAC-Remove	DP-Filter
Manufacturer	Haematex Research, Hornsby NSW Australia	5-Diagnostics, Basel Switzerland	University of Namur, Namur Belgium
Product description	Activated charcoal	Activated carbon	Single use filter
Required plasma volume	0.5–1.5 mL	1.0 mL	0.5 mL
Citrated plasma sample processing	• Add tablet to plasma • Mix for 5 min • Centrifuge for 5 min at 2000g • Remove supernatant	• Add tablet to plasma • Mix for 10 min • Centrifuge 2–5 min at 2500g • Remove supernatant	• Add plasma to upper side of device • Incubate at room temperature for 5 min • Centrifuge device for 2 min at 2000g • Remove upper filter from device
DOAC neutralizing range	Up to 1000 ng/mL	~500–700 ng/mL	Up to 1000 ng/mL

Modified from Ref.[34]

heparin-calibrated TCT with a target of 0.2 to 0.4 IU/mL or the use of either heparin neutralizing agents (ie, protamine sulfate or Dade Hepzyme, Siemens Healthcare Diagnostics, Newark, DE) or DOAC neutralizing agents (see **Table 1**) to eliminate the contribution of one class of drugs (**Fig. 3**). Any neutralizing method used should be locally verified to ensure intended effect and noninterference with assay performance in the absence of targeted drug.

FUTURE OF DIRECT ORAL ANTICOAGULANT MEASURING OPTIONS

Colleagues outside the United States enjoy more testing options to assess DOAC presence, PD or PK than we have in the United States. The top 4 international manufacturers of coagulation reagents or instruments used in the United States (Diagnostica Stago, Siemens Healthcare Diagnostics, Sysmex Corporation and Werfen) all have kits for quantifying both FIIa and FXa DOACs that are available outside the US for clinical use. A urine dipstick method (DOAC Dipstick, DOASENSE) that can differentiate between dabigatran and FXa DOAC exposure and has a high negative predictive value for ruling out significant concentrations ($\geq$30 ng/mL) of DOACs is available in some jurisdictions.[25–37] False-negative DOAC dipstick results in patients with plasma DOAC concentrations greater than 30 ng/mL have been reported,[36,37] mainly with apixaban, a drug primarily cleared by the liver with fecal excretion. Novel point of care devices are in development using various technologies including an FDA-cleared dielectric spectroscopy platform to assess whole-blood coagulation (ClotChip); a microfluidic and "Lab-on-a-Chip" technology platform (iLINE Microsystems)[38]; a point-of-care device (Perosphere PoC Coagulometer), which received European CE (Conformité Européene)-IVD (In-Vitro Diagnostic) Marking[39]; and DOAC-specific cartridges for VET testing.[21,40] How soon these novel devices or applications will become available in the US marketplace is uncertain.

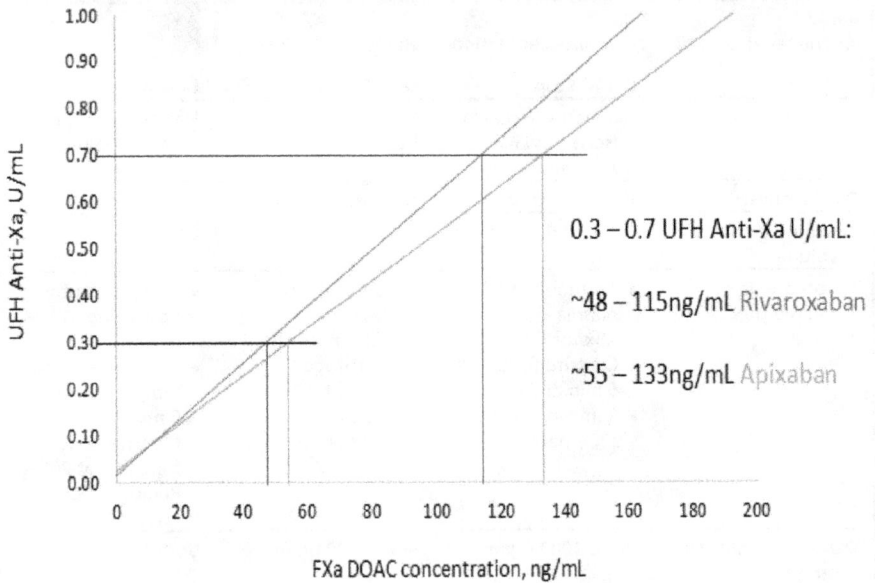

Fig. 2. Relationship of rivaroxaban or apixaban exposure to the corresponding unfractionated heparin (UFH) values in heparin naïve samples. The therapeutic target for UFH infusion is 0.3 to 0.7 U/mL. FXa DOAC concentration measured using tandem mass spectrometry.

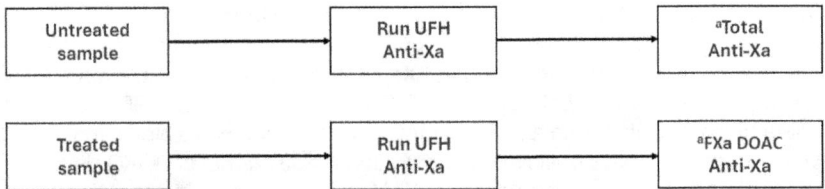

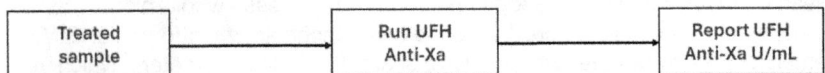

Fig. 3. Potential options for unfractionated heparin (UFH) monitoring in patients with concomitant FXa DOAC exposure. Heparin and DOAC neutralizing agents are described in the manuscript. [a]Calculation: Total Anti-Xa–FXa DOAC Anti-Xa = Anti-Xa.

SUMMARY

DOACs have revolutionized the prevention and treatment of thrombotic disorders such as VTE and atrial fibrillation. Unlike older anticoagulants such as UFH and VKAs, they do not require routine laboratory monitoring. Nevertheless, there are special clinical situations in which DOAC measurement may be important for guiding clinical management, particularly emergency situations such as major bleeding, acute stroke, or need for an urgent invasive procedure. The PT and APTT are not sufficiently sensitive to exclude the presence of clinically relevant DOAC concentrations. A normal TCT and an UFH or LMWH anti-Xa concentration below the LLOQ typically excludes the presence of clinically relevant concentrations of dabigatran and FXa DOAC, respectively. If DOAC are detected, quantification of DOAC exposure may be helpful in guiding management (eg, determining the need for a reversal agent). LC-MS/MS is the gold standard method for DOAC quantification but is not widely available and has a slow TAT. More rapid tests including the dTT, ecarin-based assays, and chromogenic FIIa assay for quantification of dabigatran and anti-Xa assay with drug-specific calibrators for quantification of FXa DOACs show excellent agreement with LC-MS/MS. Point-of-care tests for DOAC screening and quantification are in development but are not yet available in the United States.

CLINICS CARE POINTS

- All clinical laboratories that provide services to patients on DOAC therapies should have a testing strategy or algorithm for determining DOAC exposure in emergent settings.
- The PT and APTT are not reliable methods for determining DOAC exposure.
- A normal TCT rules out dabigatran presence.
- A heparin calibrated anti-Xa can be used to estimate FXa DOAC exposure.
- Dabigatran calibrated dTT, ECT, ECA, and anti-IIa assay have demonstrated equivalence to gold standard method, tandem mass spectrometry, and could be used to quantify dabigatran after local validation.
- FXa DOAC drug calibrated anti-Xa assays have demonstrated equivalence to the gold standard method, tandem mass spectrometry, and could be used to quantify FXa DOACs after local validation.
- Trough DOAC blood collections (just before next dose) do not guarantee the absence of interference on coagulation testing used for bleeding or thrombophilia evaluations.
- DOAC neutralizing products are available and should be considered for local use after validation, as permitted by regulatory authorities.
- Unless there is sample modification, the chromogenic anti-Xa assays cannot differentiate between heparin or DOACs and caution must be used when interpreting these results.
- Clinical laboratories that provide services to patients on DOAC therapies should have a monitoring strategy for concomitant (bridging) heparin anticoagulation.
- Most test methods for estimating or quantifying DOACs are either modifications to existing FDA cleared methods or laboratory developed assays. It is unclear whether future regulatory oversight and restrictions will limit the use of these types of assays and readers are encouraged to seek guidance before implementing any non-FDA cleared tests.

DISCLOSURE

R. C. Gosselin received consulting fees from Sysmex America, Inc. A. Cuker served as a consultant for MingSight, Sanofi, and Synergy and has received authorship royalties from UpToDate. There was no funders or funding sources for this article.

REFERENCES

1. Connolly SJ, Ezekowitz MD, Yusuf S, et al, RE-LY Steering Committee and Investigators. Dabigatran versus warfarin in patients with atrial fibrillation. N Engl J Med 2009;361(12):1139–51.
2. Roca B, Roca M. The new oral anticoagulants: reasonable alternatives to warfarin. Cleve Clin J Med 2015;82(12):847–54.
3. Ortel TL, Neumann I, Ageno W, et al. American Society of Hematology 2020 guidelines for management of venous thromboembolism: treatment of deep vein thrombosis and pulmonary embolism. Blood Adv 2020;4(19):4693–738.
4. US Food & Drug Administration. Bevyxxa portola pharmaceutical inc. Response to the notification of Non-Compliance with PREA, NDA 208383. Available at: https://www.fda.gov/media/143144/download.
5. Cuker A. Laboratory measurement of the non-vitamin K antagonist oral anticoagulants: selecting the optimal assay based on drug, assay availability, and clinical indication. J Thromb Thrombolysis 2016;41(2):241–7.
6. Cuker A, Burnett A, Triller D, et al. Reversal of direct oral anticoagulants: guidance from the anticoagulation forum. Am J Hematol 2019;94(6):697–709.
7. Hirsh J, Poller L. The international normalized ratio. A guide to understanding and correcting its problems. Arch Intern Med 1994;154(3):282–8.
8. Gosselin RC, Adcock DM. The laboratory's 2015 perspective on direct oral anticoagulant testing. J Thromb Haemostasis 2016;14(5):886–93.
9. Gosselin RC, Francart SJ, Hawes EM, et al. Heparin-calibrated chromogenic anti-Xa activity measurements in patients receiving rivaroxaban: can this test be used to quantify drug level? Ann Pharmacother 2015;49(7):777–83.
10. Billoir P, Barbay V, Joly LM, et al. Anti-Xa oral anticoagulant plasma concentration assay in real life: rivaroxaban and apixaban quantification in emergency with LMWH calibrator. Ann Pharmacother 2019;53(4):341–7.
11. Gosselin R, Grant RP, Adcock DM. Comparison of the effect of the anti-Xa direct oral anticoagulants apixaban, edoxaban, and rivaroxaban on coagulation assays. Int J Lab Hematol 2016;38(5):505–13.
12. Pradaxa prescribing information. Boehringer ingelheim pharmaceuticals inc. Rev june 2021 ridgefield, CT. Available at: https://content.boehringer-ingelheim.com/DAM/c669f898-0c4e-45a2-ba55-af1e011fdf63/pradaxa%20capsules-us-pi.pdf. [Accessed 7 November 2023].
13. Gosselin RC, Favaloro EJ, Douxfils J. The myths behind DOAC measurement: analyses of prescribing information from different regulatory bodies and a call for harmonization. J Thromb Haemostasis 2022;20(11):2494–506.
14. US Federal Register Medical Device. Laboratory developed tests. a proposed rule by the food and drug administration. Oct 10. 2023. Available at: https://www.federalregister.gov/documents/2023/10/03/2023-21662/medical-devices-laboratory-developed-tests. [Accessed 22 November 2023].
15. Adcock DM, Gosselin RC. The danger of relying on the APTT and PT in patients on DOAC therapy, a potential patient safety issue. Int J Lab Hematol 2017;39(Suppl 1):37–40.

16. Gosselin RC, Adcock DM, Bates SM, et al. International council for standardization in haematology (ICSH) recommendations for laboratory measurement of direct oral anticoagulants. Thromb Haemostasis 2018;118(3):437–50.
17. Gosselin RC, Adcock D, Hawes EM, et al. Evaluating the use of commercial drug-specific calibrators for determining PT and APTT reagent sensitivity to dabigatran and rivaroxaban. Thromb Haemostasis 2015;113(1):77–84.
18. Lim MS, Chapman K, Swanepoel P, et al. Sensitivity of routine coagulation assays to direct oral anticoagulants: patient samples versus commercial drug-specific calibrators. Pathology 2016;48(7):712–9.
19. Gosselin RC, Moore GW, Kershaw GW, et al. International Council for Standardization in Haematology field study evaluating optimal interpretation methods for activated partial thromboplastin time and prothrombin time mixing studies. Arch Pathol Lab Med 2023. https://doi.org/10.5858/arpa.2023-0030-OA.
20. Douxfils J, Adcock DM, Bates SM, et al. 2021 Update of the international council for standardization in haematology recommendations for laboratory measurement of direct oral anticoagulants. Thromb Haemostasis 2021;121(8):1008–20.
21. Sahli SD, Castellucci C, Roche TR, et al. The impact of direct oral anticoagulants on viscoelastic testing - a systematic review. Front Cardiovasc Med 2022;9: 991675.
22. Mani H, Rohde G, Stratmann G, et al. Accurate determination of rivaroxaban levels requires different calibrator sets but not addition of antithrombin. Thromb Haemostasis 2012;108(01):191–8.
23. Gosselin RC, Adcock Funk DM, Taylor JM, et al. Comparison of anti-Xa and dilute Russell viper venom time assays in quantifying drug levels in patients on therapeutic doses of rivaroxaban. Arch Pathol Lab Med 2014;138(12):1680–4.
24. Douxfils J, Gosselin RC. Laboratory assessment of direct oral anticoagulants. Semin Thromb Hemost 2017;43(3):277–90.
25. Rimsans J, Douxfils J, Smythe MA, et al. Overview and practical application of coagulation assays in managing anticoagulation with direct oral anticoagulants (DOACs). Curr Pharmacol Rep 2020;6:241–59.
26. Samuelson BT, Cuker A, Siegal DM, et al. Laboratory assessment of the anticoagulant activity of direct oral anticoagulants: a systematic review. Chest 2017; 151(1):127–38.
27. Gosselin R, Hawes E, Moll S, et al. Performance of various laboratory assays in the measurement of dabigatran in patients receiving therapeutic doses: a prospective study based on peak and trough plasma levels. Am J Clin Pathol 2014;141(2):262–7.
28. Brunetti L, Sanchez-Catanese B, Kagan L, et al. Evaluation of the chromogenic anti-factor IIa assay to assess dabigatran exposure in geriatric patients with atrial fibrillation in an outpatient setting. Thromb J 2016;14:10.
29. Gosselin RC, Douxfils J. Ecarin based coagulation testing. Am J Hematol 2020; 95(7):863–9.
30. Gosselin RC, Douxfils J. Measuring direct oral anticoagulants. Methods Mol Biol 2017;1646:217–25.
31. US food and drug administration reclassification order DEN190032 Sep 17. 2020. Available at: https://www.accessdata.fda.gov/cdrh_docs/pdf19/DEN190032.pdf. [Accessed 22 November 2023].
32. Gosselin RC, Adcock DM, Douxfils J. An update on laboratory assessment for direct oral anticoagulants (DOACs). Int J Lab Hematol 2019;41(Suppl 1):33–9.
33. Adelhelm JBH, Christensen R, Balbi GGM, et al. Therapy with direct oral anticoagulants for secondary prevention of thromboembolic events in the

antiphospholipid syndrome: a systematic review and meta-analysis of randomised trials. Lupus Sci Med 2023;10(2):e001018.

34. Gosselin RC. Review of coagulation preanalytical variables with update on the effect of direct oral anticoagulants. Int J Lab Hematol 2021;43(Suppl 1):109–16.

35. Margetić S, Ćelap I, Huzjan AL, et al. DOAC dipstick testing can reliably exclude the presence of clinically relevant DOAC concentrations in circulation. Thromb Haemostasis 2022;122(9):1542–8.

36. Merrelaar AE, Bögl MS, Buchtele N, et al. Performance of a qualitative point-of-care strip test to detect DOAC exposure at the emergency department: a cohort-type cross-sectional diagnostic accuracy study. Thromb Haemostasis 2022;122(10):1723–31.

37. Papageorgiou L, Hetjens S, Auge S, et al. Comparison of the DOAC Dipstick test on urine samples with chromogenic substrate methods on plasma samples in outpatients treated with direct oral anticoagulants. Clin Appl Thromb Hemost 2023;29. https://doi.org/10.1177/10760296231179684. 10760296231179684.

38. Cuker A, Santiago M, Tubia I, et al. QC.15: a novel point-of-care whole blood portable analyzer for direct oral anticoagulant monitoring. Res Pract Thromb Haemosta 2023;7(Supplement 2):75–6.

39. Ansell J, Zappe S, Jiang X, et al. A novel whole blood point-of-care coagulometer to measure the effect of direct oral anticoagulants and heparins. Semin Thromb Hemost 2019;45(3):259–63.

40. Bliden KP, Chaudhary R, Mohammed N, et al. Determination of non-Vitamin K oral anticoagulant (NOAC) effects using a new-generation thrombelastography TEG 6s system. J Thromb Thrombolysis 2017;43(4):437–45.